Library of
Davidson College

Neurology and Neurobiology

EDITORS

Victoria Chan-Palay
University Hospital, Zurich

Sanford L. Palay
The Harvard Medical School

ADVISORY BOARD

Albert J. Aguayo
McGill University

Tong H. Joh
Cornell University Medical College, New York

Günter Baumgartner
University Hospital, Zurich

Bruce McEwen
Rockefeller University

Masao Ito
Tokyo University

William D. Willis, Jr.
The University of Texas, Galveston

---

1 • **Cytochemical Methods in Neuroanatomy,** Victoria Chan-Palay and Sanford L. Palay, *Editors*

2 • **Basic Mechanisms of Neuronal Hyperexcitability,** Herbert H. Jasper and Nico M. van Gelder, *Editors*

3 • **Anorexia Nervosa: Recent Developments in Research,** Padraig L. Darby, Paul E. Garfinkel, David M. Garner, and Donald V. Coscina, *Editors*

4 • **Clinical and Biological Aspects of Peripheral Nerve Diseases,** Leontino Battistin, George A. Hashim, and Abel Lajtha, *Editors*

5 • **The Physiology of Excitable Cells,** Alan D. Grinnell and William J. Moody, Jr., *Editors*

6 • **Developing and Regenerating Vertebrate Nervous Systems,** Penelope W. Coates, Roger R. Markwald, and Alexander D. Kenny, *Editors*

7 • **Glutamine, Glutamate, and GABA in the Central Nervous System,** Leif Hertz, Elling Kvamme, Edith G. McGeer, and Arne Schousboe, *Editors*

8 • **Catecholamines,** Earl Usdin, Arvid Carlsson, Annica Dahlström, and Jörgen Engel, *Editors*. Published in three volumes: *Part A: Basic and Peripheral Mechanisms; Part B: Neuropharmacology and Central Nervous System—Theoretical Aspects; Part C: Neuropharmacology and Central Nervous System—Therapeutic Aspects*

9 • **Development of Visual Pathways in Mammals,** Jonathan Stone, Bogdan Dreher, and David H. Rapaport, *Editors*

10 • **Monoamine Innervation of Cerebral Cortex,** Laurent Descarries, Tomás R. Reader, and Herbert H. Jasper, *Editors*

11 • **The Neurobiology of Zinc,** C.J. Frederickson, G.A. Howell, and E.J. Kasarskis, *Editors*. Published in two volumes: *Part A: Physiochemistry, Anatomy, and Techniques; Part B: Deficiency, Toxicity, and Pathology*

12 • **Modulation of Sensorimotor Activity During Alterations in Behavioral States,** Richard Bandler, *Editor*

13 • **Behavioral Pharmacology: The Current Status,** Lewis S. Seiden and Robert L. Balster, *Editors*

14 • **Development, Organization, and Processing in Somatosensory Pathways,** Mark Rowe and William D. Willis, Jr., *Editors*

15 • **Metal Ions in Neurology and Psychiatry,** Sabit Gabay, Joseph Harris, and Beng T. Ho, *Editors*

16 • **Neurohistochemistry: Modern Methods and Applications,** Pertti Panula, Heikki Päivärinta, and Seppo Soinila, *Editors*

17 • **Two Hemispheres—One Brain: Functions of the Corpus Callosum,** Franco Leporé, Maurice Ptito, and Herbert H. Jasper, *Editors*

18 • **Senile Dementia of the Alzheimer Type,** J. Thomas Hutton and Alexander D. Kenny, *Editors*

19 • **Quantitative Receptor Autoradiography,** Carl A. Boast, Elaine W. Snowhill, and C. Anthony Altar, *Editors*

20 • **Ion Channels in Neural Membranes,** J. Murdoch Ritchie, Richard D. Keynes, and Liana Bolis, *Editors*

21 • **PET and NMR: New Perspectives in Neuroimaging and in Clinical Neurochemistry,** Leontino Battistin and Franz Gerstenbrand, *Editors*

22 • **New Concepts in Cerebellar Neurobiology,** James S. King, *Editor*

23 • **The Vertebrate Neuromuscular Junction,** Miriam M. Salpeter, *Editor*

24 • **Excitatory Amino Acid Transmission,** T. Philip Hicks, David Lodge, and Hugh McLennan, *Editors*

25 • **Axonal Transport,** Richard S. Smith and Mark A. Bisby, *Editors*

26 • **Respiratory Muscles and Their Neuromotor Control,** Gary C. Sieck, Simon C. Gandevia, and William E. Cameron, *Editors*

27 • **Epilepsy and the Reticular Formation: The Role of the Reticular Core in Convulsive Seizures,** Gerhard H. Fromm, Carl L. Faingold, Ronald A. Browning, and W.M. Burnham, *Editors*

28 • **Inactivation of Hypersensitive Neurons,** N. Chalazonitis and Maurice Gola, *Editors*

29 • **Neuroplasticity, Learning, and Memory,** N.W. Milgram, Colin M. MacLeod, and Ted L. Petit, *Editors*

30 • **Effects of Injury on Trigeminal and Spinal Somatosensory Systems,** Lillian M. Pubols and Barry J. Sessle, *Editors*

31 • **Organization of the Autonomic Nervous System: Central and Peripheral Mechanisms,** John Ciriello, Franco R. Calaresu, Leo P. Renaud, and Canio Polosa, *Editors*

32 • **Neurotrophic Activity of GABA During Development,** Dianna A. Redburn and Arne Schousboe, *Editors*

33 • **Animal Models of Dementia: A Synaptic Neurochemical Perspective,** Joseph T. Coyle, *Editor*

34 • **Molecular Neuroscience: Expression of Neural Genes,** Fulton Wong, Douglas C. Eaton, David A. Konkel, and J. Regino Perez-Polo, *Editors*

35 • **Long-Term Potentiation: From Biophysics to Behavior,** Philip W. Landfield and Sam A. Deadwyler, *Editors*

36 • **Neural Plasticity: A Lifespan Approach,** Ted L. Petit and Gwen O. Ivy, *Editors*

37 • **Intrinsic Determinants of Neuronal Form and Function,** Raymond J. Lasek and Mark M. Black, *Editors*

38 • **The Current Status of Peripheral Nerve Regeneration,** Tessa Gordon, Richard B. Stein, and Peter A. Smith, *Editors*

39 • **The Biochemical Pathology of Astrocytes,** Michael D. Norenberg, Leif Hertz, and Arne Schousboe, *Editors*

40 • **Perspectives in Psychopharmacology: A Collection of Papers in Honor of Earl Usdin,** Jack D. Barchas and William E. Bunney, Jr., *Editors*

41 • **Non-Invasive Stimulation of Brain and Spinal Cord: Fundamentals and Clinical Applications,** Paolo M. Rossini and Charles D. Marsden, *Editors*

42A • **Progress in Catecholamine Research, Part A: Basic Aspects and Peripheral Mechanisms,** Annica Dahlström, Haim Belmaker, and Merton Sandler, *Editors*

42B • **Progress in Catecholamine Research, Part B: Central Aspects,** Merton Sandler, Annica Dahlström, and Haim Belmaker, *Editors*

42C • **Progress in Catecholamine Research, Part C: Clinical Aspects,** Haim Belmaker, Merton Sandler, and Annica Dahlström, *Editors*

43 • **Dopaminergic Mechanisms in Vision,** Ivan Bodis-Wollner and Marco Piccolino, *Editors*

44 • **Developmental Neurobiology of the Frog,** Emanuel D. Pollack and Harold D. Bibb, *Editors*

45 • **The Lennox-Gastaut Syndrome,** Ernst Niedermeyer and Rolf Degen, *Editors*

46 • **Frontiers in Excitatory Amino Acid Research,** Esper A. Cavalheiro, John Lehmann, and Lechoslaw Turski, *Editors*

DEVELOPMENTAL NEUROBIOLOGY OF THE FROG

DEVELOPMENTAL NEUROBIOLOGY OF THE FROG

Proceedings of a Symposium in Honor of Jerry J. Kollros, Held in
New Orleans, Louisiana, December 27–30, 1987

Editors

Emanuel D. Pollack

Institute for the Study
of Developmental Disabilities
University of Illinois at Chicago
Chicago, Illinois

Harold D. Bibb

Department of Zoology
University of Rhode Island
Kingston, Rhode Island

ALAN R. LISS, INC., NEW YORK

Address all Inquiries to the Publisher
Alan R. Liss, Inc., 41 East 11th Street, New York, NY 10003

Copyright © 1988 Alan R. Liss, Inc.

Printed in the United States of America

Under the conditions stated below the owner of copyright for this book hereby grants permission to users to make photocopy reproductions of any part or all of its contents for personal or internal organizational use, or for personal or internal use of specific clients. This consent is given on the condition that the copier pay the stated per-copy fee through the Copyright Clearance Center, Incorporated, 27 Congress Street, Salem, MA 01970, as listed in the most current issue of "Permissions to Photocopy" (Publisher's Fee List, distributed by CCC, Inc.), for copying beyond that permitted by sections 107 or 108 of the US Copyright Law. This consent does not extend to other kinds of copying, such as copying for general distribution, for advertising or promotional purposes, for creating new collective works, or for resale.

Library of Congress Cataloging-in-Publication Data

Developmental neurobiology of the frog : proceedings of a symposium,
   held at New Orleans, Louisiana, on December 27–30, 1987 / editors,
   Emanuel D. Pollack, Harold D. Bibb.
      p. cm. — (Neurology and neurobiology : v. 44)
   Sponsored by the American Society of Zoologists, Division of
Developmental and Cell Biology.
   Includes index.
   ISBN 0-8451-2748-9
   1. Frogs—Development—
Congresses. 2. Developmental neurology-
-Congresses. 3. Amphibians—Development—Congresses. I. Pollack,
Emanuel D. II. Bibb, Harold D. III. American Society of
Zoologists. Division of Developmental and Cell Biology.
IV. Series.
QL668.E2D49
597.8—dc19   88-19783
                                                                                   CIP

Contents

Contributors ix
Preface
Emanuel D. Pollack and Harold D. Bibb xi

I. REGULATION OF A NEURONAL POPULATION: THE LATERAL MOTOR COLUMN

INTRODUCTION 3

Perspectives on the Development of the Lateral Motor Column
Emanuel D. Pollack 5

The Origin of Interindividual Variation in Motoneuron Number in the Lumbar Lateral Motor Column of *Xenopus laevis*
David G. Sperry 29

Meritocratic Selection Hypothesis in the Control of Motoneuron Death During Development
Alan H. Lamb, Philip W. Sheard, and Michael J. Ferns 53

II. SPECIFICITY IN NEURAL DEVELOPMENT AND REGENERATION

INTRODUCTION 79

Regulation of Spinal Nerve Fiber Growth and Neuronal Maturation In Vitro
William L. Muhlach 81

Mechanisms of Neuromuscular Junction Development Studied in Tissue Culture
H. Benjamin Peng, Qiming Chen, M. William Rochlin, Dingliang Zhu, and Brian Kay 103

Hindlimb Innervation Patterns of Bullfrog Motor Axons During Development and Regeneration
Matt T. Lee and Paul B. Farel 121

The Development of Spinal Ganglia
Harold D. Bibb 139

Specification of Spinal Sensory Neurons During Development
Carolyn Smith and Eric Frank 161

III. NEURONAL ORDER, DIFFERENTIATION, AND POPULATION ADJUSTMENTS

INTRODUCTION 189

The Early Development of Neurons in *Xenopus* Embryos Revealed by Transmitter Immunocytochemistry for Serotonin, GABA, and Glycine
Alan Roberts 191

Toward an Understanding of Tectal Development in Frogs
Jerry J. Kollros 207

A Neural Pattern Unfolding: Properties of Retinotectal Differentiation in Frog Tadpoles
Martha Constantine-Paton 231

Neurogenesis of the Frog Cerebellum
Amos G. Gona, Nándor J. Uray, and Kurt F. Hauser 255

Index 277

Contributors

Harold D. Bibb, Department of Zoology, University of Rhode Island, Kingston, RI 02881 **[xi,139]**

Qiming Chen, Department of Cell Biology and Anatomy, University of North Carolina, Chapel Hill, NC 27599 **[103]**

Martha Constantine-Paton, Department of Biology, Yale University, New Haven, CT 06511 **[231]**

Paul B. Farel, Department of Physiology, University of North Carolina, Chapel Hill, NC 27514 **[121]**

Michael J. Ferns, Department of Pathology, Neuromuscular Research Institute, University of Western Australia, Nedlands, 6009, Western Australia **[53]**

Eric Frank, Department of Neurobiology, Anatomy, and Cell Biology, University of Pittsburgh School of Medicine, Pittsburgh, PA 15261 **[161]**

Amos G. Gona, Department of Anatomy, University of Medicine and Dentistry of New Jersey, Newark, NJ 07103 **[255]**

Kurt F. Hauser, Department of Anatomy and Neurobiology, University of Kentucky, Lexington, KY 40536 **[255]**

Brian Kay, Department of Biology, University of North Carolina, Chapel Hill, NC 27599 **[103]**

Jerry J. Kollros, Department of Biology, University of Iowa, Iowa City, IA 52242 **[207]**

Alan H. Lamb, Department of Pathology, Neuromuscular Research Institute, University of Western Australia, Nedlands, 6009, Western Australia **[53]**

Matt T. Lee, Department of Physiology and Biophysics, University of Iowa, Iowa City, IA 52242 **[121]**

William L. Muhlach, Department of Zoology, Southern Illinois University at Carbondale, Carbondale, IL 62901 **[81]**

H. Benjamin Peng, Department of Cell Biology and Anatomy, University of North Carolina, Chapel Hill, NC 27599 **[103]**

Emanuel D. Pollack, Institute for the Study of Developmental Disabilities, Department of Biological Sciences, and Committee on Neuroscience, University of Illinois at Chicago, Chicago, IL 60680 **[xi,5]**

Alan Roberts, Department of Zoology, University of Bristol, Bristol, BS8 1UG, England **[191]**

The numbers in brackets are the opening page numbers of the contributors' articles.

M. William Rochlin, Department of Cell Biology and Anatomy, University of North Carolina, Chapel Hill, NC 27599 **[103]**

Philip W. Sheard, Department of Pathology, Neuromuscular Research Institute, University of Western Australia, Nedlands, 6009, Western Australia **[53]**

Carolyn Smith, Department of Neurobiology, Anatomy, and Cell Biology, University of Pittsburgh School of Medicine, Pittsburgh, PA 15261 **[161]**

David G. Sperry, School of Life and Health Sciences, University of Delaware, Newark, DE 19716 **[29]**

Nándor J. Uray, Department of Anatomy, Kirksville College of Osteopathic Medicine, Kirksville, MO 63501 **[255]**

Dingliang Zhu, Department of Cell Biology and Anatomy, University of North Carolina, Chapel Hill, NC 27599 **[103]**

Preface

This volume is the outcome of a symposium on the developmental neurobiology of the frog held under the auspices of the Division of Developmental and Cell Biology of the American Society of Zoologists, December 1987. Both the symposium and this book were planned with two primary purposes in mind: to redirect attention to the usefulness of the frog as a model for the study of nervous system development, particularly as it continues to serve as a framework for understanding much of vertebrate neural development, and to honor Professor Jerry J. Kollros, whose contributions to the study of amphibian development have been of primary significance. Dr. Kollros has contributed most emphatically to the understanding of metamorphosis and the role of thyroid hormone in forming the foundation for the study of developmental neurobiology of the frog.

Although the uninitiated might have come to believe that the primary history and advances in developmental neurobiology reside in the study of the chick embryo, it is clear that the amphibian has served as the model for neural development for most of this century. Probably Ross Granville Harrison comes to mind first for his use of the frog embryo in a series of classical neuroembryological experiments. Santiago Ramón y Cajal (1929) took advantage of the frog tadpole to observe the growth of nerve fibers in the highly transparent tail fin of the tadpole, and we need look no further than the elegant studies of Speidel (e.g., 1932) to realize the excellence of the frog as a model of neural development.

Major contributions to our understanding of neural development have come through the use of the frog by Spemann, Weiss, and Sperry. It is from this coterie of distinguished neuroembryologists that the modern leaders in the field emerged, among them Jerry Kollros. Kollros gave us the critical information that nervous system maturation, as exemplified in his early studies on the corneal reflex (Kollros, 1942, 1943a,b, 1958), depends on thyroid hormone for its functional development. This theme was developed further in the elaborate analyses of the mesencephalic Vth nucleus (Kollros and McMurrray, 1955, 1956; Kollros, 1977, 1984; Kollros and Thiesse, 1985). He made us aware that the metamorphic events of the tadpole are dependent on thyroid hormone in a rigorous sequence that invokes the notion of thresholds in tissue response, hormone action, and time (Kollros, 1968; 1981). And although his study of larval *Xenopus* has been a boon to developmental neurobiology, few realize that Kollros was the first to rigorously describe the development of the lateral motor columns and spinal ganglia in *Xenopus* with his contributions to the "Normal Tables of *Xenopus laevis*" published in 1956 under the editorship of Nieuwkoop and Faber. Among developmental neurobiologists, few are unacquainted with the stages of the tadpole of *Rana pipiens*, as described by Taylor and Kollros in 1946, which has served as a developmental standard for forty years. A substantial part of Kollros' time these past several years has been spent in studying various developmental phenomena associated with the visual system, some of which are reported in this volume.

The topics selected are representative of the primary issues in developmental neurobiology to which studies of the frog have made significant contributions. This volume has been organized as a continuum from aspects of spinal cord development to peripheral nervous system and target relationships on to differentiation of CNS neurons and mechanisms of development of brain components. Overlapping of topics and, therefore, particular problem-oriented issues is intentional so as to emphasize particular themes. From the initial chapters, it will become apparent that long-standing and yet to be resolved problems surround the issues of neuron death and survival and the incumbent control of neuronal populations. This theme arises again as we move along the neuraxis and subsequently deal with several aspects of neuronal specificity and differentiation. No doubt the reader will recognize that a common thread running through frog development is the developmental dependency on thyroid hormone. And finally, it will be noted that the majority of the chapters focus on the larval, or tadpole, period of development. In this sense, we must apologize to those whose endeavors deal with the primacy of neuroembryology. But the excitement accompanying the unraveling of mechanisms that account for the development of neuron sets and their relationships to other cellular configurations has largely set the framework for this book.

We recognize that only a fraction of what has come to be known or speculated about neural development, even in the frog, is covered in these pages. If, however, some of the ideas and findings reported here stimulate a degree of excitement or reawaken interest in amphibian nervous system development as a means of adding to developmental neurobiology, then we shall be pleased.

The editors take pleasure in thanking the contributors for their endeavors in assuring the successful outcome of both the symposium and this volume. Special recognition is due the American Society of Zoologists for both financial and logistical support, most notably Mrs. Mary Adams-Wiley, Dr. Bruce M. Carlson, and Dr. Joanne Cameron. The resources of the Institute for the Study of Developmental Disabilities of the University of Illinois at

Chicago assisted in the production of this publication. We thank Mrs. Veronica Liebig for her expert assistance in proofreading and compiling the manuscripts, and we are indebted to Alan R. Liss, Inc., and staff for enthusiastically agreeing to and promoting this publication. No small appreciation is due our families, who have tolerated extended absences during the time of the symposium and the preparation of this volume and who cheerfully provided the necessary moral support.

Emanuel D. Pollack
Harold D. Bibb

REFERENCES

Kollros JJ (1942) Experimental studies on the development of the corneal reflex in Amphibia. I. The onset of the reflex and its relationship to metamorphosis. J Exp Zool 89:37–67.

Kollros JJ (1943a) Experimental studies in the development of the corneal reflex in Amphibia. II. Localized maturation of the reflex mechanism effected by thyroxin-agar implants into the hindbrain. Physiol Zool 16:269–275.

Kollros JJ (1943b) Experimental studies in the development of the corneal reflex in Amphibia. III. The influence of the periphery upon the reflex center. J Exp Zool 92:121–142.

Kollros JJ (1958) Hormonal control of onset of the corneal reflex in frogs. Science 128:1505.

Kollros JJ (1968) Endocrine influences in neural development. In Wolstenholme GEW, O'Connor M (eds): "Ciba Foundation Symposium on Growth of the Nervous System," London: Churchill, Ltd., pp 179–192.

Kollros JJ (1977) Hormonal control of the mesencephalic fifth nucleus in amphibians. In Grave GD (ed): "Thyroid Hormones and Brain Development." New York: Raven Press, pp 119–136.

Kollros JJ (1981) Transitions in the nervous system during amphibian metamorphosis. In Gilbert LI, Frieden E (eds): "Metamorphosis: A Problem in Developmental Biology." New York: Plenum, pp 445–459.

Kollros JJ (1984) Growth and death of cells of the mesencephalic fifth nucleus in *Rana pipiens* larvae. J Comp Neurol 224:386–394.

Kollros JJ, McMurray VM (1955) The mesencephalic V nucleus—anurans. I. Normal development in *Rana pipiens* tadpoles. J Comp Neurol 102:47–64.

Kollros JJ, McMurray VM (1956) The mesencephalic V nucleus—anurans. II. The influence of thyroid hormone on cell size and cell number. J Exp Zool 131:1–26.

Kollros JJ, Thiesse ML (1985) Growth and death of cells of the mesencephalic fifth nucleus in *Xenopus laevis* larvae. J Comp Neurol 233:481–489.

Ramón y Cajal S (1929) Etude sur la neurogenese de quelques vertèbrés. (L Guth, 1960, transl: "Studies on Vertebrate Neurogenesis.") Springfield, IL: Charles C Thomas, p 10.

Speidel CC (1932) Studies of living nerves. I. The movements of individual sheath cells and nerve sprouts correlated with the process of myelin sheath formation in amphibian larvae. J Exp Zool 61:279–331.

Taylor AC, Kollros JJ (1946) Stages in the normal development of *Rana pipiens* larvae. Anat Rec 94:7–23.

SECTION I

REGULATION OF A NEURONAL POPULATION: THE LATERAL MOTOR COLUMN

SECTION I. REGULATION OF A NEURONAL POPULATION: THE LATERAL MOTOR COLUMN

Among the long term problems of neural development have been those related to the means by which a neuron set comes to have its finite population determined. One functional group of nerve cells that has engendered substantial attention is the lateral motor column of the spinal cord. Because its component motor neurons are responsible for the efferent innervation of the limbs it has been a system amenable to peripheral target manipulation. Although there is little argument that the limb periphery is an essential ingredient in the determination of the final population size of the lateral motor columns, the mechanisms by which the periphery might regulate neuron number and influence the progression of naturally-occurring neuron death have remained open to investigation. Quite clearly, any consideration of neuron population size must, in addition to the target, take into account the potential for inherent or genetic roles, the pervasive role of thyroid hormone as a major determinant in larval frog development, and the likelihood that in a system where the concept of trophic requirements is often invoked there is a role for the afferents to the motor neurons.

The following three chapters provide a wide-ranging consideration of the various elements that may be involved in determining the size of the spinal motor neuron population. Although one can envision other alternatives to those discussed, or even unique experimental approaches, the focus is on where we stand in light of what is known relative to frog development. It is, after all, the processes leading to the establishment of a definitive neuron set that prepares the groundwork for the specificity of interactions that follows or accompanies nerve cell differentiation and provides plasticity. These interactions between a neuron and its target, or with its environment, are in themselves a very likely component of population regulation and are exemplified by the lateral motor column.

PERSPECTIVES ON THE DEVELOPMENT OF THE LATERAL MOTOR COLUMN

Emanuel D. Pollack

Institute for the Study of Developmental Disabilities, Department of Biological Sciences, and Committee on Neuroscience, University of Illinois at Chicago, Chicago, Illinois 60680

INTRODUCTION

As a result of tissue interactions on a background of permissive and instructive genetic information, a region of the embryonic ectoderm signals the onset of formation of the nervous system, first identifiable as the thickened neuroectoderm and the neural plate. Subsequently, complex morphogenetic movements result in the elevation of neural folds and eventually the fused neural tube. Once the neural tube has formed, the specific regions of the central nervous system appear as the result of timed cell divisions and migrations in what seems to be spatially ordered sequences. These early embryonic events are generalized to all vertebrates and with reference to the frog have been detailed by Rugh (1951).

Although the adult frog has served the field of neurobiology in an exemplary manner, developmental neurobiologists have increasingly turned to the chick embryo in attempting to elucidate neurodevelopmental processes. With due acknowledgment to colleagues who have contributed much to developmental neurobiology through their studies on non-amphibian species, I hope to demonstrate that the larval frog spinal cord, and specifically, its motor components are a suitable model for trying to understand the mechanisms contributing to much of neural development.

AN INTERACTIVE APPROACH

Let us first consider the spinal cord as the center of interactive tissues in development. Within it, accumulations of motor neurons give rise to efferent axons that extend to peripheral targets, the developing limbs (Fig. 1). This periphery also receives sensory nerve fibers from the sensory ganglia, or dorsal root ganglia. The ganglionic neurons additionally send centripetal nerve fibers to the spinal cord, thus establishing a crude reflex arc. At the outset, we can consider several of the problems with which this system is faced from a developmental perspective, a number of which will be considered further in this volume. How for instance do growing nerve fibers find their targets? What might account for the specificity, not only of oriented growth, but of the matching of the neuron to its appropriate postsynaptic cell? What role does the simultaneously differentiating target, neuronal or non-neuronal, play? Where can we separate the genetic from the epigenetic controls? What accounts for the establishment of determinate neuron numbers in any neuron set? Are there different rules for the development of

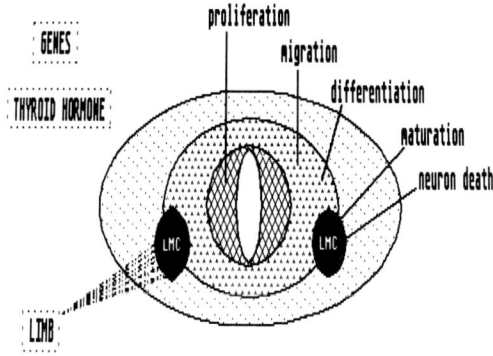

Figure 1. Schematic diagram of the larval frog spinal cord in cross-section indicating the primary mechanisms contributing to the formation of the lateral motor column (LMC). The three boxed influences act to different degrees upon these mechanisms in determining the final LMC configuration.

afferent inputs than for efferents? When we refer to specific neuronal populations, to what degree are they truly homogenous? And how do we reconcile the potential mechanistic roles for non-neuronal cells, particularly glia, with the increasingly known influences of the extracellular environment? As a definitive neuron set residing within the central nervous system, yet with axons that are a part of the peripheral nervous system as they extend to their limb targets, the lateral motor column (LMC) and its component neurons are a suitable model for resolving some of these and other issues. An excellent overview of central nervous system development in the amphibian can be found in Fox (1984), while comprehensive reviews of the anuran LMC have been reported earlier by Hughes (1968) and Kollros (1968a).

The LMCs exist as two pairs of longitudinal columns, also known as the ventral, or anterior, horns (Fig. 2). The rostral pair, or brachial lateral motor columns, are responsible for the motor innervation of the forelimb musculature, while the more caudal, or lumbosacral, pair innervate the hindlimbs. Their formation and subsequent development take place entirely during the larval period.

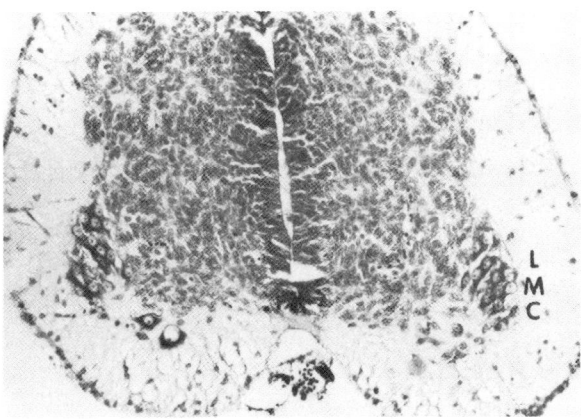

Figure 2. Typical cross-section through the lumbosacral spinal cord of a stage XI _Rana pipiens_ tadpole demonstrating the characteristic appearance of the LMC pair during the midst of the period of naturally-occurring neuron loss.

MECHANISMS OF LMC FORMATION

From consideration of the primary mechanisms that result in the formation of definitive motor columns, it will be obvious that the same processes are involved in the development of most all neurons sets (Fig. 1). Presumptive motor neurons arise in the proliferative ventricular zone adjacent to the spinal canal and subsequently migrate through the intermediate zone coming to rest in a ventrolateral position as a protrusion into the marginal zone. During their migrations, the neurons begin to elaborate axons (Farel and Bemelmans, 1980; Chu-Wang et al., 1981) so that virtually all neurons that ultimately reside in the LMC have extended axons into the periphery (Lamb, 1974; Prestige and Wilson, 1974). Cell differentiation and maturation continue within the definitively formed LMC; yet not long after the maximum number of neurons has arrived, the population of the LMC begins a reduction through what is commonly thought of as naturally-occurring neuron death (Beaudoin, 1955; Prestige, 1967; Pollack, 1969a; Lamb, 1985). As will become apparent, assorted interactions between cells and between cells and their environment are critical components of motor neuron development. It is upon these mechanisms (proliferation, migration, differentiation and maturation, neuron death, interactions) that external influences are exerted to eventually shape the system. When we view a system such as this, our attention inevitably is drawn to the regulation of the cellular configuration.

The generalized developmental transition of the LMC from a densely populated group of neurons to its more characteristic appearance as a set of large motor neurons signals questions regarding the reduction in neuron number at the same time that the remaining cells increase in size and take on the cytology of mature neurons (Fig. 3). We think of the decrease in cell number as being the result of neuron death. Yet, some question exists as to whether alternative processes might be at work in the developmental adjustment of neuron number. These might take the form of cell shrinkage without degeneration or reverse migration out of the LMC.

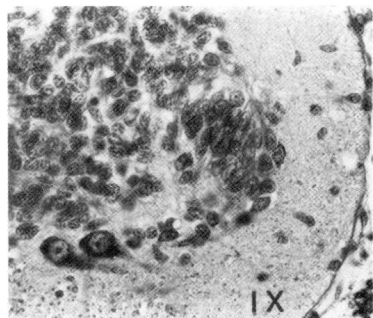 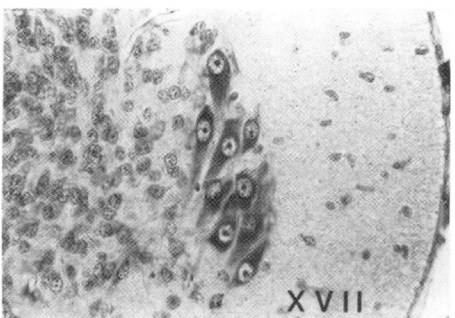

Figure 3. Typical appearance of the lumbosacral LMC prior to the onset of the period of greatest neuron loss (stage IX) and following this period (stage XVII). Note the reduced neuron population and density, but well-differentiated motor neurons in the older cord.

DEVELOPMENTAL PATTERN OF THE LMC

The two pairs of lateral motor columns (LMCs), brachial and lumbosacral, differ in several respects (Pollack, 1976; Fig. 4). First, it is now apparent that the brachial pair lags slightly behind the comparable milestones for the lumbosacral LMC. For instance, the onset of the period of greatest reduction in cell number (50% or more) occurs first in the lumbosacral LMC beginning at stage IX in Rana pipiens and continuing to stage XIII (the stages of Taylor and Kollros, 1946, are followed throughout). Stages XI through XV define the greatest neuron loss in the brachial cord. The same pattern is true of Xenopus laevis (Kollros, 1956). This caudal-rostral sequence occurs as well for the frequency of tritiated-thymidine labeled cells that represents the continuing migration of newly-formed motor neurons from the proliferative ventricular zone to the ventrolaterally positioned LMC into the midlarval stages (Pollack and Kollros, 1975). A similar relationship holds for the presence of mitotically active cells in the ventricular zone which in itself corresponds nicely with cell migration data.

Quantitatively, the brachial LMC is comprised of greater numbers of neurons of smaller size than the lumbosacral LMC, a characteristic that is probably related to the relative size and functional demands of the respective limbs. Of primary significance is the fact that new LMC neurons are entering the LMC at the same time that others are being lost (Pollack, 1972; Pollack and Kollros, 1975).

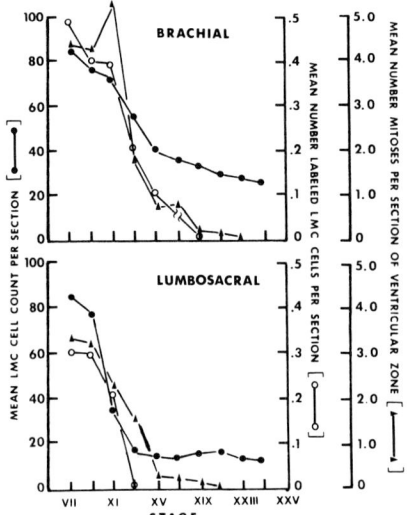

Figure 4. Comparison of the development of the brachial LMC with the lumbosacral LMC in R. pipiens. The brachial column consistently lags behind the lumbosacral with respect to cell loss, labeling index and mitotic activity. (From Pollack, 1976.)

NON-TARGET INFLUENCES ON LMC DEVELOPMENT

On the face of it, it would appear that the formation of the LMC and the controls imparted to it are relatively straightforward, and perhaps minimally altered by external factors. In fact, this is not so. If, for instance, one takes advantage of the embryonically hypophysectomized tadpole that, for lack of circulating thyroid hormone, fails to differentiate beyond stage VII or VIII (Kollros, 1961; Kollros, 1968b), the events that take place within the formed LMC are quite informative. Such tadpoles can be maintained for extended periods of time, far beyond the time it normally takes to complete metamorphosis.

Thyroid Hormone and the Hypophysectomized Tadpole

Compared to normal stage VII R. pipiens tadpoles, the LMC of the same stage, yet chronologically older, hypophysectomized tadpole has substantially more neurons (Fig. 5). In fact, the number of nerve cells continues to increase in the LMC up to a point, suggesting that new neurons continue to migrate into the LMC for a vastly extended period. Following a peak in cell number, a decline occurs that is coincident with the virtual cessation of mitotic activity in the ventricular zone.

It appears, therefore, that in the hypophysectomized frog larva, cells continue to migrate into the LMC over a protracted period, mechanistically perhaps not unlike the normal situation, except that cell loss is probably taking place at an extraordinarily slow pace. When cell production stops, the otherwise slow reduction in cell number becomes obvious. It is feasible that in this system, cell proliferation eventually works itself out as though the need to accomplish a finite number of cell divisions is programmed into the putative motor neuron progenitor cells.

Recently, J. Goldberg (personal communication) in our laboratory has shown that the removal of a hindlimb at stage IX not only inhibits the normal progression of LMC cell loss (a finding already known for earlier stages; Kett and Pollack, 1985), but continued exposure to thyroid hormone (DL-thyroxine; 25 µgm/l) results in a lumbosacral LMC at metamorphic climax with at least as many neurons, and often substantially more, than are normally present at stage IX. This unexpected finding

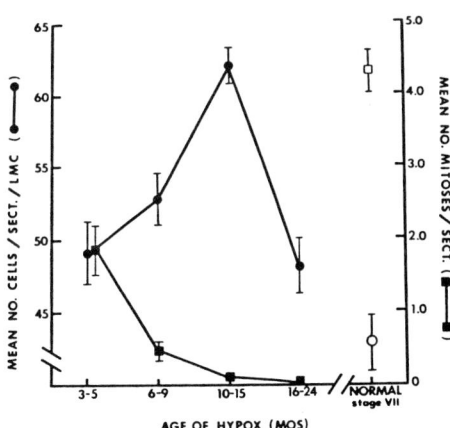

Figure 5. Changes in neuron and ventricular mitotic counts over time in the brachial LMC of hypophysectomized R. pipiens tadpoles in comparison with normal same-stage tadpoles (±s.e.m.).

is in contrast to the results for earlier amputations reported by Beaudoin (1956) that would have predicted that LMC cell death would be accelerated by the thyroid hormone. We have interpreted this to mean that LMC neurons are being produced through a thyroxine-stimulated increase in mitotic activity with subsequent migration into the LMC at a time when cell loss is being inhibited. Tritiated-thymidine labeling studies ought to verify or refute this possibility.

We do know that the spinal cord, at early stages at least, is capable of generating substantially more mitoses than would be apparent from simple observations, since the addition of thyroid hormone to the tadpole water greatly enhances mitotic number (Reynolds, 1966; Fig. 6). Together, this information suggests that a direct relationship exists between ventricular mitotic activity and the number of motor neurons that come to reside in the LMC at any particular time. Subsequently, the quantity of produced neurons is regulated by thyroid hormone, while the new numerical outcome is controlled by elimination of some neurons, the latter related, in part at least, to the peripheral targets for the motor axons.

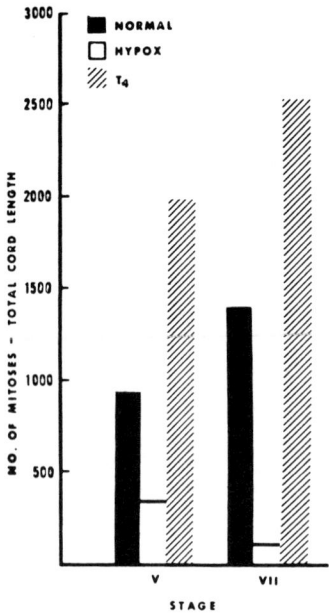

Figure 6. Increased mitotic activity in the ventricular zone of the early larval brachial spinal cord can be induced by treating normal tadpoles with dl-thyroxine (T_4). Mitotic counts in normal animals far exceed those of hypophysectomized tadpoles fixed as soon as they reached stages equivalent to normal.

Chromosomal Balance and the LMC of the Triploid Tadpole

The quantitative configuration of the LMC can also be altered for each stage of development through increasing the ploidy of the animal. A standard method of creating triploid frog embryos is to expose newly fertilized eggs to high pressure forcing the retention of the second polar body (Dasgupta, 1962). The result is normal appearing tadpoles whose LMCs contain far fewer neurons of much larger average sizes than diploid counterparts (Pollack and Koves, 1977; Fig. 7, Table 1).

Because of the implications for the control of cell number through cell loss, it is worth noting that both the diploid and triploid lumbosacral LMC lose an average of 65% of the full complement of neurons present at early stages. Interestingly, the percentage loss of neurons in the triploid brachial LMC is much less than for the diploid (37% vs. 61%; Pollack, 1977; unpublished data courtesy of H. Maheras). Preliminary information shows that the skeletal muscle fibers of triploid R. pipiens tadpoles are of normal (i.e., diploid) size and

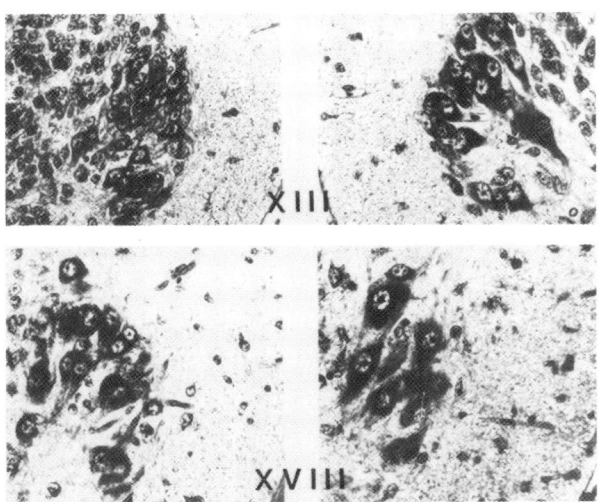

Figure 7. Comparison of diploid (left column) and triploid (right column) LMCs at two stages of R. pipiens development. Larger and fewer motor neurons are apparent in the LMC of triploid tadpoles.

Table 1. Comparison of brachial and lumbosacral lateral motor columns in triploid R. pipiens tadpoles.

	% Difference in mn Neuron Number from Diploid	% Difference in mn Nuclear Area from Diploid
Mid-larval stages		
Brachial LMC	60%	40%
Lumbosacral LMC	34%	13%
Late-larval stages		
Brachial LMC	37%	28%
Lumbosacral LMC	41%	18%

number. This further suggests that the relationship between motor neuron number and peripheral muscle characteristics is not necessarily straightforward (see Sperry, this volume).

THE PERIPHERAL TARGET AND THE LMC

Because the primary innervation target for the motor neurons of the LMC is the developing limb, it is most appropriate to consider the role that the limb plays in regulating LMC development. Of course, it has long been known that various limb manipulations can alter the outcome of the LMC. It is relatively recent, however, that we have come to realize that the ongoing differentiation of the limb can be the critical corollary to LMC progression (Pollack and Kollros, 1972; Pollack and Richmond, 1981). Although some evidence tends to be circumstantial, other lines are more definitive. Above all, we need to recognize that motor nerves enter the limb bud in advance of the presence of skeletal muscle, and thus if there is to be an early influence of the limb on the LMC it is while the limb bud is largely mesenchymal. Indeed, in vitro studies demonstrate the importance of the pre-muscle tissue in controlling elements of nerve growth (Pollack and Liebig, 1977; Pollack et al., 1981). Further, the transition of mesenchyme to muscle may be an element regulating neuron survival (Pollack, 1980; Pollack and Muhlach, 1982).

As much as we have come to accept as dogma that the elimination of the limb from a tadpole will result in the eventual depletion of the LMC neurons, the overloading of the target field by adding limbs has been less clear. For instance, we would expect that a R. pipiens tadpole with three functional forelimbs where only one ought to be should result in perhaps three times the number of motor neurons to provide the proper innervation; if not three times, then at least some increase. But what has been found in this one instance is that the number of motor neurons on the side of the spinal cord with the extra limbs did not differ from the contralateral side with one forelimb (Pollack, 1969b).

On the other hand, in an animal with four hindlimbs a difference did occur between the two sides (Maheras and Pollack, 1985). Substantially more neurons appeared in the LMC of the supernumerary side, but still not in expected numbers based on the increased peripheral territory. However, what additionally had transpired was that the LMC associated with the extra limbs had many more very large neurons than its counterpart. In fact, this is exactly what occurred in the first case except that excess neurons were not present. We do not know how these large neurons might have subserved the functional innervation of the supernumerary limbs (but see Hollyday and Mendell, 1976, for an analysis of the movement of transplanted supernumerary limbs in X. laevis). Nor can we readily attribute the limited 'rescuing' of neurons to territorial competition, a concept most developed by Prestige and Willshaw (1975) and countered by the work of Lamb (e.g. 1981 and this volume). Yet, what is important is the recognition that this particular neuron set has alternative means of responding to peripheral manipulations, an indication of developmental plasticity.

Because we have come to recognize that most adjustments in LMC cell number following manipulation of the peripheral field is in actuality an adjustment among those cells that survive the period of normal cell reduction, or naturally-occurring neuron death, we also realize that the onset of LMC cell loss is coincident with the maturation of the limb (Pollack and Richmond, 1981). That is, it seems that the limb tissue can no longer support the massive numbers of neurons it could earlier, prior to complete transformation of the mesenchyme. In the slowly developing bullfrog, however, the period of greatest lumbosacral LMC neuron reduction takes place at earlier stages than for R. pipiens and before myotube formation begins in the hindlimb (Farel, 1987).

Just as limb absence leads to an eventual elimination of most LMC neurons, so the limb is also required for the normal onset of cell loss. If the hindlimb is removed just at the time that cell loss begins in earnest, neuron reduction fails to continue at the normal pace. In effect, the absence of the limb results in a sparing of motor neurons, at least for a period of time (Kett and Pollack, 1985). It is as though the neurons have not received that information from the periphery necessary for a life or death decision.

If, in fact, the state of differentiation of the limb is important in regulating the LMC, then we ought to be able to test this notion by producing in the same animal one LMC that is at a different stage from its partner by dissynchronizing the limbs associated with each. This has been done in one study by partially amputating an early limb bud and allowing it to completely regenerate so that it would consistently lag behind its normal counterpart (Stebbins and Pollack, 1986). The LMC corresponding to each limb was appropriate for the stage of the limb, except that it was necessary to account for contralateral effects that altered the intact side of the animal and for the proximal limb that was not ablated. In a somewhat different type of preliminary experiment (Pollack, unpublished), the hindlimb bud of stage II tadpoles was transplanted to a same-stage host tadpole that was then maintained in the cold so as to retard development. When the donor tadpole reached a two to three stage differential, the grafted limb was returned to its original position. The tadpole then advanced to a stage where a cell count differential in the two LMCs could be expected based on the stages of the limbs. Preliminary results have yielded several successful animals to demonstrate that the stage of differentiation of the limb is a primary determinant in the size of the LMC cell population rather than the overall stage of the animal as indicated by the unoperated contralateral limb (for example, Fig. 8).

In most instances, we are faced with severe surgical manipulation in order to question the nature of center-periphery relationships. Recently, we have found that X. laevis tadpoles raised in a nutrient-deficient environment exhibit a high incidence of an outward defect of the forelimbs, such that they are largely immotile (Fig. 9). In these cases, the brachial LMC typically is cell-deficient and disorganized (Fig. 10). Further, the ventral roots are absent or very small, while the forelimbs are of normal overall length and gross muscle anatomy. Although we do not yet know if the LMC appearance is primary or secondary to a peripheral disorder, this may be a useful non-invasive means

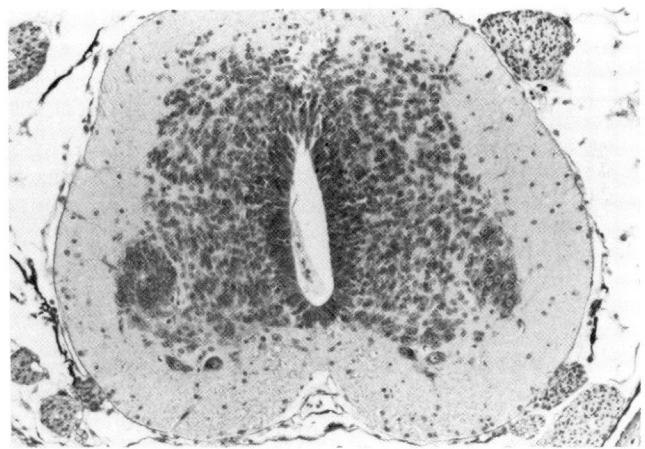

Figure 8. Cross-section through the lumbosacral spinal cord demonstrating the differential neuron density and maturation among the LMCs, one of which (left LMC) innervated a hindlimb that was two stages behind its counterpart as a result of the grafting procedure discussed in the text.

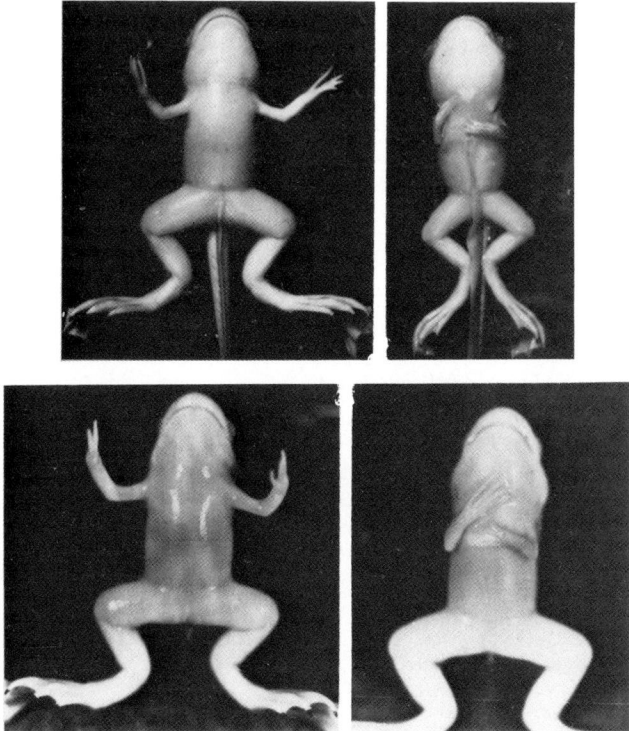

Figure 9. Xenopus raised under nutrient-deficient conditions often develop "forelimb immotility" as seen in the two animals on the right (top: stage 67; bottom: froglet) in comparison to normal animals at the same stages on the left.

of perturbing the motor neuron-target relationship during development. Additionally, there are virtually no known focal neurological lesions of development associated with specific nutritional deficits.

LMC NEURON SURVIVAL IN VITRO

Target regulation of the LMC most frequently focuses on the population size outcome, particularly

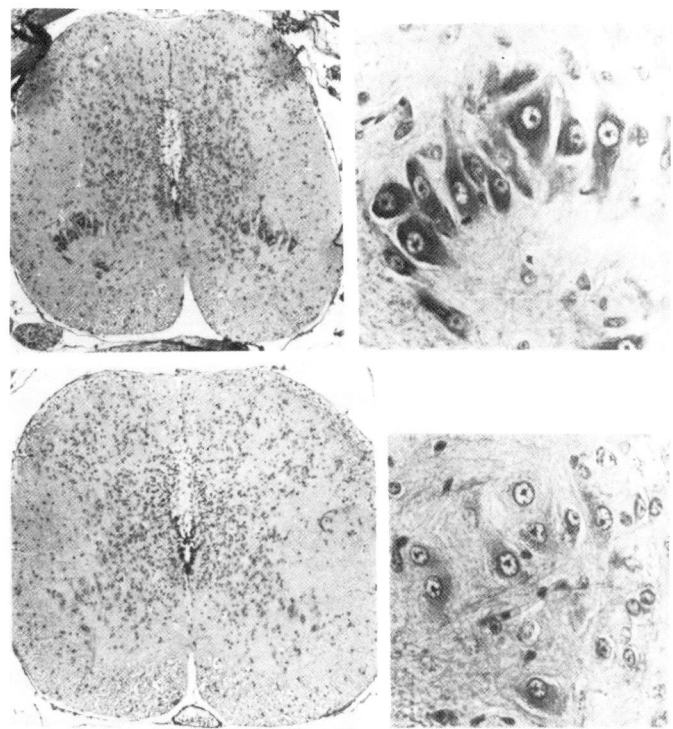

Figure 10. Low and high power views of the normal brachial LMC (top) of larval Xenopus in contrast to the disorganized and neuron-deficient LMC (bottom) of the stage 67 defective tadpole of Fig. 9.

expressed in terms of the survival or loss of neurons. In vitro analyses of the tadpole LMC may be particularly informative in these respects since explants of spinal cord placed in tissue culture are clearly deprived of their longitudinal tract inputs and dorsal root ganglion associations (see Davis et al., 1983 for the in vivo effect of ganglia removal on the LMC in R. pipiens). Further, in that they maintain organotypic architecture, the LMC is readily identifiable in histological section, and there is little doubt as to the type of cell being identified.

Explants of tadpole spinal cord can be grown in tissue culture in a defined medium and are particularly successful if co-cultured with the appropriate staged limb tissue (Pollack and Koves, 1975; Muhlach and Pollack, 1978; Pollack and Muhlach, 1981). Importantly, the limb tissue must be pre-muscle mesenchyme to elicit the most extensive directed outgrowth. The aspects of nerve fiber extension and neuronal maturation in this type of system have been described elsewhere (see Muhlach, this volume).

In the presence of limb mesenchyme, the lumbosacral LMC of stage V tadpoles can be maintained intact for extended periods (up to six weeks) in contrast to explants cultured in the absence of target tissue that survive no longer than an average of two weeks. Survival is further enhanced by using the polycationic surface, polylysine, for explant attachment. The combination of limb mesenchyme and polylysine effectively maintains the LMC neuron count at the level of in vivo controls for at least twenty-one days (Fig. 11). Although skeletal muscle also is effective in promoting motor neuron

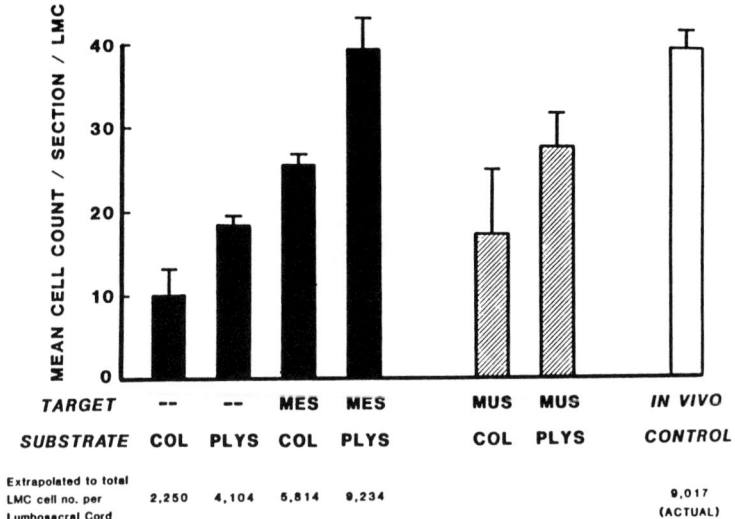

Figure 11. Graph demonstrating lumbosacral LMC neuron counts in stage V spinal cord explants at 21 days in vitro under alternative co-culturing and substratum conditions. COL = collagen; PLYS = polylysine; MES = mesencyhme; MUS = muscle.

survival, its effectiveness is much reduced from that of mesenchyme and is probably related to its denervated status.

Thus, at least for the period just after the LMC has formed, the target tissue, as well as the surface to which the nerve fibers attach, is important to motor neuron survival in vitro. These results along with other experiments in our laboratory, have led us to propose that the target tissue is the source of a motor neuron growth factor or factors, associated with parameters of growth and survival. And further, that young limb tissue is the most active source of this material which diminishes with progressive development.

Using medium that had been conditioned over limb mesenchyme, it has become clear that substantial growth- and survival-promoting effects directed to spinal nerve fibers and motor neurons are produced by this target tissue. Counts of LMC neurons in spinal cord explants

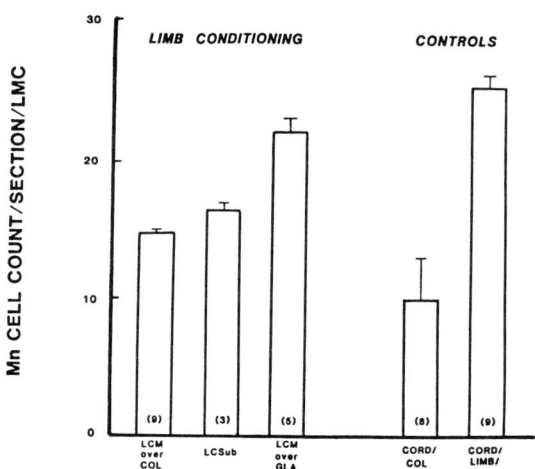

Figure 12. Stage V lumbosacral spinal cord explants were maintained to 21 days in vitro in defined medium that had been conditioned by limb mesenchyme. The mode of conditioning makes some difference, but always results in significantly more neurons in the LMC than in its absence. LCM = limb conditioned medium; LCSub = limb conditioned substratum (collagen); COL = collagen; GLA = glass.

that had been exposed to the conditioned medium provide evidence that a component of the mesenchyme promotes the survival of motor neurons in vitro (Fig. 12), and that the active component binds to surfaces such as collagen.

NEURITE SURVIVAL RELATED TO ATTACHMENT SURFACES

Because some surfaces act as enhancers of nerve growth in vitro, it is worth knowing if any of these, particularly those that are likely extracellular matrix components, have survival-promoting capabilities. Up to now we have examined only the nerve fibers themselves. As shown in Table 2, several surfaces do enhance spinal nerve fiber survival either in concert with, or independent of, the target tissue and not necessarily in association with nerve fiber growth promotion. Putative growth and survival promoters are viewed as acting directly on neurons or via an intermediary, particularly

Table 2. Stage V spinal cord explant neurite survival on assorted substrata.

Extracellular Matrix Components	Enhanced Survival
Fibronectin	With Target
Laminin	Yes
Heparan Sulfate	Yes
Chondroitin Sulfate A	No
Chondroitin Sulfate B	No*
Chondroitin Sulfate C	No
Hyaluronic Acid	Yes*
Collagen (Type I)	With Target*
Artificial Substrata	
Glass	No
HEMA Gel	No
Polylysine	Yes*

* Enhanced neuritic outgrowth in the presence of the limb target tissue.

a surface. Although some surfaces to which nerve fibers attach may promote their survival, perhaps by a stabilizing action, an effect resulting from a factor alone or interactively with a substratum is most representative of target-derived influences and probable in vivo events.

As our studies have drawn us more into the realization that motor neuron-directed growth factors can explain many of the phenomena associated with the differentiation and population control of the LMC, we have initiated studies to relate the products of the mesenchymal limb in vitro to the developmental events observed in vitro and in vivo. At this point, we have been able to identify through SDS gel electrophoresis of conditioned media three potential candidate protein molecules of 59 kD, 300 kD and 620 kD released by limb mesenchyme that meet criteria related to substratum binding and developmental uniqueness (Kaminski and Pollack, in preparation). The primary consideration is that the limb mesenchyme can in fact produce and release unique proteins that are not normally released by skeletal muscle in vitro. One or more motor neuron growth factors, once unequivocally identified, can explain many of the results obtained in in vivo manipulations of the periphery.

CONCLUSION

It is important to recognize that the lateral motor column of the frog is subject to the same mechanisms and influences that developmentally control the nervous system in general. The perspective that several primary processes are the inherent regulators of nervous system development, upon which may be imposed extrinsic influences, has provided a framework for building an integrated picture from which more critical analyses can proceed. The LMC itself provides a well-defined central nervous system nucleus with easily manipulatable targets in an animal whose protracted development permits careful dissection of events. Through both in vivo and in vitro approaches, a comprehensive pattern of LMC development, including a system of interactions, is emerging that will be amenable to study at increasingly refined levels.

ACKNOWLEDGMENT

Although a number of individuals have variously contributed to the work in this laboratory, the author is particularly indebted to Veronica Liebig for her extensive contributions to its many phases. William L. Muhlach was a significant contributor to the in vitro studies while associated with the laboratory. The ongoing support of the Institute for the Study of Developmental Disabilities is gratefully acknowledged. And above all, the author is particularly indebted to his longstanding and inspirational association with Professor Jerry J. Kollros.

REFERENCES

Beaudoin AR (1955). The development of the lateral motor column cells in the lumbo-sacral cord in Rana pipiens. I. Normal development and development following unilateral limb amputation. Anat Rec 121:81-95.
Beaudoin AR (1956). The development of the lateral motor column cells in the lumbo-sacral cord in Rana pipiens. II. Development under the influence of thyroxine. Anat Rec 125:247-254.
Chu-Wang I-W, Oppenheim RW, Farel PB (1981). Ultrastructure of migrating spinal motoneurons in anuran larvae. Brain Res 213:307-318.
Dasgupta S (1962). Induction of triploidy by hydrostatic pressure in the leopard frog, Rana pipiens. J Exp Zool 151:105-121.
Davis MR, Constantine-Paton M, Schorr D (1983). Dorsal root ganglion removal in Rana pipiens produces fewer motoneurons. Brain Res 265:283-288.
Farel PB (1987). Motoneuron number in the lumbar lateral motor column of larval and adult bullfrogs. J Comp Neurol 261:266-276.
Farel PB, Bemelmans SE (1980). Retrograde labeling of migrating spinal motoneurons in bullfrog larvae. Neurosci Lett 18:133-136.
Fox H (1984). "Amphibian Metamorphosis." Clifton NJ: Humana, pp 81-89.
Hollyday M, Mendell L (1976). Analysis of moving supernumerary limbs of Xenopus laevis. Exp Neurol 51:316-324.

Hughes AFW (1968). "Aspects of Neural Ontogeny." London: Logos Press.

Kett NA, Pollack ED (1985). Retention of lateral motor column neurons during the phase of rapid cell loss after limb amputation in Rana pipiens tadpoles. J Exp Zool 236:59-66.

Kollros JJ (1956). The further development of the spinal cord, ganglia and nerves. In Nieuwkoop PD, Faber J (eds): "Normal Table of Xenopus laevis (Daudin)." Amsterdam: North-Holland, pp 63-73.

Kollros JJ (1961). Mechanisms of amphibian metamorphosis: hormones. Am Zool 1:107-114.

Kollros JJ (1968a). Order and control of neurogenesis (as exemplified by the lateral motor column. Develop Biol Suppl 2:274-305.

Kollros JJ (1968b). Endocrine influences in neural development. In Wolstenholme GEW, O'Connor M (eds): "Ciba Foundation Symposium on Growth of the Nervous System." Boston: Little Brown, pp 179-192.

Lamb AH (1981). The timing of the earliest motor innervation to the hind limb bud in the Xenopus tadpole. Brain Res 67: 527-530.

Lamb AH (1981). Selective bilateral motor innervation in Xenopus tadpoles with one hind limb. J Embryol Exp Morphol 65:149-163.

Lamb AH (1985). Motoneuron death in the embryo. CRC Crit Rev Clin Neurobiol 1:141-197.

Maheras HM, Pollack ED (1985). Quantitative compensation by lateral motor column neurons in response to four functional hindlimbs in a frog tadpole. Develop Brain Res 19:150-154.

Muhlach WL, Pollack ED (1978). Improved method for the in vitro study of amphibian neural development utilizing Sykes-Moore chambers. Tiss Cult Assoc Man 4:875-879.

Pollack ED (1969a). Normal development of the lateral motor column in the brachial cord in Rana pipiens. Anat Rec 163:111-120.

Pollack ED (1969b). Response of the lateral motor column to multiple forelimbs in Rana pipiens. Teratol 2:159-162.

Pollack ED (1972). Cell migration into the "established" lateral motor column in Rana pipiens larvae. I. Brachial spinal cord. J Exp Zool 179:183-190.

Pollack ED (1976). Presumptive relationships between ventricular proliferation and development of the lateral motor columns in the spinal cord of <u>Rana pipiens</u> larvae. Am J Anat 147:183-192.

Pollack ED (1980). Target-dependent survival of tadpole spinal cord neurites in tissue culture. Neurosci Lett 16:269-274.

Pollack ED, Kollros JJ (1975). Cell migration into the "established" lateral motor column in <u>Rana pipiens</u> larvae. II. Lumbosacral spinal cord and comparative aspects. J Exp Zool 192:299-306.

Pollack ED, Koves J (1975). In vitro cultivation of larval frog spinal cord. Tiss Cult Assoc Man 1:193-197.

Pollack ED, Koves J (1977). Compensatory responses in the development of the brachial lateral motor column in triploid <u>Rana pipiens</u>. Anat Rec 188:173-180.

Pollack ED, <u>Liebig V</u> (1977). Differentiating limb tissue affects nerve growth in spinal cord cultures. Science 197:899-900.

Pollack ED, Muhlach WL (1981). Stage dependency in eliciting target-dependent enhanced neurite outgrowth from spinal cord explants in vitro. Develop Biol 86:259-263.

Pollack ED, Muhlach WL (1982). Target control of neuronal development during formation of the spinal reflex arc: an operant model. J Neurosci Res 8:343-355.

Pollack ED, Muhlach WL, Liebig V (1981). Neurotropic influence of mesenchymal limb target tissue on spinal cord neurite growth in vitro. J Comp Neurol 200:393-405.

Pollack ED, Richmond M (1981). Analysis of mesenchyme in the developing hind limb of <u>Rana pipiens</u> larvae with implications for neural development. J Morphol 169:253-257.

Prestige MC (1967). The control of cell number in the lumbar ventral horns during the development of <u>Xenopus laevis</u> tadpoles. J Embryol Exp Morphol 18:359-387.

Prestige MC, Willshaw DJ (1975). On a role for competition in the formation of patterned neural connexions. Proc Roy Soc Lond B 190:77-98.

Prestige MC, Wilson MA (1974). A quantitative study of the growth and development of the ventral root in normal and experimental conditions. J Embryol Exp Morphol 32:819-833.

Reynolds WA (1966). Mitotic activity in the lumbosacral cord of <u>Rana pipiens</u> larvae after thyroxine and thiourea treatment. Gen Comp Endocrinol 6:453-465.

Rugh R (1951). "The Frog: Its Reproduction and Development." New York:McGraw-Hill.

Stebbins CA, Pollack ED (1986). Neuron number and asynchronous hindlimb development during the period of profound cell loss in the lateral motor column of Rana pipiens larvae. J Exp. Zool 237:79-85.

Taylor AC, Kollros JJ (1946). Stages in the normal development of Rana pipiens larvae. Anat Rec 94:7-23.

THE ORIGIN OF INTERINDIVIDUAL VARIATION IN MOTONEURON NUMBER IN THE LUMBAR LATERAL MOTOR COLUMN OF XENOPUS LAEVIS

David G. Sperry

School of Life and Health Sciences, University of Delaware, Newark, Delaware 19716

INTRODUCTION

The various mechanisms operating during normal development to ensure that a functional nervous system is produced in the frog are the underlying subjects of this volume. Two questions pertaining to these mechanisms in general are how the size of the developing nervous system is determined and how the developing nervous system responds to size differences that emerge during the time when neuron populations and their interconnections are established. Interest in the answers to these questions is heightened by knowing that the final size of many neuron populations is not the end of a progressive series of cell additions, but rather the result of an early period of overproduction followed by cell death (for reviews see Hamburger and Oppenheim, 1982; Cowan et al., 1984; Lamb, 1984). The process of neuron proliferation appears to be intrinsically or genetically controlled, and information regarding interindividual size differences is not generally thought to be incorporated into the production process. On the other hand, neuron survival is conspicuously target dependent, very sensitive to the presence or absence of the appropriate target, and therefore likely capable of responding to information about differences in size.

Why the nervous system incorporates overproduction and cell death into its development is not fully understood, but one role for target-dependent survival may be to effect a size match between a developing neuron population and its appropriate postsynaptic target. Implied in a systems-matching hypothesis such as the one articulated by Hamburger and Oppenheim (1982), is the idea that adequate innervation of a tissue whose size might vary unpredictably could be provided quite simply by altering the magnitude of cell death in relation to the innervation opportunities presented to the ingrowing neuronal processes. The results from experimental attempts to identify numerical relationships between neuron populations and their postsynaptic targets have been mixed, and whether a competition-based, cell death-related, size-matching process operates during normal development and regulates the size of a neuron population is uncertain. The uncertainty regarding normal development may be even greater because most studies that focus on the issue of size matching do so by comparing the magnitude of cell death between populations of experimental and control animals.

The anuran lateral motor column has already been introduced in the preceding chapter as a model system for studying neuronal development in general, and certainly this cell population has been used extensively to study the specific question of how neuron number and the postsynaptic target's size are related. In one species of anuran, Xenopus laevis (the African clawed frog), the question of how neuron number is controlled has been readdressed using a different approach (Sperry, 1987, and in prep.). Rather than creating differences in neuron number by experimentally altering the magnitude of cell death, the naturally occurring interindividual differences in motoneuron number were used. Both normally developing diploid and triploid Xenopus have been studied, and the observations have demonstrated how differences in muscle size, how differences in neuron production, and how the process of cell death contribute to producing the naturally occurring interindividual variation in motoneuron number within the lumbar lateral motor column (L-LMC).

DEVELOPMENT OF THE L-LMC AND CHARACTERISTICS OF THE MOTONEURON POPULATION AT THE COMPLETION OF CELL DEATH

The development of the lumbar lateral motor column

in Xenopus, as in other anuran amphibians, clearly coincides with the normal development of the hindlimb (Kollros, 1968). L-LMC motoneurons are proliferated, and they migrate into their characteristic ventrolateral positions during the time that the hindlimb bud elongates and forms digits on the foot paddle (Hughes, 1961; Prestige, 1967, 1973). The total number of motoneurons counted in the motor column peaks in animals at stages of development when the hindlimb digits are formed and when the first limb movements occur (stages 53/54, Nieuwkoop and Faber, 1965; Hughes and Prestige, 1967; Fig. 1). Neuron number subsequently declines, and by the completion of metamorphosis, neuronal cell death reduces neuron number by roughly 70% (Hughes, 1961; Prestige, 1967; Sperry, 1987). At metamorphosis (stage 66), the lateral motor columns are easily recognized histologically as cell clusters composed of significantly fewer, but larger, cells than were present at stages prior to cell death (Fig. 1).

In a large heterogeneous sample of stage 66 Xenopus representing 15 groups of siblings reared under similar conditions, the motoneurons of the right and left lateral motor columns were counted (Sperry, 1987). Two characteristics of the motoneuron population were apparent and they are demonstrated in Fig. 2. First, there was a very high degree of bilateral symmetry of motoneuron number in the animals. Second, while motoneuron number within an individual was highly symmetrical, there was significant interindividual variation in neuron number, ranging from extreme values of roughly 750 to 2100 motoneurons, although most counts varied from 1000 to 1800 motoneurons.

The symmetry and interindividual variation in neuron number in Xenopus were not unexpected. Previously published L-LMC motoneuron counts from Xenopus demonstrated a high degree of bilateral symmetry and total cell number varied from author to author, a difference of concern to Prestige (1967) and again commented on by Kollros (1968). Bilateral symmetry and equally large interindividual variation in the total number of L-LMC motoneurons have also been observed among newly metamorphosed Bufo americanus (the common American toad, Sperry and Grobstein, 1983; Sperry, unpublished obervations). Symmetry and large interindividual variation may, in fact, prove to be general characteristics of the lateral motor column motoneuron population of anuran amphibians if sufficient numbers of individuals of other species are examined.

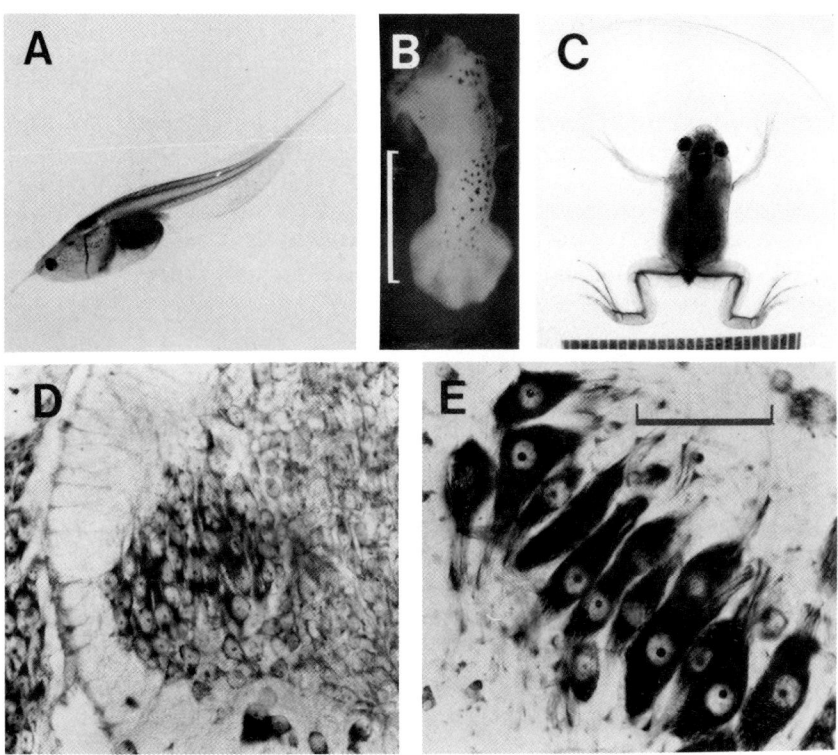

Figure 1. A and B) a stage 54 tadpole and hindlimb. C) a stage 66 frog. D and E) representative sections through the L-LMC of stage 54 and 66 animals, respectively. Photographs of animals and motoneurons are to same scale for comparison (A, B, and C scale bar = 1 mm; D and E scale bar = 50 µm).

The striking bilateral symmetry is evidence that neuron number in an individual animal is very precisely controlled. Presumably, an equally precise process produces the interindividual differences as well. Whether the bilateral symmetry and the interindividual variation are produced by the same or different mechanisms is, however, uncertain.

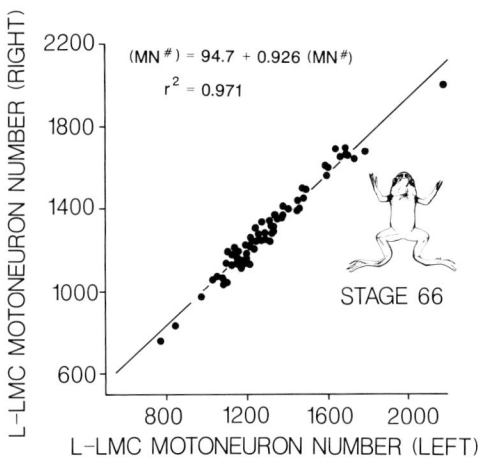

Figure 2. Plot of L-LMC motoneuron number on left versus right sides of the spinal cord of stage 66 Xenopus from 15 sibling groups.

THE RELATIONSHIP BETWEEN MOTONEURON NUMBER AND METAMORPHIC BODY SIZE: EVIDENCE FOR SIZE MATCHING

The interindividual variation in motoneuron number at the end of cell death should be related to variation in body size or to variation in the postsynaptic target's size if a size-matching process operates during normal development. Metamorphic body sizes of amphibians in general are quite variable, even among siblings that are reared under uniform conditions (whether reared individually or in groups; Wilbur and Collins, 1973; Wilbur, 1977; Duellman and Trueb, 1986). The size differences are greatly accentuated by changing environmental temperature (the effect on Rana pipiens was demonstrated by Decker and Kollros, 1969), by reversibly

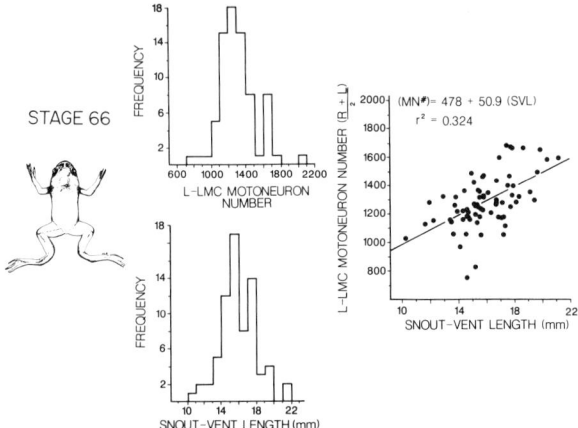

Figure 3. Frequency histograms of motoneuron number and snout-vent length and a plot of motoneuron number versus snout-vent length of stage 66 Xenopus from 15 sibling groups.

blocking the production or release of thyroxine (the effect on Xenopus was demonstrated using a goitrogen by Sperry and Grobstein, 1985) and by interindividual competition for food resources (density-dependent effects demonstrated by Wilbur, 1976, 1977). Certainly, a size-matching process that regulates neuron number would appear appropriate for meeting the demands of variation in body size that are easily produced in amphibians by unpredictable environmental conditions.

For the stage 66 Xenopus whose motoneurons were counted, the variation in body size was also large (Fig. 3). As might be expected, motoneuron number and body size were significantly correlated. Therefore, even in a heterogeneous sample of animals reared under roughly similar conditions, the interindividual variation in motoneuron number appeared to be at least partly size-related. To investigate further how the size-related interindividual variation in motoneurons might be produced, the size of the postsynaptic target was measured in a more homogeneous sample of animals (representing only two sibling groups). Within this more homogeneous sample, the variation in motoneuron number and the variation in body size were large and highly correlated with one another (Fig. 4A).

Variation in Hindlimb Muscle Fiber Number

Muscle fibers were counted in two representative thigh muscles (the gracilis major and the semimembranosus; Noble, 1922) from both the right and left hindlimbs. Four characteristics of the muscle fiber populations that appeared to be particularly relevant to the size-matching issue were noted.

First, intraindividual bilateral symmetry in muscle fiber number was very high (Fig. 4B). Second, interindividual variation in muscle fiber number in each of the two muscles was about two-fold: a difference about equal to the interindividual variation in motoneuron number. Presumably, the process controlling the number of muscle fibers produced is also very precise: maintaining a high degree of intraindividual symmetry while producing large interindividual differences.

Third, the interindividual differences in muscle fiber number in the two muscles were significantly positively correlated (Fig. 4C). Therefore, large and small fiber populations were produced proportionally in these muscles, and perhaps proportional changes in muscle fiber number occurred throughout the hindlimb muscles in general. Observing the proportional relationship strengthens any comparison made between the numbers of muscle fibers counted in representative muscles and the number of motoneurons in the entire motor column. Fourth, interindividual variation in fiber number was itself size-related (although the equation best fitting the data may not be that of a straight line; Fig. 4D).

The Relationship Between Motoneuron Number and Muscle Fiber Number

The relationships between body size, the size of the postsynaptic target and the size of the motoneuron

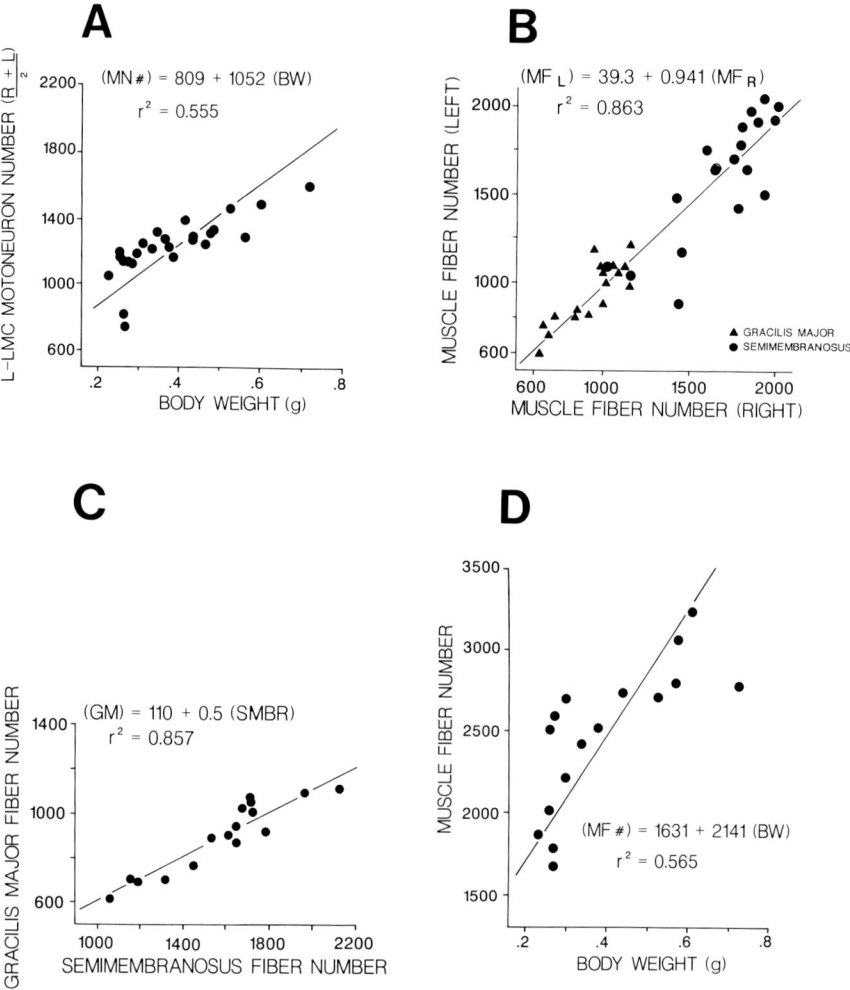

Figure 4. Characteristics of the L-LMC motoneuron population and the muscle fiber populations of representative hindlimb muscles of stage 66 animals from two sibling groups. A) plot of motoneuron number versus body weight. B) plot of muscle fiber number from left versus right hindlimb muscles. C) plot of fiber number in the gracilis major versus the semimembranosus muscles. D) plot of muscle fiber number (gracilis major and semimembranosus) versus body weight.

population in the homogeneous sample of stage 66 Xenopus are illustrated in Fig. 5. In this diagram, the correlation coefficients representing the level of relatedness between various components are included (r^2 values for simple linear regressions). Body weight and snout-vent length were highly correlated and could be used interchangeably as body size in the analyses. Within the nervous system, the variation in motoneuron number was significantly correlated with the variation in motor column length and with the variation in body size (as already described). Within the postsynaptic target, the numbers of muscle fibers in the two muscles were highly correlated, and total muscle fiber number (gracilis major + semimembranosus) was highly correlated with body size. As might be expected, the size-related variation in muscle fiber number and the size-related variation in motoneuron number were significantly correlated as shown.

Overall, normally developing stage 66 animals were composed of parts that were very appropriately sized for one another. Both the motoneuron population and the hindlimb muscle fiber population were highly bilaterally symmetrical, and the interindividual differences in cell numbers were significantly correlated. Therefore, both the bilateral symmetry and the variation in motoneuron number at the end of cell death could have been produced by a competition-based, systems-matching process that altered neuronal cell death to match the interindividual differences in the postsynaptic target's size.

THE L-LMC MOTONEURON POPULATION PRIOR TO CELL DEATH

The characteristics of the motoneuron population in animals at a stage before cell death were also determined in an effort to identify any that might have contributed to the interindividual variation observed at the end of cell death. Motoneuron number, body size and hindlimb size were measured in stage 54 tadpoles which were collected from the same groups of siblings that composed the heterogeneous sample of stage 66 Xenopus. Motoneuron proliferation has ended by stage 54 (Prestige, 1973) and the massive motoneuronal cell death occurs after this stage, although small numbers of

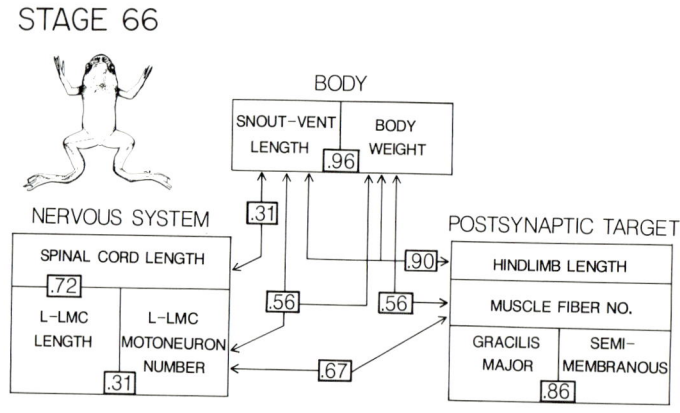

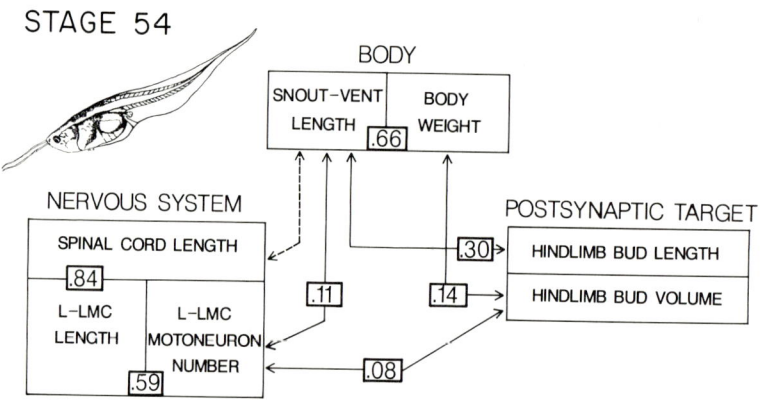

Figure 5. Summary of correlations between components of stage 66 (upper) and stage 54 (lower) <u>Xenopus</u>. See text for description.

degenerating cells in the motor column cell clusters of younger animals have been reported by other investigators (Hughes, 1961; Prestige, 1967).

The relationships between body size, the size of the postsynaptic target and the size of the motoneuron population of stage 54 animals are illustrated in Fig. 5. Again, the correlation coefficients representing the level of relatedness between various components are included. The stage 54 animals were very different from their stage 66 siblings. Prior to cell death, body size, hindlimb size and the size of the developing nervous system were remarkably unrelated. The apparent absence of significant size correlations before cell death is consistent with the explanation that a systems-matching process sensitive to variation in postsynaptic target size established the size-related variation observed after cell death.

However, there were several other observations from the stage 54 animals less consistent with the interpretation that a size-matching process produced the variation in motoneuron number at the end of cell death. Both a high degree of bilateral symmetry in motoneuron number and very large interindividual differences in neuron number were already present in the stage 54 animals (Fig. 6), and both were created by the process of cell proliferation. It is possible, therefore, that the variability in motoneuron number at stage 54 was actually causal to the variability at stage 66. To explore this possibility, sibling groups were compared.

THE RELATIONSHIP BETWEEN VARIATION IN MOTONEURON NUMBER BEFORE AND AFTER CELL DEATH: SIBLING GROUP COMPARISONS

For 12 sibling groups, motoneurons were counted in animals at both stage 54 and stage 66, and the mean number of motoneurons for each stage in each sibling group was calculated. When the mean values were compared, significant sibling group differences were obvious (Fig. 7). In addition to the sibling group differences at either stage (i.e., some groups had larger or smaller motoneuron populations), the differences in the number of motoneurons at stage 54

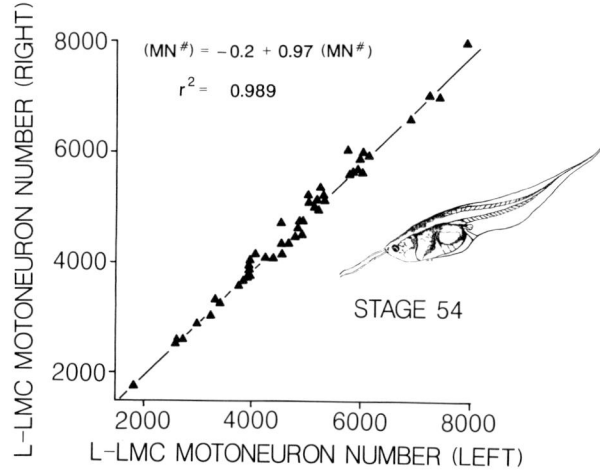

Figure 6. Plot of motoneuron number on the right versus left sides of the spinal cord of stage 54 Xenopus.

significantly influenced the differences in the number of motoneurons at the end of cell death. On the basis of comparing mean values, the process of neuronal cell death eliminated a very constant percentage of the motoneuron population in the different sibling groups (about 70%), even though the absolute numbers of cells eliminated in different groups varied from 2000 to 4000 cells. Consequently, the numbers of neurons in siblings at stage 66 (the stage after cell death) were highly correlated with the numbers of neurons in their siblings at stage 54 (the stage prior to cell death); the process that produced the symmetry and variation in the L-LMC motoneuron population was an excellent predictor of the symmetry and variation present at the end of cell death. The correlations across cell death would not be predicted if a systems-matching process involving postsynaptic target size variation was regulating motoneuron number and producing the interindividual variation in motoneuron number after cell death.

The observations from sibling group comparisons are

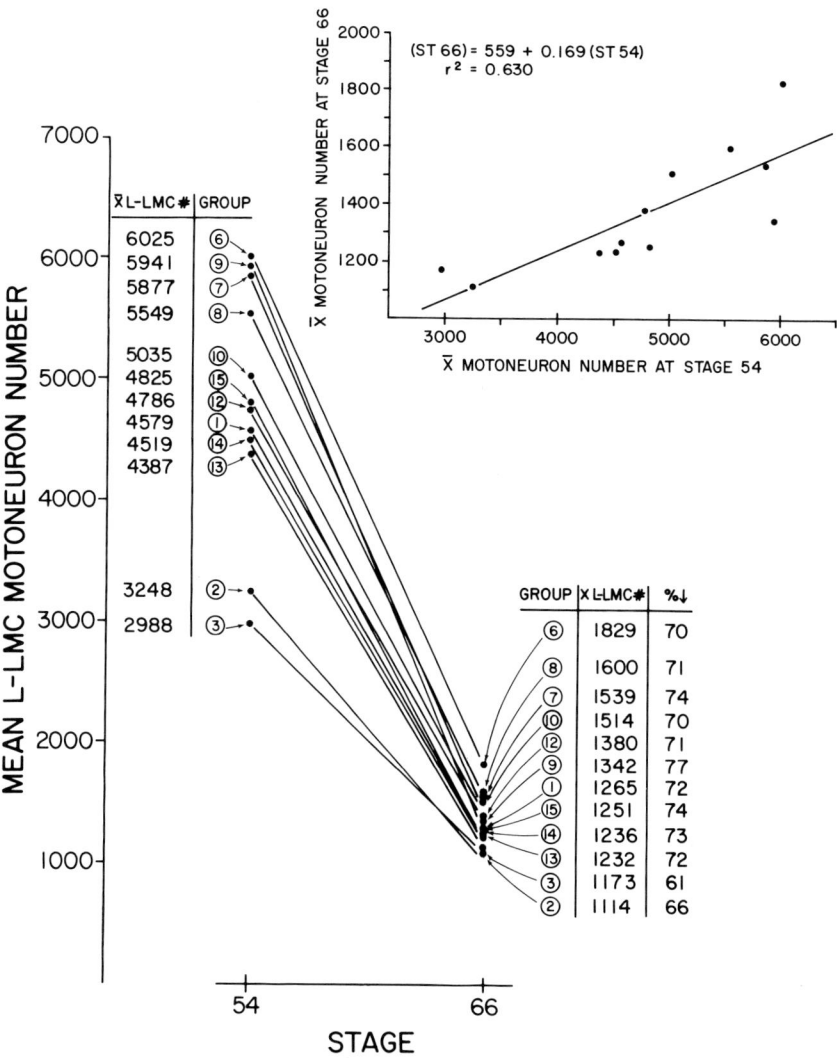

Figure 7. Mean motoneuron number for stage 54 and stage 66 animals from 12 groups of siblings. Group numbers (identifying egg batches) and motoneuron numbers are indicated, and the percent decrease from stage 54 to stage 66 is also indicated (far right). The inset (upper right) is a plot of mean motoneuron number at stage 66 versus mean motoneuron number at stage 54 for the 12 sibling groups. (From Sperry, 1987).

summarized in Fig. 8. Among groups of siblings, the intraindividual symmetry and the variation in the L-LMC motoneuron population are created during the process of motoneuron proliferation. The variation in motoneuron number at stages 53/54 is represented by a hypothetical frequency histogram placed at the upper end of the vertical scale. During normal development, the neuronal cell death occurring between stages 53/54 and 66 is not a highly variable event producing large differences in motoneuron number. To the contrary, neuronal cell death appears to be largely responsible for retaining the variation originally present, a point represented in Fig. 8 by the same hypothetical frequency histogram appearing at the lower end of the vertical scale after cell death (stage 66). Because variation in neuron number within a sibling group is also large at stage 53/54, the same process (variable cell production followed by a constant magnitude of cell death) might produce the interindividual variation at the end of cell death as well.

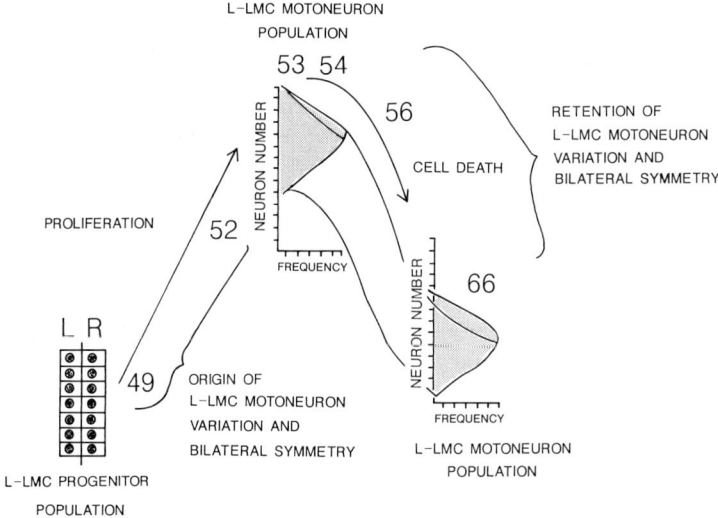

Figure 8. Schematic summary of L-LMC development. See text for explanation.

EXPLANATIONS FOR THE CORRELATION BETWEEN MOTONEURON NUMBER AND POSTSYNAPTIC TARGET SIZE AT THE END OF CELL DEATH

Since the interindividual variation in neuron number at the end of cell death can be related to an event occurring long before the cell death process, it follows that the variation in the postsynaptic target's size is not likely to be causal to the differences in motoneuron number observed in normally developing animals. If postsynaptic target size variation is not causing the variation in motoneuron number through a systems-matching process, then alternate explanations for the observed correlation must be considered.

Two possibilities are recognized. First, the correlation could be produced by the reverse of what has generally been assumed to happen. The variation in the number of neurons originally produced may be causal to the variation in the postsynaptic target's size (i.e., muscle fiber number). This possibility is similar to an explanation proposed earlier by Purves (neurons regulate the target property for which they compete; 1980) and it is consistent with the more recent findings that one phase of the process of muscle differentiation, the production of secondary myotubes, is dependent on innervation (McLennan, 1983; Ferns and Lamb, 1987; Ross et al., 1987).

A second possibility is that both the neuron population and the postsynaptic target receive size signals very early in development, and that the correlation observed at the end of cell death in normally developing animals is simply the outcome of two independent developmental programs that do not pass size-related information back and forth. A comparison of diploid and experimentally produced triploid Xenopus help to distinguish which of these two explanations is likely correct.

MOTONEURON NUMBER, MUSCLE FIBER NUMBER, AND CELL DEATH IN TRIPLOID XENOPUS

In anurans, triploid siblings can be produced by subjecting fertilized diploid eggs to increased hydrostatic pressure for a brief period after sperm entry (Dasgupta, 1962; Tompkins, 1978). At the tissue level, an increase in ploidy generally results in an increase in cell size with a compensatory decrease in cell number to retain the same overall size (Fankhauser, 1945; Gurdon, 1959). This type of compensatory response was observed in the brachial lateral motor column of triploid R. pipiens by Pollack and Koves (1977).

The lumbar lateral motor column motoneurons and the fibers in the gracilis major and semimembranosus muscles of stage 66 diploid and triploid Xenopus siblings were counted (Sperry, in prep.). Motoneurons were also counted in stage 54 animals (both diploid and triploid; Sperry, personal observations).

Ploidy-Related Effects on Motoneuron Number and Muscle Fiber Number: Stage 66 Animals

At stage 66, triploid Xenopus had significantly fewer, but larger, motoneurons than diploids (Fig. 9). The intraindividual symmetry and the interindividual variation in motoneuron number were not affected by the change in ploidy. The total size of the motor column (whether measured as column length or total motoneuron nuclear area) in triploids and diploids was roughly equal, and the ploidy-related differences in total neuron number were caused by significant differences in motoneuron density throughout the length of the motor column (mean number of cells per section in each sixth of the motor column; Fig 10). The interindividual differences in motoneuron number in diploids and triploids were significantly size related (Fig. 11). In general, all of these results were expected from the previous observations on triploid anurans.

The findings from the postsynaptic target were not what might have been expected. While the muscles of triploids demonstrated the same characteristics described for muscles of normally developing diploid animals (i.e., intraindividual symmetry, interindividual size-related variation, and a proportional change in fiber number in the two muscles), the numbers of muscle fibers in these two thigh muscles were not significantly different in diploids and triploids (Fig. 12). In fact,

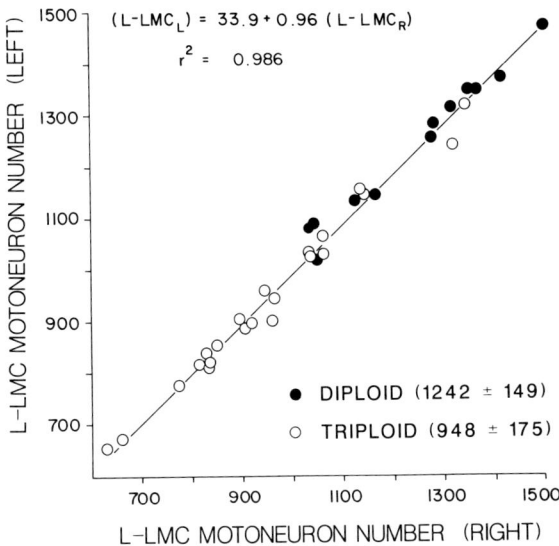

Figure 9. Plot of motoneuron number on the left versus right sides of the spinal cord of diploid and triploid stage 66 Xenopus siblings. Mean ± S.D. are included in the figure.

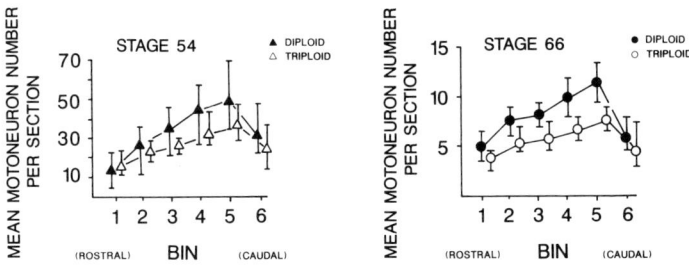

Figure 10. Plot of the mean number of motoneurons per 10 μm section in each sixth of the L-LMC (BIN) for all diploid and triploid siblings at stage 54 (left) and stage 66 (right). Each symbol represents the mean of individual mean values and each vertical line represents the range of individual mean values.

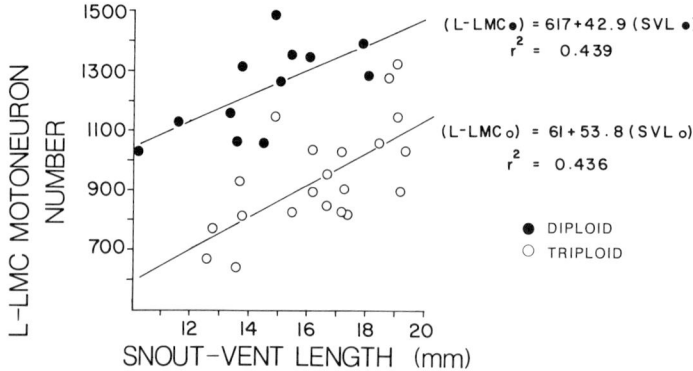

Figure 11. Plot of motoneuron number versus snout-vent length for diploid and triploid stage 66 Xenopus siblings.

the values for triploids fell completely within the range of values for diploids. While motoneuron number and muscle fiber number were significantly correlated in diploids, motoneuron number and muscle fiber number were not significantly correlated in triploids. Therefore, the decrease in motoneuron number produced by the increase in ploidy was not caused by, nor did it cause a ploidy-related decrease in muscle fiber number, observations interpreted as being inconsistent with an active size-matching process operating in either direction.

Ploidy-Related Effects on Motoneuron Number at Stage 54 and on Cell Death

At stage 54, total motoneuron numbers in diploids and triploids were bilaterally symmetrical (although not illustrated) and highly variable. Motoneuron number in triploids was reduced, but the values for diploids and triploids overlapped considerably (Fig. 13). The ploidy-related differences in motoneuron number were, as in stage 66 animals, the result of significant ploidy-

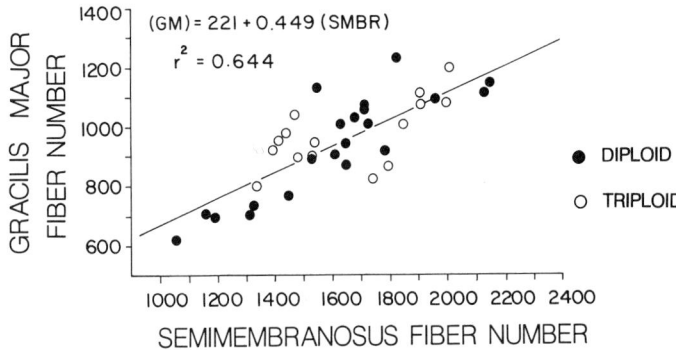

Figure 12. Plot of muscle fiber number in the gracilis major versus fiber number in the semimembranosus for diploid and triploid stage 66 Xenopus.

related differences in motoneuron density throughout motor columns of roughly equal lengths (mean motoneuron number per section in each sixth of the column; Fig. 10).

Finally, on the basis of differences in mean values, neuronal cell death eliminated equal percentages of the motoneuron population in diploids and triploids (66% and 70%, respectively; Fig. 13). Therefore, the ploidy-related differences in motoneuron number at the end of cell death, while not apparently related to variation in muscle fiber number, appeared to have been produced in the same way that differences in motoneuron number between groups of normally developing diploid siblings were produced: variation in cell production followed by equal magnitudes of cell death.

SUMMARY: A COMMON DENOMINATOR IN L-LMC DEVELOPMENT

The interindividual differences in neuron number after cell death in normally developing Xenopus are largely, if not wholly, the result of events that

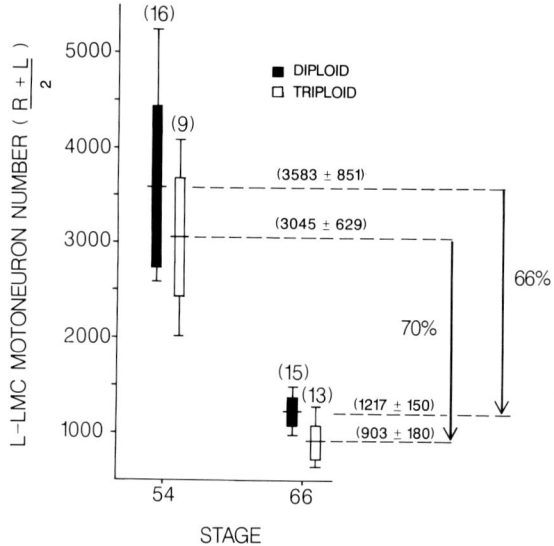

Figure 13. Bar plot (mean, standard deviation and range) of motoneuron number of diploid and triploid siblings at stages 54 and 66. Mean values (± S.D.) for each group and the percent decrease from stage 54 to stage 66 are illustrated.

produce large differences in the motoneuron population prior to cell death. This conclusion is consistent with the observations made between groups of siblings of the same ploidy as well as between siblings of different ploidy. Presumably, the differences in motoneuron number between individual animals in a particular sibling group might also be produced in the same manner. This assumption is supported by the observations from triploids; siblings in which an experimentally induced increase in neuron size resulted in a decrease in neuron number.

Relating the naturally occurring variation in neuron number after cell death to a cell production event implies that the significant correlation between the final number of motoneurons and the postsynaptic target's size (muscle fiber number for example) was not likely created by imposing target variation onto the neuron population through a variable cell death process. In fact, if cell death is measured in terms of the fraction of motoneurons removed, cell death is remarkably consistent. Likewise, the converse explanation, that the significant correlation between neuron number and target size was produced by imposing the variation in the neuron population onto the target by differential production of muscle fibers also was not likely. Diploid and triploid siblings demonstrated ploidy-related differences in neuron number before and after cell death, but only size-related differences in muscle fiber number.

It appears very likely, therefore, that the size of the motoneuron population and the size of the postsynaptic target are being determined by signals that they both receive early in development. These signals establish the interindividual variation in motoneuron number and the interindividual variation in muscle fiber number with a very high degree of bilateral symmetry. During subsequent normal development, when neuronal cell death acts uniformly on motoneuron populations of highly variable size, size-related signals that significantly alter the relative size of the lumbar lateral motor column or the postsynaptic target probably do not pass between these cell populations. The correlation between motoneuron number and the size of the postsynaptic target after cell death may largely reflect the level of the correlation between the size signals that were originally received rather than any size match that occurred late in development.

The available data are insufficient to conclude that no size signals affecting the magnitude of cell death, and therefore adjusting cell number during normal development, pass from the L-LMC to the hindlimb muscles or from the hindlimb muscles to the L-LMC. However, any such signals would only act in addition to the significant interindividual variation that was established when motoneurons were proliferated, since the naturally occurring variation in the number of neurons produced probably is causal to the naturally occurring variation in the number of neurons at the end of cell death in the L-LMC of Xenopus laevis.

ACKNOWLEDGMENTS

I wish to thank Mr. Christopher Whitney and Ms. Kathryn Bostock for their technical assistance. Mrs. Margie Barrett prepared the figures. I am grateful to Drs. Margaret Hollyday, Paul Grobstein and Ray Guillery for their many suggestions, criticisms and discussions. The research reported and the preparation of this manuscript was supported by NIH grant NS21878.

REFERENCES

Cowan WM, Fawcett JW, O'Leary DDM, Stanfield BB (1984). Regressive events in neurogenesis. Science 225:1258-1265.
Dasgupta S (1962). Induction of triploidy by hydrostatic pressure in the leopard frog, Rana pipiens. J Exp Zool 151:105-121.
Decker RS, Kollros JJ (1969). The effect of cold on hind-limb growth and lateral motor column development in Rana pipiens. J Embryol Exp Morphol 21:219-233.
Duellman WE, Trueb L (1986). "Biology of Amphibians." New York: McGraw-Hill.
Ferns MJ, Lamb AH (1987). Regulation of cell numbers in the developing neuromuscular system in Xenopus laevis. Neurosci Lett Suppl 27:S72.
Fankhauser G (1945). The effects of changes in chromosome number on amphibian development. Quart Rev Biol 20:20-78.
Gurdon JB (1959). Tetraploid frogs. J Exp Zool 141:519-543.
Hamburger V, Oppenheim RW (1982). Naturally occurring neuronal death in vertebrates. Neurosci Commentaries 1:39-55.
Hughes A (1961). Cell degeneration in the larval ventral horn of Xenopus laevis (Daudin). J Embryol Exp Morphol 9:269-284.
Hughes A, Prestige MC (1967). Development of behaviour in the hindlimb of Xenopus laevis. J Zool 152:347-359.
Kollros JJ (1968). Order and control of neurogenesis (as exemplified by the lateral motor column). Develop Biol Suppl 2:274-305.
Lamb AH (1984). Motoneuron death in the embryo. CRC Crit Rev Clin Neurobiol 1:141-179.
McLennan IS (1983). Neural dependence and independence

of myotube production in chicken hindlimb muscles. Develop Biol 98:287-294.

Nieuwkoop PD, Faber J (1965). "Normal Table of Xenopus laevis (Daudin)." Amsterdam: North-Holland.

Noble GK (1922). The phylogeny of the Salientia. I. The osteology and the thigh musculature; their bearing on classification and phylogeny. Bull Amer Mus Nat Hist 46:2-133.

Pollack ED, Koves J (1977). Compensatory responses in the development of the brachial lateral motor column in triploid Rana pipiens. Anat Rec 188:173-180.

Prestige MC (1967). The control of cell number in the ventral horns during the development of Xenopus laevis tadpoles. J Embryol Exp Morphol 18:359-387.

Prestige MC (1973). Gradients in time of origin of tadpole motor neurons. Brain Res 59:400-404.

Purves D (1980). Neuronal competition. Nature 287:585-586.

Ross JJ, Duxson MJ, Harris AJ (1987). Neural determination of muscle fibre numbers in embryonic rat lumbrical muscles. Development 100:395-409.

Sperry DG (1987). Relationship between natural variations in motoneuron number and body size in Xenopus laevis: A test for size matching. J Comp Neurol 264:250-267.

Sperry DG, Grobstein P (1983). Postmetamorphic changes in the lumbar lateral motor column in relation to muscle growth in the toad, Bufo americanus. J Comp Neurol 216:104-114.

Sperry DG, Grobstein P (1985). Regulation of neuron numbers in Xenopus: Effects of hormonal manipulation altering size at metamorphosis. J Comp Neurol 232:287-298.

Tompkins R (1978). Triploid and gynogenetic diploid Xenopus laevis. J Exp Zool 203:251-256.

Wilbur HM (1976). Density-dependent aspects of metamorphosis in Ambystoma and Rana sylvatica. Ecology 57:1289-1296.

Wilbur HM (1977). Density-dependent aspects of growth and metamorphosis in Bufo americanus. Ecology 58:196-200.

Wilbur HM, Collins JP (1973). Ecological aspects of amphibian metamorphosis. Science 182:1305-1314.

MERITOCRATIC SELECTION HYPOTHESIS IN THE CONTROL OF MOTONEURON DEATH DURING DEVELOPMENT

Alan H. Lamb, Philip W. Sheard and Michael J. Ferns

Neuromuscular Research Institute, Department of Pathology, University of Western Australia, Nedlands, 6009, Western Australia

INTRODUCTION

Although the occurrence of neuronal death in the developing nervous system has been described intermittently since the turn of the century, it has become widely recognised only recently with publication of several reviews drawing attention to the magnitude of the phenomenon (Hughes, 1968; Kollros, 1968; Prestige, 1970, 1974; Cowan, 1973). Since, neuronal death has been observed in nearly all parts of the developing nervous system, in vertebrates and invertebrates (Oppenheim, 1981a), and a considerable amount of experimentation and speculation has been applied to understanding the purpose and control mechanisms involved (Cunningham, 1980; Clarke, 1982; Lamb, 1984). The majority of authors have assumed, tacitly or explicitly, that a common function is served by neuronal death in all systems, although Clarke (1982), among others, has emphasised for some time that the evidence suggests varying functions and control mechanisms depending on the developmental needs of the system in question. Newer evidence in a variety of systems, including some described here, amplifies Clarke's view.

THE PERIPHERAL COMPETITION HYPOTHESIS

The most widely held "common-function" view has been the peripheral competition hypothesis which proposes that neuronal death is a reflection of a fail-safe mechanism to ensure numerical balance between the numbers of neurons and the size of the peripheral field. A strategy of generating an excess of neurons has evolved, so the argument goes, to ensure that the peripheral field is adequately innervated. The final number of neurons surviving is regulated by a limited availability of some target factor such as synaptic sites, or trophic factor, forcing the neurons to compete for survival. Several variants of the hypothesis have been proposed (see Lamb, 1984 for review), but in all, target regulation of neuronal number is the common theme.

The peripheral competition hypothesis arose gradually from the thinking of several authors (Hamburger and Levi-Montalcini, 1949; Hamburger, 1958, 1975; Prestige, 1967, 1970, 1974; Cowan, 1973) that it was the most parsimonious of several hypotheses examined to explain the early experimental affects on the peripheral motor and sensory systems of developing chick and frog of complete or partial removal of the limb bud. Particular emphasis was given to the correlation between the quantity of developing musculature and the number of surviving motoneurons. However, later work began to raise doubts about the validity of target regulation, at least as a sole mechanism. First, experiments involving implantation of supernumerary target organs prior to innervation did not result in the increases in motoneuron survival predicted by the hypothesis (Hollyday and Mendell, 1975; Hollyday and Hamburger, 1976; Narayanan and Narayanan, 1978; Boydston and Sohal, 1979). Even under the best conditions, such as in frogs with naturally occurring supernumerary limbs (Bueker, 1945; Pollack, 1969; Lamb, 1979a), the increases tended to be much smaller (approximately 20%) than the 100% increase predicted. Second, removal of segments of the developing spinal cord in both frog (Lamb, 1979b) and chick (Lance-Jones and Landmesser, 1980a) did not result in significantly increased motoneuron survival rates within the remaining segments as predicted. Lance-Jones and Landmesser did observe, however, specific increases of survival in certain motor pools in a few isolated instances suggesting a more complex mechanism than proposed thus far.

A TEST OF THE COMPETITION HYPOTHESIS

A very direct test of the peripheral competition hypothesis was carried out in Xenopus tadpoles (Lamb, 1980) by inducing both sides of the spinal cord (and the dorsal root ganglia) to innervate one of the hindlimb buds, the other having been removed just as motor axon outgrowth from the spinal cord begins (monopodal frogs). In a proportion of animals operated on at the optimal moment, the whole ventral horn cell population from both sides could be made to project into a single limb bud, in effect doubling the competition pressure within the limb. The result was surprising in that an almost normal population of motoneurons survived on the contralateral side, in addition to the normal population on the ipsilateral side. No numerical effect of the contralateral population could be observed on the ipsilateral population; i.e., the ispilateral population was always normal regardless of the numbers of contralateral motoneurons. These results suggested that there was no peripheral interaction between the motoneurons on the two sides. More important, since it was assumed that the quantity of target available to the ipsilateral motoneurons must be compromised by the presence of the contralateral motoneurons, it was concluded that there could not be any peripheral competition taking place among the ipsilateral motoneurons themselves. However, in order to be rigorous about such a conclusion, information about how the motoneurons terminate in the limb, and how the musculature was affected by the double innervation was needed. These aspects have been examined in a series of further studies.

MOTONEURONS AND MUSCULATURE IN MONOPODAL FROGS

The somatotopic projections from the contralateral side were shown to be normal using horseradish peroxidase uptake (Lamb, 1981a) and electrical stimulation of the spinal nerve roots (Denton et al.,1985). Nerve root stimulation also showed that the contralateral motoneurons were as effective as ipsilateral motoneurons at causing muscle contractions, while stimulation of single motor axons indicated that contralateral motoneurons had the same chance as ipsilateral motoneurons of innervating a given muscle fibre (allowing for any disparity in

the quantity of motor innervation from the two sides). In normal Xenopus, the muscle fibres have multiple synapses distributed along their length and are polyneuronally innervated, although any given synapse is innervated by only one motoneuron. No alterations to this arrangement were observed in monopodal animals.
In many instances, individual muscle fibres were polyneuronally innervated by motoneurons from both sides, while the rule of one motoneuron per synapse remained unchanged. The numbers of synapses per muscle fibre were counted using a cholinesterase stain and found not to be increased in the monopodal frogs (Denton et al., 1985). Assuming that the number of muscle fibres was not changed (see below) and knowing that the number of synapses per fibre was not increased, it could be inferred that the number of synapses per motoneuron must be diminished in inverse proportion to the increased number of innervating motoneurons. Although this was not directly analyzed, a marked increase in the average voltage of the mini-end-plate potentials of motoneurons on both sides was observed, consistent with the expectation that a smaller number of synapses per motoneuron would result in larger quantal release by the terminal vesicles (Denton et al., 1985).

Despite the fact that the numbers of synapses per motoneuron were probably reduced, the effect on motor unit size could not be directly inferred because of the polyneuronal and distributed character of Xenopus motor innervation. Conflicting results were obtained using two different methods to analyze this question. Twitch and tetanic tensions of single motor units tended to be smaller in monopodal frogs, suggesting smaller average unit sizes (Denton et al., 1985). In a later study (Sheard and Lamb, unpublished), the glycogen depletion method was used to assess motor unit sizes. Single axons were stimulated by teasing out a small bundle of axons, drawing the bundle into a suction pipette and raising the stimulus voltage until a single unit twitch was observed. Stimulation was then continued at the same voltage (usually about 2 V) using 3 msec pulses at 1 Hz until twitch activity ceased (usually at 2-6 hrs.), followed by short bursts of stimuli at 50 Hz until tetanic activity ceased. No difference was observed between normal and monopodal frogs in the average number of glycogen depleted muscle fibres per motor unit.

It is difficult to know how much significance to attach to either set of data. In the first place, the two studies were not performed on exactly equivalent animals; unfortunately, in the glycogen depletion study none of the monopodal frogs showed high levels of contralateral innervation, and thus motor unit sizes may begin to diminish only when the amount of contralateral innervation is above a certain level. On the other hand, a problem of interpretation is raised by the fact that the polyneuronal, distributed character of motor innervation in Xenopus is associated with local, non-propagated depolarization of the muscle fibres, which would tend to give lower than expected tensions in any given motor unit (in fact, the motor unit itself, as a discrete entity, cannot be defined precisely in Xenopus). This variable may be affected independently in the monopodal frog. A clear answer to the question of the effect of bilateral innervation on motor unit size may come only from another genus such as Rana, in which case the muscle fibres are mono-neuronally innervated.

An important source of uncertainty concerned the number of muscle fibres in the monopodal limb. Qualitatively, the remaining limb appeared normal in size and function, while histologically, no obvious differences in muscle fibre size or number could be seen. In the first of two studies to examine this question, the light microscope was used to count the number of muscle fibres and myonuclei in transverse sections of the gastrocnemius and tibialis anterior (medial belly) of juvenile frogs (Sheard and Lamb, 1986). These were chosen to represent muscles of embryonic origin from the ventral and dorsal pre-muscle masses, respectively, each of which is innervated by medial/early-generated and lateral/late-generated motoneurons respectively, to exclude the possibility of different responses depending on developmental history. The sections were taken from positions in each muscle through which all the fibres of the muscle pass. Because of the anatomical arrangements of the myotendinous junctions, particularly in the gastrocnemius, great care was exercised in selecting an appropriate section to ensure that all fibres of the muscles were included. To facilitate counting, 5% sucrose was added to 5% phosphate buffered glutaraldehyde to separate the fibres by shrinkage.

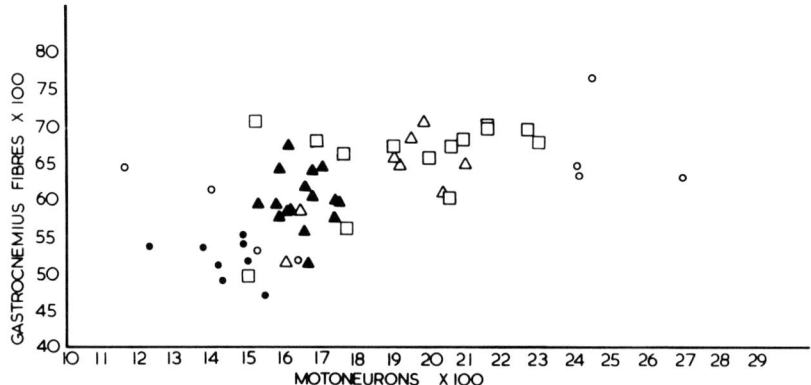

Figure 1. Numbers of muscle fibres in gastrocnemius muscle of normal (solid symbols) and monopodal (open symbols) juvenile frogs plotted against the total number of motoneurons innervating the limb (i.e., ipsilateral plus contralateral in monopodal frogs). Symbols indicate parental origin.

Surprisingly, the muscle fibre numbers were increased by up to 30% in the monopodal frogs depending on the amount of innervation received from the contralateral side. When the number of muscle fibres was plotted against the total number of contralateral plus ipsilateral motoneurons (Figs. 1, 2), the 30% average increase in muscle fibre number was found to be a ceiling value corresponding to total motoneuron counts of approximately 1,800, or about the upper limit of the range of motoneuron numbers on one side of the normal control animals used in this study. Any increases in innervation over this value, regardless of the proportion on the contralateral and ipsilateral sides were not associated with any further increase in muscle fibre number.

Counts of myonuclei showed a similar pattern, as shown by the strong correlation ($r = 0.77$, $p < 0.001$) between the number of myonuclei and the number of myofibres in tibialis anterior (Fig. 3), indicating that the increase in fibres was due to an increase of myogenic cell production, not to the formation of smaller muscle fibres each from a lesser number of progenitor cells.

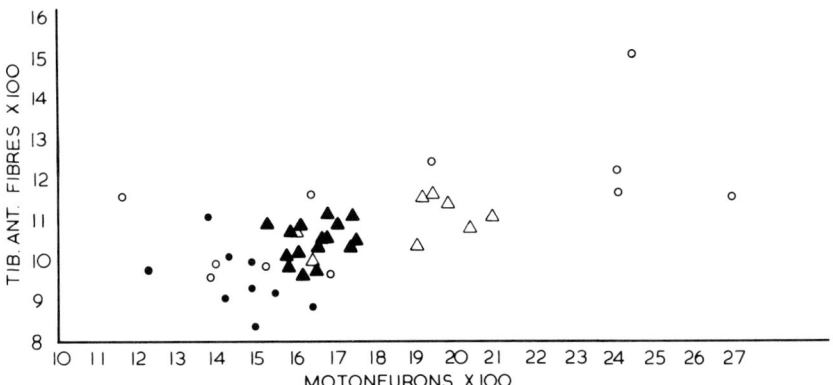

Figure 2. Muscle fibre numbers in the medial belly of tibialis anterior plotted against motoneuron numbers in the same animals as Fig. 1.

Because of the limitations and uncertainty arising from the use of light microscopy, the study was repeated and extended to include early developmental stages using electron microscopy (Ferns and Lamb, 1986, 1987). Individual muscle cells were identified and counted on adjacent thick and thin sections of tibialis anterior (Fig. 4). Both the medial and lateral bellies were counted, in contrast to the earlier study, to provide greater accuracy. An added advantage of this method was that proper fixation without shrinkage allowed an assessment of the muscle fibre sizes. Extra care was taken in this study to use match-paired controls for age, maturity and rearing conditions (experimental and control animals reared together in common aquaria). Muscle fibre areas

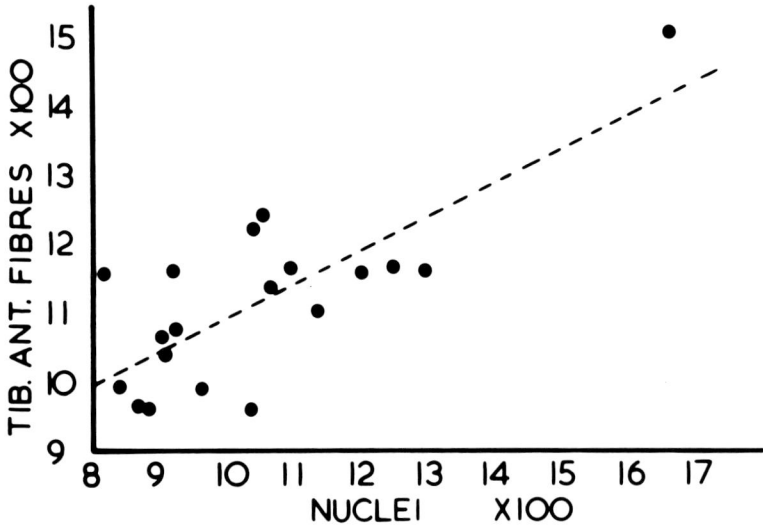

Figure 3. Comparison between the numbers of muscle fibres and myonuclei counted in a single transverse section of the medial belly of tibialis anterior in each monopodal frog represented in Figs. 1 and 2.

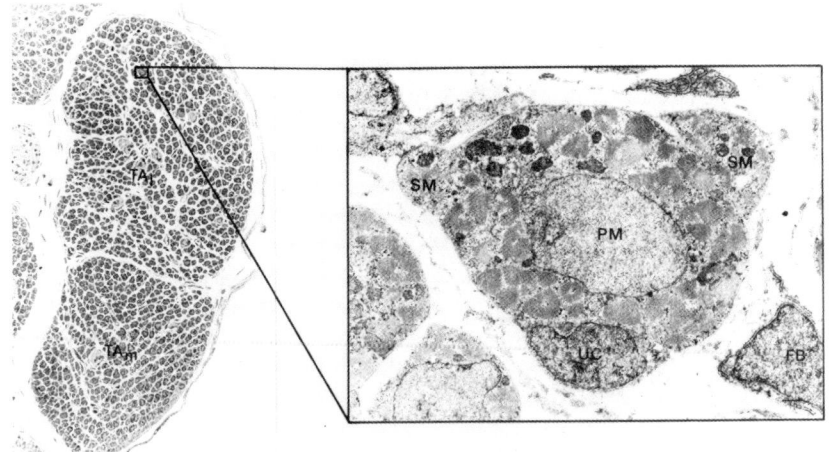

Figure 4. Light and electron micrographs of tibialis anterior, medial (TA_m) and lateral (TA_l) bellies, at stage 58, showing primary (PM) and secondary (SM) myotubes and a myoblast (UC) within a common basal lamina. FB = fibroblast.

in the juvenile frogs are shown as frequency plots in Fig. 5 and indicate that apart from a small number of extra-large muscle fibres in the monopodal animals, the muscle fibre sizes are essentially no different from normal (Lamb et al., 1987). The cause of the few large fibres is uncertain, but may indicate an inductive

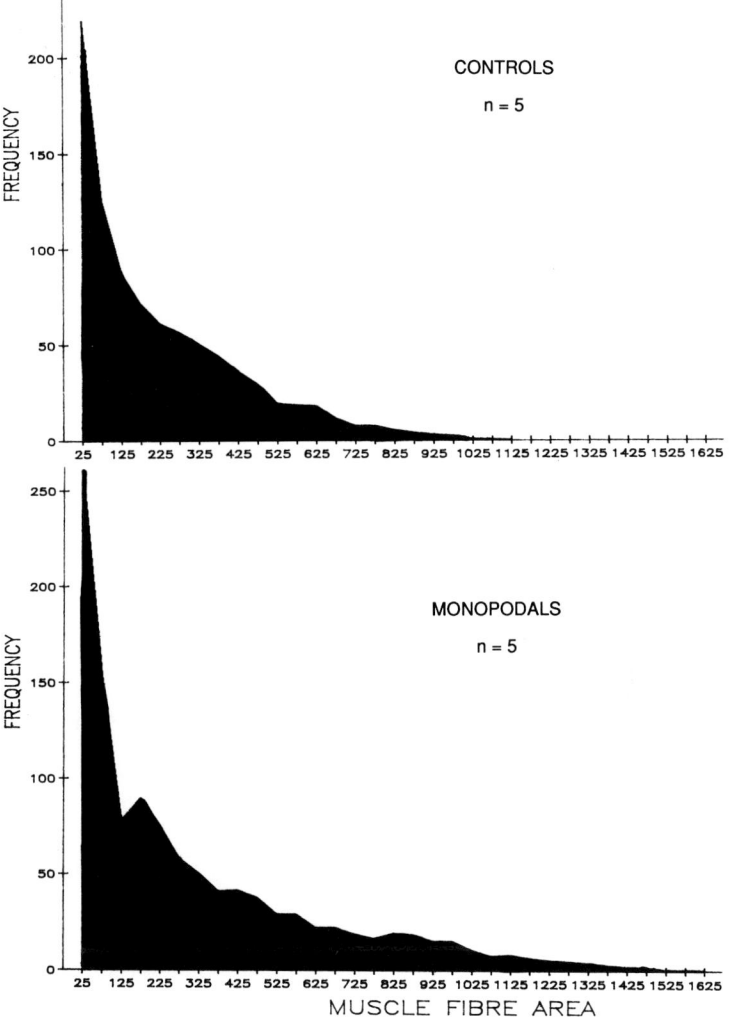

Figure 5. Graphs of average numbers of muscle fibres per fibre area in tibialis anterior of control and monopodal juvenile frogs one week after metamorphosis.

effect of the increased innervation, or a degree of work hypertrophy resulting from increased activity of the single limb.

Muscle fibre numbers in the juveniles (Fig. 6) showed very similar results to the earlier study; i.e., once the total number of motoneurons innervating the limb exceeded a level slightly above normal, no further increases in muscle fibre number above approximately 130% of normal were observed. (Nb: In the batch of animals used in this study, the average motoneuron count in normal animals was about 2,300, which is higher than previously reported. However, this does not affect the interpretation of the results which depends on relative ratios between normal and monopodal animals. Presumably genetic differences between adult breeding stock account for such variations.) (See Sperry, this volume.)

The most crucial question now was when, during development, the increase of muscle fibre numbers in the monopodal animals took place. McLennan (1982) has proposed a very precise version of the peripheral

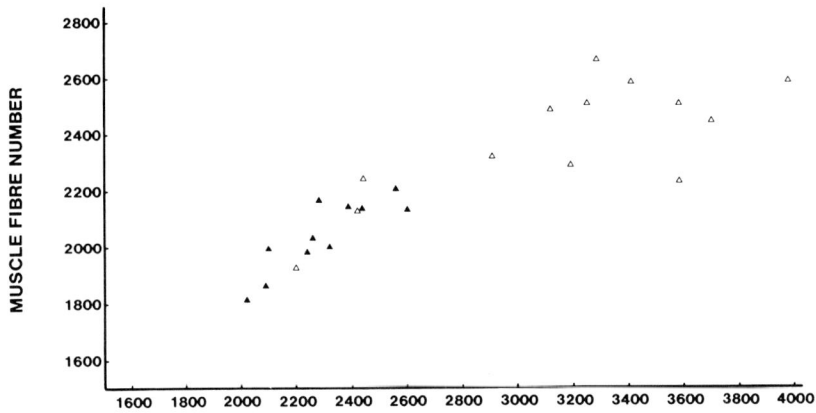

Figure 6. Muscle fibre counts using electron microscopy in tibialis anterior (medial plus lateral bellies) of monopodal (open) and control (filled) juvenile frogs compared with the total number of motoneurons innervating the limb (ipsilateral plus contralateral in monopodals).

competition hypothesis on the basis of a transient one-to-one correlation between the number of developing primary myotubes during the period of motoneuron death and the final number of motoneurons. That such a correlation occurs is not in itself surprising since the two populations must cross each other in opposite directions during this period, the one rising from zero while the other is falling from a maximum. Nevertheless, the monopodal frog has provided an excellent model for testing this notion directly.

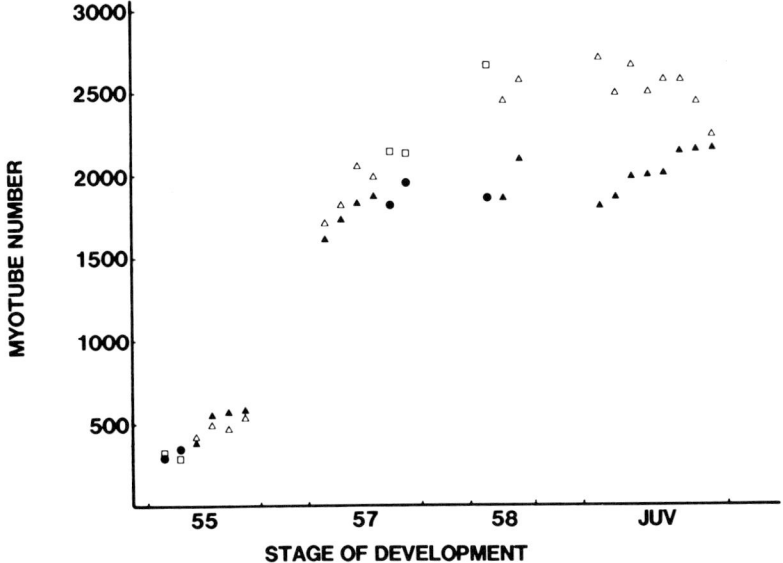

Figure 7. Number of myotubes in tibialis anterior (both bellies) of tadpoles and frogs from stage 55 to juvenile in pair-matched monopodals (open) and controls (filled). Triangles: siblings reared together; Squares, circles: siblings reared apart. Monopodals were chosen with good levels of contralateral innervation judged from the thickness of the spinal nerves in cross-section (tadpoles) or from motoneuron counts (juveniles).

Fig. 7 shows a plot of the total number of myotubes and/or myofibres in the developing tibialis anterior muscle from stage 55 tadpoles to the juvenile frog. Motoneuron death begins at stage 53, reaches its maximum rate at stage 55, and then rapidly tails off to a lower rate by stage 57 and to zero by stage 60 during metamorphic climax. Myotube formation begins in early stage 54, but they cannot be counted reliably until stage 55 because of their haphazard orientation until then. No difference in myotube numbers between normal and monopodal animals was observed until stage 58 when significant increases in number leading to the 30% increases noted earlier in juvenile monopodals were observed. These increases at stage 58 were accompanied by a marked increase in the number of mononuclear myogenic cells (Fig. 8); whereas prior to stage 58 the myogenic cells were normal. This indicates that the increased production of myotubes is consequent on an increase in myogenic cell proliferation at stage 58.

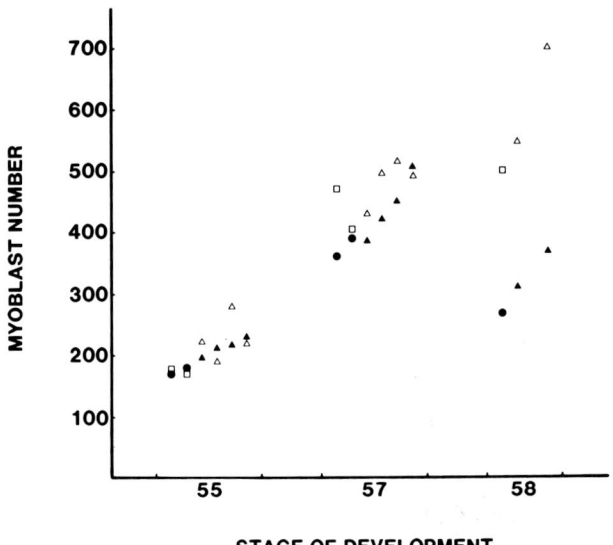

Figure 8. Myoblast numbers in tibialis anterior in the same animals as in Fig. 7.

Using ultrastructural criteria (Fig. 4), myotubes were classified as primary or secondary. Prior to stage 57 only primary myotubes can be observed, whereas secondary myotubes start to appear from stage 57 onwards. Thus, during the period when the bulk of motoneuron death takes place, there are only primary myotubes present, and their numbers are unaffected by the increased innervation.

This observation is in accord with the conclusion of Harris (1981) for the rat that primary myotube formation is not dependent on motor innervation, i.e., it is intrinsically determined by the limb. Secondary myotube production in the rat, however, is dependent on the presence of motor innervation and does not take place in its absence. The results from the monopodal frog suggest that Harris' conclusion can be extended to state that the number of secondary myotubes produced is controlled at least in part by the quantity of motor innervation. A reasonable interpretation is that in normal animals the number of secondary myotubes is regulated linearly by the number of motoneurons surviving the cell death period. The monopodal animals suggest that the mechanism can be saturated at a level of motor innervation just above the normal range. Thus the monopodal animals lead to the conclusion that in the case of motoneurons the numbers are not determined by peripheral regulation, i.e., the peripheral competition hypothesis is wrong. Rather, the opposite is true: the final number of muscle fibres is determined by the number of motoneurons surviving through some influence on myogenic cell proliferation.

MERITOCRATIC COMPETITION

The question therefore arises: what does control motoneuron death and the resultant mature numbers? Hughes (1965) suggested that neuronal death could be a mechanism for establishing precise patterns of neuronal connections if the initial patterns of axonal outgrowth and termination in the target were random, or "fuzzy". Neuronal death would serve as the means of removing inappropriate projections. This idea has been investigated in the motor projections to the limb in the chick (Landmesser and Morris, 1975: Landmesser, 1978; Lance-Jones and Landmesser, 1981a; Hollyday, 1983) and frog (Lamb, 1976; Farel and Bemelmans, 1985). In general, the initial axonal projections conform closely with the future adult projections. Several studies have demonstrated that this comes about by active navigation of the motor axons to predetermined target regions of the limb (Lance-Jones and Landmesser, 1980b, 1981b; Lamb, 1981a; Laing, 1984). The mechanism of navigation is sufficiently powerful to be able to compensate for surprisingly drastic experimental disturbances to the normal pathways, well in excess of any variations which would be expected to occur naturally in normal animals. Even in normal animals, however, a small minority of axons (5-10%) make "aberrant" projections for one reason or another (Lamb, 1976; Hollyday, 1983), and in the case of Xenopus these aberrant projections have been shown to be removed specifically by neuronal death (Lamb, 1977). It was found that the death of these motoneurons could not be prevented by removing the motoneurons that normally innervate the limb regions to which the aberrant projections are made (Lamb, 1979b), suggesting that different populations of motoneurons within the motor column are specified in some genetically determined sense to be compatible only with certain regions of the limb (Lamb, 1981b).

The size of these regions in relation to the accuracy of the initial axon invasion is a matter of debate. There is some evidence from developing frogs that the initial motor projections into individual muscles are randomly distributed and become refined later, although whether by neuronal death is unclear (Bennett and Lavidis, 1981). This raises the possibility that predetermined regions of compatibility may be quite small and beneath the resolution of most techniques for determining developing motor projections (see Lamb, 1984 for detailed argument). A study by Laing (1982) on the chick embryo provides strong circumstantial evidence in favour of small regions. He made use of the fact that paralysis by cholinergic blockade prevents motoneuron death (Laing and Prestige, 1978; Pittman and Oppenheim, 1979). However, Laing (1982) noticed that paralysis will not prevent motoneuron death if the limb bud previously has been removed, i.e., the target must be present for paralysis to be effective. By comparing the effects of partial limb bud deletions in paralysed and normal embryos, Laing was able to show that the target regions of individual motoneurons must be defined rather narrowly since the distributions of surviving motoneurons were only marginally expanded in paralysed embryos, i.e., only motoneurons determined for nearby removed regions and not distant removed regions could "compress" into remaining regions. By the same token, one should not expect to rescue by paralysis those motoneurons making initial projections to distant aberrant locations, and thus experiments setting out to demonstrate aberrant projections using paralysis must fail (Oppenheim, 1981b).

Laing's observations also raise the possibility that motoneurons might be selected on the basis of relative compatibility within small and restricted fields. The term meritocratic competition has been coined to include such a notion (Lamb, 1984). It is important to note that this concept of competition is quite different from that of the peripheral competition hypothesis. Whereas peripheral competition is essentially a means for attaining numerical balance of pre- and post-synaptic cell populations, the purpose of meritocratic competition is to attain optimal patterns of connectivity. Any numerical effects would be secondary. Meritocratic competition, in effect, would constitute an epigenetic mechanism for arriving at a precision of connectivity beyond the encoding capacity of the genome. Whereas in small nervous systems such as the insect, it is probable that the precision of connectivity necessary for optimal performance can be encoded entirely in the genome, the size and complexity of the vertebrate nervous system precludes such an option since the information requirement rises as a power function of the number of constituents (e.g., neurons).

Recent evidence on the fine structure of muscle (Lazarides et al., 1982) and the precise coordination of motor unit firing (Burke, 1980) suggests a need for resolution of ordering of the motor system, perhaps as precise as the visual system, in order to avoid shear-stress damage to muscle fibres of neighboring motor units, and to maximize the efficiency of muscle contraction (Lamb, 1984). Although relative compatibility could provide an epigenetic mechanism for attaining such precision, there are lines of evidence which suggest that the function of the system itself might underlie a meritocratic selection, possibly as an additional and sequential fine-tuning mechanism.

It is well known that early interference with the

cholinergic function of the motor system can prevent motoneuron death (Laing and Prestige, 1978; Pittman and Oppenheim, 1979; Creazzo and Sohal, 1979). While most authors have assumed that the neuromuscular junction is the site at which the cholinergic antagonists (e.g., curare, bungarotoxin) exert their action, the possibility that cholinergic synapses within the spinal cord are also involved has not been excluded. It is clear that the mechanism is quite complex since some agents (e.g., myasthenia gravis serum, Sohal et al., 1983) can produce the effect without causing paralysis.

During normal development, on about day six in the chick embryo, the motoneurons of the lateral motor column begin to fire in orderly rostral to caudal sequential waves which sweep repeatedly through the motor columns (Provine, 1986) and activate the limb musculature in the phasic movements characteristic of the embryo (Beckoff, 1981). Although the patterns of activation and contraction are not precisely identical from one cycle to the next (Landmesser and Szente, 1986), nevertheless there is a probability bias that ensures that the order of motoneuron firing is statistically non-random. This in turn must impart a statistical ordering to the firing of the motor terminals within the limb. By coupling the firing order to some mechanism conferring a competitive asymmetry, it can be seen how motoneurons may be selected on the basis of functional merit (e.g., coherent activation of adjacent motor units). Such coupling mechanisms have been proposed previously (Nelson and Brenneman, 1982; and see Constantine-Paton, this volume).

Recent efforts to test the functional merit hypothesis in this laboratory by attempting to alter the normal ordering of motoneuron firing have, so far, been unsuccessful due to methodological difficulties. However, it is interesting to note that Landmesser and Szente (1986) have reported that curare disrupts the normal activation patterns of the motoneurons, presumably as an independent effect from its peripheral action on the neuromuscular junction. We also have found (Renshaw and Lamb, unpublished), using iodinated bungarotoxin, that nicotinic cholinergic receptors which bind alpha-bungarotoxin administered in ovo are present in high concentration in the lateral motor column of

chick embryos from day six onwards. There is, therefore, a route by which cholinergic antagonists could exert their action by disrupting a central firing pattern necessary for selecting optimal motoneurons.
A similar rationale could be used to explain how a double population of motoneurons can survive in monopodal Xenopus, since the firing patterns on the two sides of the cord are not likely to be strongly coupled in the absence of direct synaptic links (Lamb, 1984).

According to the hypothesis of meritocratic competition, or selection, the actual number of motoneurons surviving the period of cell death is relatively unimportant. What is important is that selection is needed to choose the motoneurons of best fit following axon invasion. It would be reasonable to expect that the proportion of best-fit motoneurons must be constant since it should be a function of an "uncertainty factor" inherent in each individual motoneuron's initial projection. This prediction appears to have been met according to recent data obtained in Xenopus by Sperry (this volume) who has found, using normal and triploid animals, that final motoneuron numbers are closely correlated with initial numbers, but only poorly correlated, if at all, to parameters such as body size and muscle fibre number.

At least in Xenopus, it seems appropriate to give consideration to meritocratic selection as a more accurate model of motoneuron death, and perhaps to discard the older notion of peripheral competition. However, it is pertinent to observe that whilst the purpose of neuron death in the peripheral motor system is perhaps to select a population of optimally connected motoneurons, the same need not necessarily be true for all neuronal classes. Counts of surviving dorsal root ganglion cells in juvenile monopodal frogs (Table 1), combined with horseradish peroxidase labeling, gave the somewhat surprising result that the total number of sensory neurons innervating the single limb is probably no greater than for one limb of normal animals (Lamb et al., in preparation). The slightly increased average totals in the monopodal frogs probably reflects the survival of about 800 dorsal root ganglion cells innervating the skin over the amputation site (i.e., not innervating the remaining limb). Furthermore, there was a significant negative

Table 1. Sensory neuron counts from dorsal root ganglia 8, 9 and 10 of control and monopodal juvenile frogs. Sensory axons appear to be about 40% less successful than motoneurons at crossing over, perhaps because many are attracted to residual limb-type skin regenerating over the amputation site.

	Right (Ipsilateral)	Left	Total (Contralateral)
Monopodals			
XL 739	5274	3063	8337
XL 730	5553	2742	8295
XL 756	4953	2606	7560
XL 793	6636	2196	8832
XL 782	6852	2313	9165
XL 737	6912	1800	8712
XL 778	5901	1560	7461
XL 731	5112	1956	7068
XL 740	6474	915	7389
XL 745	6018	828	6846
XL 795	9360	1098	10458
XL 726	7350	852	8202
Controls			
XL 747	7314	6888	14202
XL 746	7194	7065	14259
XL 764	6996	6996	13992
XL 797	8247	7761	16008
XL 765	7734	6891	14625
XL 750	8154	8487	16641

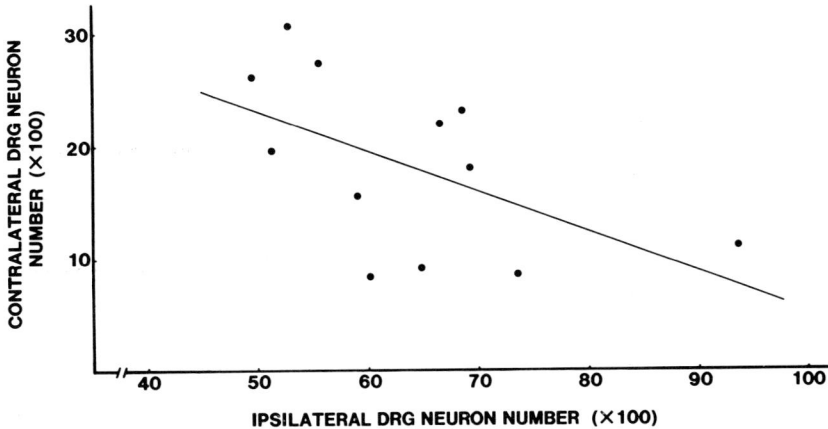

Figure 9. Contralateral dorsal root ganglion cell numbers plotted against ipsilateral dorsal root ganglion cell numbers showing a negative correlation as would be expected if the cells were competing peripherally for a target factor.

correlation ($p < 0.05$) between the numbers of surviving ipsilateral and contralateral dorsal root ganglion cells (Fig. 9). These results strongly suggest that in contrast to motoneurons, sensory ganglia cell numbers are determined by competitive peripheral target regulation. It is tempting to speculate that peripheral regulation is the best strategy for bringing the sensory system into register with the motor system, the motor system being the first to develop and having already done the work of determining the optimal patterns of connectivity.

ACKNOWLEDGMENTS

This work is supported by the National Health and Medical Research Council of Australia, the Muscular Dystrophy Research Association and the Neuromuscular Foundation of Western Australia, and the Australian Brain Foundation.

REFERENCES

Beckoff A (1981). Embryonic development of chick motor behaviour. Trends Neurosci 4:181-184.

Bennett MR, Lavidis NA (1981). Development of the topographical projection of motor neurons to an amphibian muscle accompanies motor neuron death. Develop Brain Res 2:448-452.

Boydston WR, Sohal GS (1979). Grafting of additional periphery reduces embryonic loss of neurons. Brain Res. 178:403-410.

Bueker ED (1945). Hyperplastic changes in the nervous system of a frog (Rana) as associated with multiple functional limbs. Anat Rec 93:323-331.

Burke RE (1980). Motor unit types: functional specializations in motor control. Trends Neurosci 3:255-258.

Clarke PGH (1981). Chance, repetition and error in the development of normal nervous systems. Perspect Biol Med 25:2-19.

Cowan WM (1973). Neuronal death as a regulative mechanism in the control of cell number in the nervous system. In Rockstein M (ed): "Development and Aging in the Nervous System." New York: Academic Press, pp 19-41.

Creazzo TL, Sohal GS (1979). Effects of chronic injections of bungarotoxin on embryonic cell death. Exp Neurol 66:135-144.

Cunningham TJ (1982). Naturally occurring neuron death and its regulation by developing neural pathways. Int Rev Cytol 74:163-186.

Denton CJ, Lamb AH, Wilson P, Mark RF (1985). Innervation patterns of muscles of one-legged Xenopus laevis supplied by motoneurons from both sides of the spinal cord. Develop Brain Res 17:85-94.

Farel PB, Bemelmans SE (1985). Specificity of motoneuron projection patterns during development of the bullfrog tadpole (Rana catesbeiana). J Comp Neurol

238:128-134.
Ferns MJ, Lamb AH (1986). Muscle development in Xenopus laevis: a quantitative electron microscopic study. Neled Suppl 23:S45.
Ferns MJ, Lamb AH (1987). Regulation of cell numbers in the developing neuromuscular system in Xenopus laevis. Neled Suppl 27:S72.
Hamburger V (1958). Regression versus peripheral control of differentiation in motor hypoplasia. Am J Anat 102:365-410.
Hamburger V (1975). Cell death in the development of the lateral motor column in the chick embryo. J Comp Neurol 160:535-546.
Hamburger V, Levi-Montalcini R (1949). Proliferation, differentiation and degeneration in the spinal ganglia of chicks under normal and experimental conditions. J Exp Zool 111:457-502.
Hamburger V, Oppenheim RW (1982). Naturally occurring neuronal death in vertebrates. Neurosci Commentaries 1:39-55.
Harris AJ (1981). Embryonic growth and innervation of rat skeletal muscles. I. Neural regulation of muscle fibre numbers. Phil Trans Roy Soc Lond Ser B 293:257-277.
Hollyday M (1983). Development of motor innervation of chick limbs. In Fallon JF, Caplan AI (eds): "Limb Development and Regeneration, Part A." New York: Alan R. Liss, pp 183-193.
Hollyday M, Hamburger V (1976). Reduction of naturally occurring motoneuron loss by enlargement of the periphery. J Comp Neurol 170:311-320.
Hollyday M, Mendell L (1976). Analysis of moving supernumerary limbs of Xenopus laevis. Exp Neurol 51:316-324.
Hughes AFW (1965). A quantitative study of the development of the nerves in the hind limb of Eleutherodactylus martinicenus. J Embryol Exp Morphol 13:9-34.
Hughes AFW (1968). "Aspects of Neural Ontogeny." London: Logos.
Kollros JJ (1968). Order and control of neurogenesis as exemplified by the lateral motor column. Develop Biol Suppl 2:274-305.
Laing NG (1982). Motor projection patterns to the hind limb of normal and paralyzed chick embryos. J Embryol Exp Morphol 72:269-286.
Laing NG (1984). Motor innervation of proximally

rotated chick embryo wings. J Embryol Exp Morphol 83:213-223.
Laing NG, Prestige MC (1978). Prevention of spontaneous motoneuron death in chick embryos. J Physiol (Lond) 282:33-34.
Lamb AH (1976). The projection patterns of the ventral horn to hind limb during development. Develop Biol 54:82-99.
Lamb AH (1977). Neuronal death in the development of the somatotopic projections of the ventral horn in Xenopus. Brain Res 134:145-150.
Lamb AH (1979a). Ventral horn cell counts in a Xenopus with naturally occurring supernumerary hindlimbs. J Embryol Exp Morphol 49:13-16.
Lamb AH (1979b). Evidence that some developing motoneurons die for reasons other than peripheral competition. Develop Biol 71:8-21.
Lamb AH (1980). Motoneuron counts in Xenopus frogs reared with one bilaterally innervated hindlimb. Nature 284:347-350.
Lamb AH (1981a). Selective bilateral motor innervation in Xenopus tadpoles with one hind limb. J Embryol Exp Morphol 65:149-163.
Lamb AH (1981b). Target dependency of developing motoneurons in Xenopus laevis. J Comp Neurol 203:157-171.
Lamb AH (1984). Motoneuron death in the embryo. CRC Crit Rev Clin Neurobiol 1:141-179.
Lamb AH, Ferns MJ, Klose K (1987). Muscle fibre sizes in monopodal Xenopus laevis frogs. Neled Suppl 27:S93.
Lance-Jones C, Landmesser L (1980a). Motoneuron projection patterns in embryonic chick limbs following partial deletions of the spinal cord. J Physiol (Lond) 302:559-580.
Lance-Jones C, Landmesser L (1980b). Motoneuron projection patterns in the chick hind limb following partial reversals of the spinal cord. J Physiol (Lond) 302:581-602.
Lance-Jones C, Landmesser L (1981a). Pathway selection by chick lumbosacral motoneurons during normal development. Proc Roy Soc Lond Ser B 214:1-18.
Lance-Jones C, Landmesser L (1981b). Pathway selection by embryonic chick motoneurons in an experimentally altered environment. Proc Roy Soc Lond Ser B 214:19-52.
Landmesser L (1978). The development of motor projection patterns in the chick hind limb. J Physiol (Lond)

284:391-414.
Landmesser L, Morris DG (1975). The development of functional innervation in the hind limb of the chick embryo. J Physiol (Lond) 249:301-326.
Landmesser L, Szente M (1986). Activation patterns of embryonic chick hind-limb muscles following blockade of activity and motoneurone cell death. J Physiol (Lond) 380:157-174.
Lazarides E, Gard DL, Granger BL, O'Connor CM, Breckler J, Danto SI (1982). Regulation of the assembly of the Z-disk in muscle cells. Prog Clin Biol Res 85 part B: 317-340.
McLennan IS (1982). Size of motoneuron pool may be related to number of myotubes in developing muscle. Develop Biol 92:263-265.
Narayanan CH, Narayanan CY (1978). Neuronal adjustments in developing nuclear centres of the chick embryo following transplantation of an additional optic primordium. J Embryol Exp Morphol 44:53-70.
Nelson PG, Brenneman DE (1982). Electrical activity of neurons and development of the brain. Trends Neurosci 5:229-232.
Oppenheim RW (1981a). Neuronal cell death and some related regressive phenomena during neurogenesis: A selective historical review and progress report. In Cowan WM (ed): "Studies in Developmental Neurobiology: Essays in Honour of Viktor Hamburger." London: Oxford University Press, pp 74-133.
Oppenheim RW (1981b). Cell death of motoneurons in the chick embryo spinal cord. V. Evidence on the role of cell death and neuromuscular function in the formation of specific peripheral connections. J Neurosci 1: 141-151.
Pittman R, Oppenheim RW (1979). Cell death of motoneurons in the chick embryo spinal cord. IV. Evidence that a functional neuromuscular interaction is involved in the regulation of naturally occurring cell death and the stabilization of synapses. J Comp Neurol 187:425-446.
Pollack ED (1969). Response of the lateral motor column to multiple forelimbs in *Rana pipiens*. Teratology 2: 159-162.
Prestige MC (1967). The control of cell number in the lumbar ventral horns during the development of *Xenopus laevis* tadpoles. J Embryol Exp Morphol 18:359-387.
Prestige MC (1970). Differentiation, degeneration and

the role of the periphery: quantitative considerations. In Schmitt FO (ed): "The Neurosciences: Second Study Program." New York: Rockefeller University Press, pp 73-83.

Prestige MC (1974). Axon and cell numbers in the developing nervous system. Brit Med Bull 30:107-111.

Provine RR (1986). Behavioral neuroembryology: motor perspectives. Develop Neuropsychobiol 593:213.

Sheard PW, Lamb AH (1986). The regulation of motoneuron and muscle fibre numbers in normal and bilaterally innervated Xenopus hindlimbs. Neled Suppl 23:S81.

Sohal GS, Leshner RT, Swift TR (1983). Myasthenia gravis immunoglobin augments motor neuron survival without producing muscle paralysis. Musc Nerve 6: 122-127.

Stehouwer DJ, Farel PB (1985). Development of locomotor mechanisms in the frog. J Neurophysiol 53: 1453-1466.

SECTION II

SPECIFICITY IN NEURAL DEVELOPMENT AND REGENERATION

SECTION II. SPECIFICITY IN NEURAL DEVELOPMENT AND REGENERATION

Just as the previous chapters were directed toward spinal motor neurons and the control of their numbers, this section turns outward to the peripheral nervous system and issues of specificity. On the one hand, there is concern for how nerve fibers reach their target locale and how specific synapses finally are effected. As a part of understanding what cues might be involved in connectivity, an examination of nerve-target specificity in a regenerating system can be enlightening, particularly when differences between developing and mature stages are considered.

The chapters that follow deal with these issues by approaching questions on the regulatory roles played by target tissues and the environment in directed nerve growth and neuronal maturation, the signals that mediate the formation of a neuromuscular synapse, and the specificity of neuromuscular connections following nerve regeneration. Furthermore, attention is given to the specification of connections between sensory ganglion neurons and the spinal cord neurons, again with some focus on the peripheral target. Here functional specification becomes as important as morphological specificity and, from a philosophical viewpoint, perhaps the most important element. Since the periphery in the spinal cord-spinal ganglion-limb axis arises continually as a theme in the mechanisms of growth control, a view of the periphery, i.e., the developing limb, as it might be a reflection of, or a retrograde influence on neural development, is provided.

In the following five chapters, it will become apparent that specificity codes of whatever nature and from whatever source ultimately will need to be determined in order to formulate an integrated notion as to the mechanisms that bring about an ordered nervous system.

REGULATION OF SPINAL NERVE FIBER GROWTH AND NEURONAL MATURATION IN VITRO

William L. Muhlach

Department of Zoology, Southern Illinois University at Carbondale, Carbondale, Illinois 62901

INTRODUCTION

As many as one hundred billion neurons, some of which form thousands of synaptic connections, can comprise the vertebrate nervous system (Black, 1983). The best information indicates that the development of neural connections is quite accurate from the beginning and involves relatively little trial and error. Given the complexity and diversity of the nervous system, together with its developmental accuracy and plasticity, many questions remain regarding the mechanisms that regulate the formation of its functional architecture, the ultimate goal of neural development.

During development, the commitment of a cell to a particular differentiated fate involves a combination of influences from both intrinsic and extracellular determinants and from the topographical location of embryonic cells (reviewed in Stent, 1985). Similarly, complex interactions between genetic and epigenetic factors provide a framework for the spatial and temporal coordination necessary for nervous system development. This concept is emphasized, for example, when considering coordinated cell and tissue interactions as determinative events in development.

In recent years, there has been an increasing awareness of the role that specific chemical factors might play in directing developmental events. Collectively, these factors represent a class of biologically active molecules defined as "growth factors". With respect to the topic of this chapter, a significant amount of evidence points toward peripheral target tissues as a potential source of neuronal growth factors (Pollack and Liebig, 1977; Pollack and Muhlach, 1981, 1982; Heaton and Paiva, 1986; Heaton and Wayne, 1986; Davies et al., 1986) that may represent "extracellular neuronal determinants". The target tissue is defined as the postsynaptic site for a particular neuron or population of neurons, this being in the present instance the presumptive limb musculature. A major focus of the work described in this chapter is on the role that peripheral target tissues play in the development of spinal motor neurons that project to the limb periphery. The initial studies using cultured spinal cord and limb tissue from Rana pipiens tadpoles described target tissue effects on morphological characteristics of spinal cord neuron development, whereas more recent investigations have been aimed at establishing whether such interactions also can influence the functional development of target-affected motor neurons.

Spinal Cord-Target Specificity

Motor neurons of the spinal cord that make topographical synaptic connections in the limb (Landmesser, 1978; Lance-Jones and Landmesser, 1981; Hollyday, 1983; Farel and Bemelmans, 1985) provide a convenient model for the study of neuron-target interactions during development. The general hypothesis being examined is that the target tissue control of parameters of neuronal development is a major contributor to the high degree of specificity that develops between the neuron and its target. Two major aspects of the specificity required for a functional nervous system are: 1) the establishment and maintenance of appropriate connections which would involve such processes as pathway selection, target recognition, synaptogenesis and survival, and 2) the appropriate differentiation of the neuron to suit its function, which would include neurotransmitter production. The former involves aspects of development that could, for the most part, represent morphogenesis, while the latter can be defined by biochemical differentiation. These general categories will be addressed with respect to neuron-target interactions in development.

AXON EXTENSION AND LIMB DEVELOPMENT

While migrating through the spinal cord to the lateral motor columns, the young motor neurons extend axons that pass through the cord basal lamina and into the mesenchyme of the somites on their way to the limb buds. (See previous chapters by Pollack, Sperry and Lamb for considerations of the in vivo development of the motor neuron and lateral motor columns.) As the axons exit the spinal cord there is an important switch in the environment, and thus a problem arises as to whether the intra-cord surround of the neuronal soma or the extra-cord environment of the axon predominates as a growth influence. The axonal environment is probably most critical in consideration of pathway selection, synaptogenesis and target-related trophic influences on the neuron. Nevertheless, pathway selection and neuronal differentiation are likely to be dependent on spatially and temporally coordinated neuron-target interactions.

The Neuronal Growth Cone

Late in the nineteenth century, Ramón y Cajal (1929) became the first to recognize that the nerve growth cone at the axon terminus was the searching organelle of the neuron. More recently, Letourneau (1987) has called the growth cone a "sensory-effector" system that senses local cues and responds accordingly. The navigational activities of the growth cone are directly responsible for establishing the pathway taken by an elongating axon, and therefore ultimately influence its contact with a potential target. Interestingly, the growth cone has many characteristics in common with migratory cell types (Bray, 1987), including filopodial and lamellipodial extensions that range from the apex to the base of the cone thereby permitting the continuous sampling of the micro-environment of the growth cone. As described by Bray (1979), growth cones are capable of producing mechanical pull based upon adhesion to the attachment substratum, and as is the case for migrating cell types (Carter, 1967), neuronal growth cones respond positively to the more adhesive substratum when provided with a choice (Letourneau, 1975). Further, they respond to substrata in an apparent hierarchical manner. As would be predicted, the growth cone contains actin components that support both its locomotive behavior and steering movements (Bray, 1987).

The sensory function of the growth cone appears to be subserved by membrane surface components that recognize or interact with adhesive ligands, extracellular matrix components, growth factors, neurotransmitters, or surface components of other cells (for example, see recent volume edited by Kater and Letourneau, 1985). Pfenninger et al. (1984) have suggested that neuronal growth cones contain type-specific plasma membrane glycoconjugates or a "surface carbohydrate signature". Might not this signature play a discriminatory role in target recognition (Lockerbie, 1987) as well as in pathway selection and extracellular signal responsiveness?

The growth cone effector system might then involve a transmembrane signal transduction pathway. Such a system has been described by Ruoslahti and Pierschbacher (1987) in which adhesion proteins (RGD-containing proteins) and their receptors (integrins) provide a recognition complex that has the potential of providing a cell with information regarding adhesion, migration, polarity, position, differentiation and growth.

Limb Innervation Patterning

During the period of initial motor axon outgrowth in avians, myogenic stem cells migrate from the ventrolateral edge of the somites along the somatopleure to the region of the prospective limb (Jacob et al., 1979). Here the stem cells produce a mesenchymal limb bud that proceeds to differentiate into ventral and dorsal premuscle masses. Motor neuron neurotization in the developing amphibian hindlimb takes place when the limb bud consists of an undifferentiated mesenchymal sac (Taylor, 1943; see Bibb, this volume). Thus, the true target for the extending motor neuron axon is the undifferentiated mesenchyme of the early limb bud.

Motor neuron groups within the lateral motor column (LMC) project to particular regions of the limb musculature with no significant overlap in territories (reviewed in Bennett, 1983) and is a pattern that is consistent for amphibians, birds and mammals. Even during early development there is a fairly precise nerve projection from the spinal cord to the pre-muscle masses. Motor neurons in lateral regions of the LMC innervate dorsal muscle mass derivatives, while those in medial regions innervate ventral muscle mass derivatives. However, even before the initial division into ventral and dorsal pre-muscle masses, the somatotopic organization of the motor nerve projections has been established. Shortly after axons leave the spinal cord they sort out within the spinal nerves according to their segmental origins and cellular positions within the LMC (reviewed in Bennett, 1983). Axon bundles depart their respective myotomes and unite in the plexus region before converging toward the most densely packed mesenchyme in the limb bud (Bennett, 1983; Nurcombe and Bennett, 1983). Hollyday (1983) has observed a "waiting period" in the chick embryo during which spinal axons collect at the base of the myotomes and then converge at the base of the limb before entering the limb en masse. It is as though the axons await a specific developmental event before they continue their extension into the limb bud. Once the primary nerves have entered the limb, branches extend into the newly formed pre-muscle masses. Although the primary limb nerve of the chick embryo can form in the absence of limb pre-muscle, the branches do require the presence of pre-muscle cells for their development (Lewis et al., 1983).

In vivo examples of accurate early innervation patterns demonstrate that those projections are formed as a result of nerve fibers following appropriate pathways from the outset (Hollyday, 1983; Ashwell and Watson, 1983; Farel and Bemelmans, 1985; Tosney and Landmesser, 1985). Axonal growth cones of motor neurons have been reported to express specific directional preferences when they reach branch points (the "decision regions" of Lance-Jones and Landmesser, 1981; the "critical choice points" of Hollyday, 1983). Motor neuron growth cones in vivo are larger, more lamellipodial and have more complex trajectories in these decision regions than in other areas (Tosney and Landmesser, 1985) suggesting the growth cone is responding to local cues. Experimental manipulations of the neuron-target relationship in vivo have demonstrated an ability of axons to follow aberrant routes in order to reach their correct targets (Constantine-Paton and Law, 1978; Laing, 1984; Harris, 1986). Motor innervation of the chick wing can compensate for reversal of the limb axes by innervating the appropriate muscles as long as the manipulation is performed prior to nerve arrival in the limb and at a proximal level (Laing, 1984). An abnormal brachial plexus in these cases demonstrates that considerable reorganization of axonal outgrowth must have occurred distally as adjustments in the projection paths compensate for the new environment. Therefore, it appears as though the orientation of the distal target can influence the environmental cues presented to the advancing axons in the decision regions.

Clearly, two considerations help assure that the pre-muscle masses receive innervation from appropriate motor neuron groups in the spinal cord with respect to projection pathways. First is the ability of axons to sort out and then associate as spinal and limb nerves according to their cell body origin. This behavior likely involves molecules that mediate axon-to-axon associations such as the neural cell adhesion molecule, N-CAM (Rutishauser, 1984). The second aspect involves the ability of the dense, mesenchymal pre-muscle masses to attract fasciculi of axons from the primary limb nerves. It is noteworthy that sensory axons use motor axons as a growth substratum (but see Lee and Farel, this volume and Scott, 1988).

NEURON-TARGET INTERACTIONS IN VITRO

The system used to test certain aspects regarding the involvement of peripheral target tissue in the control of neuronal development has been the in vitro culture of Rana pipiens tadpole spinal cord and limb target tissues (for culturing methods see Pollack and Koves, 1975; Muhlach and Pollack, 1978). Importantly, the larval frog is particularly well-suited for studies on neuron-target developmental interactions in vitro since the relevant tissues can be cultured in totally defined medium for extended periods of time (up to three months).

Initial work with this system has supported the

notion that target tissue has a substantial influence on certain phases of neuronal development in vitro. It has now been established that the limb mesenchyme, as the developmental target for LMC neurons, is capable of enhancing and directing nerve fiber (neurite) outgrowth from larval frog spinal cord explants (Pollack and Liebig, 1977; Pollack et al., 1981). The limb tissue additionally is able to prolong the survival of the spinal nerve fibers (Pollack, 1980) and of the motor neurons in vitro (Pollack et al., 1981). Furthermore, the developmental stage-specific interactions of both the motor and sensory components of the spinal reflex arc in relationship to their target tissues have been described (Pollack and Muhlach, 1982). The data of the above studies have demonstrated that the undifferentiated limb tissue (from stage V tadpoles; Taylor-Kollros series, 1946) is quantitatively more effective in stimulating neurite growth than older stage tissues (stage XII-XIII, skeletal muscle) or non-target tissue (liver, heart). These observations correlate well with in vivo timing of limb neurotization and innervation, differentiation of the limb and timing of naturally-occuring neuron death (Pollack and Muhlach, 1982). This scheme represents a "window of development" as specified by the competency of the neuron to respond optimally at stage V and of the limb tissue to elicit an optimal response at stage V. Other investigators have since documented similar relationships between neuronal populations and their target tissues (Nurcombe and Bennett, 1983; Heaton and Paiva, 1986).

In order to gain additional information on these interactions, several growth and development features were identified as being suitable for determining the extent of extrinsic influences on the spinal neurons. These included neurite morphology, nerve fiber growth (elongation) rate, periodicity of nerve fiber growth, neuronal metabolic activity, and neurotransmitter synthesis. The in vitro analyses of these parameters took advantage of the two major variables used in the initial characterization of the spinal cord-limb interactions. The first was related to the target tissue: its presence or absence in a co-culture paradigm, the use of target-conditioned medium, and the state of development of the limb target (i.e., mesenchyme vs. skeletal muscle). The second variable was the growth substratum that consisted of either collagen (type I), a natural extracellular matrix component, or polylysine, a synthetic adhesive surface. Combinations of these two variables formed the major experimental groups. Morphological characteristics of nerve fiber outgrowth from spinal cord explants were dependent upon the target tissue and the composition of the substratum.

Morphological Responses to Target and Substratum

Neurite outgrowth (quantified as the Neurite Density Index, NDI, described by Pollack et al., 1981) from stage V spinal cord explants placed on collagen substratum is characterized by sparse, short, thin neurites that typically degenerate within seven days of culturing. Fascicles and extensively branched neurites were rare in this group. This represents the typical control cord explant on collagen (Fig. 1A). Co-culture of spinal cord on collagen with stage V limb mesenchyme (Fig. 1B) or stage XII-XIII limb tissue resulted in increased neuritic outgrowth of 2,142% and 1,475% respectively, over control outgrowth. In the presence of the limb tissue, a greater proportion of neurites could be identified with distinct, active growth cones exhibiting lamellipodial and filopodial protrusions than could be seen in control cultures. While neuritic branching and fasciculation were increased in the co-cultures, they were characteristically long, thick and wavy in appearance with trajectories indicative of a directional response toward the limb tissue.

Spinal cord explants grown on polylysine substratum showed a 7,592% increase in neurite density over controls on collagen (Fig. 1C). This group clearly demonstrates the importance of neuron-substratum adhesion for neuritic outgrowth. On polylysine, limb mesenchyme and skeletal muscle tissue elicited neurite density increases of 177% and 183%, respectively, over values in the absence of the target tissue, and increases of 21,244% and 21,642% in comparison to control cord explants on collagen. The nerve fiber features observed on collagen in the presence of target tissue were characteristic of those on polylysine as well, i.e., they tended to be long, of thick diameter, wavy, arborizing,

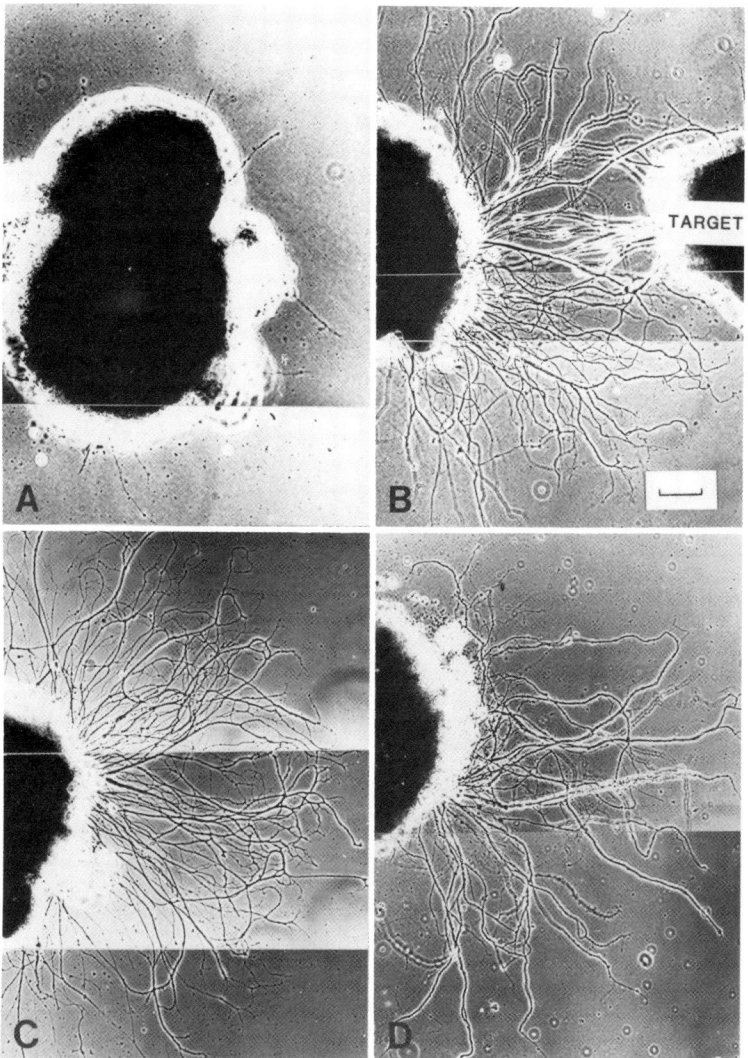

Figure 1. Neuritic outgrowth from stage V spinal cord explants: (A) control on collagen at 14 days in vitro (DIV), NDI=18; (B) cord co-cultured with stage V limb tissue on collagen at 11 DIV, NDI=1,241; (C) cord on polylysine at 10 DIV, NDI=1,551; (D) cord on collagen in presence of mesenchyme-conditioned medium at 16 DIV, NDI=1,579. Bar=100 µm.

and capable of forming fascicles. Fasciculation was enhanced in the presence of the limb tissue with directional neurite growth. Co-cultures of spinal cord with same stage liver or heart failed to enhance outgrowth beyond control levels.

Limb mesenchyme-conditioned medium (Fig. 1D) and mesenchyme-conditioned collagen substratum both were effective in eliciting enhanced neuritic outgrowth from naive spinal cord explants on collagen (3,585% and 3,284% increases respectively in NDI over control values). These data support the idea that the target tissue releases a diffusible, substratum-binding factor capable of promoting nerve fiber outgrowth. An inverse relationship between NDI and directional response with respect to distance from the target (Pollack, et al., 1981) has been interpreted as evidence of a substratum-localized, gradient-like effect of the putative target-originated neuronal growth factor.

Nerve Fiber Growth Rate

One mechanism that can account for the increased neurite outgrowth under some experimental situations is the stimulation of rapid neurite extension (Muhlach and Pollack, 1982). The rationale is provided by chemotactically responsive non-neuronal cells that increase their rate of migration when following a chemotactic signal. A test of this possibility was designed through the use of time-lapse cinemicrophotography to track the trajectories of neurite growth cones at one to two minute intervals over twenty-four hours. It is clear that the limb mesenchyme is the most potent enhancer of neurite growth rate (Fig. 2, Left). Two unique growth related characteristics became apparent during the analysis of the time-lapse data. First, individual neurites showed intermittent variations in the rate at which they elongated. Importantly, neurites did not grow continuously over 24 hours, nor did they grow synchronously within the same culture. The second characteristic was that a wider range of growth rates existed for neurites co-cultured with target tissue than for any other group (Fig. 2, Left). One possible explanation for this observation is that neurite growth rate might be affected by a target-originated gradient.

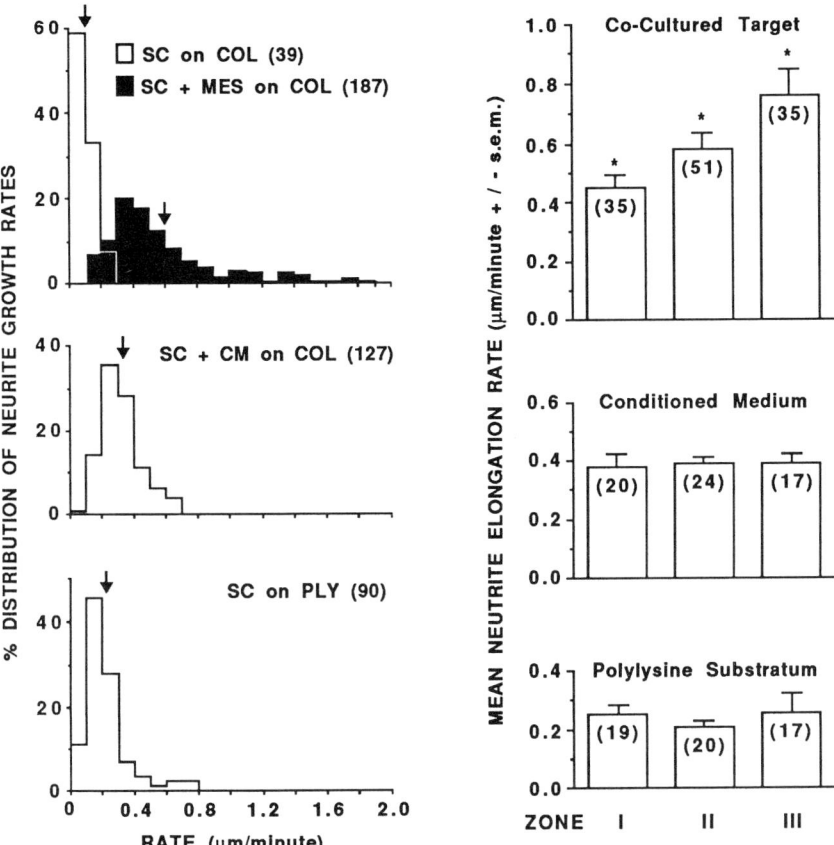

Figure 2. Left: Comparison of neurite growth rate distributions for spinal cord (SC) explants on collagen (COL), in the presence of mesenchymal target (MES) and target-conditioned medium (CM) and on polylysine (PLY). Arrows=mean values; n=number of neurites. Note the wide range of rates with a "centralized" source of target-derived factor (top). Right: Mean growth rate for neurites elongating within respective zones (see text). Top: centralized source of target factor. Middle: uniform distribution of target factor. Bottom: uniform distribution of neurite-promoting surface. *=significant difference by Student's t-test.

In order to test whether neurite elongation rates were influenced by their proximity to the target tissue, the field of neurite outgrowth was divided into three concentric zones such that zone I was closest to the explant, zone III was closest to the target (when present) and thus furthest from the cord, and zone II was intermediate. Co-cultured target tissue served as a centralized source of the growth influence, i.e., a putative growth factor (Fig. 2, Right, top). Cultures treated with the limb mesenchyme-conditioned medium are assumed to have possessed a uniform distribution of the growth factor over the substratum (Fig. 2, Right, middle), while explants on polylysine in the absence of target tissue represent cultures with a uniform distribution of a neurite growth-supporting surface (Fig. 2, Right, bottom). As is readily apparent, only the cultures with a centralized source of the target factor exhibited a significant difference in neurite elongation rates among the zones (zones I to II, $p=.05$; zones I to III, $p=.002$; zones II to III, $p=.05$). This demonstrates that as the neurite nears the target tissue, its rate of elongation accelerates. Uniform surfaces produce relatively constant rates of elongation regardless of the distance of the growth cone from the explant. (One might further suggest that these data rule out any significant growth factor output from the explant itself.)

Metabolic Responses to Target and Substratum

Non-neuronal cells respond to chemotactic gradients in part by increasing their rate of metabolism, an event referred to as a "chemokinetic response" (Snyderman and Goetzel, 1981). As an attempt to determine the basis for the increased neurite growth rates as described above, the metabolic activity of specific neuron populations was assayed to see if any relationship exists between growth rate response to the target and substratum and oxidative metabolism. Uptake by cord cultures of tritiated 2-deoxyglucose, an analog of glucose, was analyzed autoradiographically (a preliminary report is found in Muhlach and Pollack, 1984). 2-deoxyglucose is trapped in the neuron after it has been phosphorylated in the same pathway as glucose, and therefore its incorporation is an index of cellular metabolic activity (Sokoloff, 1981). This approach has permitted the identification of specific populations of spinal cord cells that metabolically respond to the various experimental variables under consideration. The analyses involved quantitation of silver grains in histological sections of spinal cord explants. Comparisons were performed among the ventricular zone, non-motor intermediate zone, marginal zone, and the left and right lateral motor column (Fig. 3). The central canal and extra-cord space served as background sources. Only one population of spinal cord cells showed a significant change in metabolic activity in response to the target or substratum. That was the lateral motor column neurons (Fig. 3). This effect is equivalent to the chemokinetic response of chemotactic leukocytes and is the first demonstration that there is a chemokinetic component in the neuronal response to target tissue. Furthermore, these results indicate that the influence of the target tissue is directed only to the motor neurons.

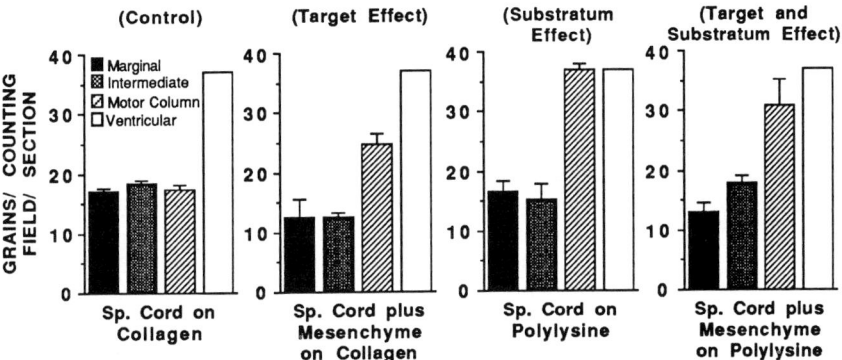

Figure 3. ^{3}H-2-deoxyglucose labeling of spinal cord regions. Striped bars (±s.e.m.) emphasize the relative increase in LMC neuron metabolism under the influence of target tissue and substratum. All other regions remained at a constant labeling level.

Differentiative Effects of Target vs. Substratum

Thus far, the evidence clearly suggests that the target tissue for spinal motor neurons can influence nerve fiber growth processes. However, growth cones of developing neurons apparently can exhibit their specific neurotransmitter as well as the uptake and release machinery before a post-synaptic contact is made (Lockerbie, 1987). The question is whether the target tissue can exert any influence on the processes related to neurotransmitter expression in the system of present concern. Functional maturation/differentiation represents an important component in any consideration of the specificity associated with innervation.

Motor neuron differentiation and function are indicated in part by the ability to synthesize neurotransmitter-related enzymes. Comparisons were carried out between protein content, as a general growth index, and the activity of a neurotransmitter specific synthetic enzyme under the variable conditions discussed previously. Since choline acetyltransferase (ChAT) is responsible for acetylcholine synthesis, it can serve as a useful marker for the development of cholinergic neurotransmitter synthetic capabilities. Because motor neurons are the predominant cholinergic neuron in the lumbosacral region of the spinal cord (Burt, 1970; Kása et al., 1970), ChAT can act as a marker for potential maturational effects of target tissue and substratum on spinal cord motor neurons.

The radiochemical method of Fonnum (1975) provided the assay for ChAT in the spinal cord explants. Homogenate samples of the explants were standardized to a cell number equivalency by DNA assay (Hill and Whatley, 1975), and protein content of the explants was determined by a micro-Lowry method (Keletti and Lederer, 1974). Protein content data paralleled both the neurite density and the neurite growth rate data discussed above (Fig. 4, left). The metabolic activation, as evidenced by the 2-deoxyglucose study, may be the basis of these protein responses. A critical finding is that the mesenchymal target tissue was the only effector in bringing ChAT activity in spinal cord explants to a stage-appropriate level (Fig. 4, right).

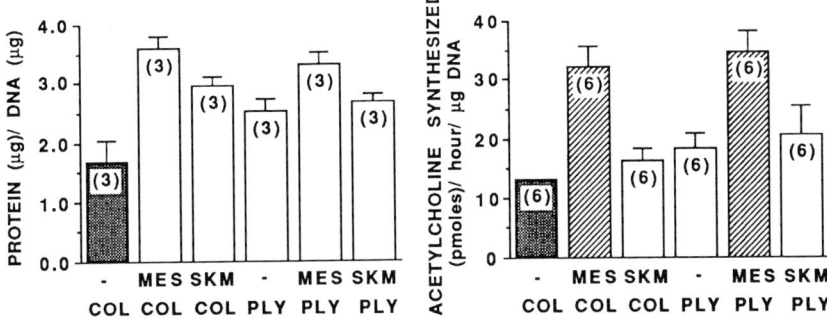

Figure 4. Left: Histogram representation of mean protein content ± s.e.m. for each group. The target tissues, limb mesenchyme (MES) and skeletal muscle (SKM), and the polylysine (PLY) all increased the protein levels in the spinal cord explants as compared to explants on collagen (COL). Note that the target tissues and PLY substratum were not additive. Right: ChAT activity is shown as acetylcholine synthesized, the baseline being explants on COL. PLY and SKM resulted in slight, non-significant increases in ChAT activity. MES produced the only significant increase in ChAT activity regardless of substratum.

The transition from an apparent young, low ChAT activity motor neuron population to a cholinergically more mature motor neuron population was in response to the limb target only at the particular developmental state in which it was largely undifferentiated mesenchyme. The target influence must be maturation-promotive since the LMC neurons have embarked substantially toward full differentiation as motor neurons by the stage at which these studies were performed. However, this interaction between the limb target and the spinal cord motor neurons appears to be an essential, specific requirement for motor neuron cholinergic maturation in vitro. In contrast, spinal cord explants on polylysine, in the absence of target, survive for long periods (one to two months), produce dense neuritic outgrowth and show dramatic increases in protein content with in vitro age; yet, they develop no enhanced cholinergic capabilities. Increases in neurite density, directional control of neurite elongation, neuronal protein content and metabolic activity all reflect substratum-related influences. These processes are, however, susceptible to modulation by specific factors such as the biologically active components released by the target. The elevation of cholinergicity in the cord explant involves the specific presence of a presumed factor derived from the mesenchymal limb tissue, the action of which may be substratum-independent. In vivo comparisons of protein content and ChAT activity indicate that in vitro target effects keep these parameters on a normal developmental course.

CONCLUSIONS

As an outcome of the numerous investigations centered around the larval frog motor neuron-limb target interaction model, the mesenchymal target-derived factor(s) is tentatively designated as a "motor neuron growth factor" or "MNGF" (see Pollack et al., 1985; Muhlach and Pollack, 1986). Similarly, both mesenchyme-conditioned medium and mesenchyme-conditioned substratum can be considered to contain the target-derived "MNGF". Laminin, fibronectin, Nerve Growth Factor and assorted extracellular matrix components have been experimentally eliminated as candidates for the biologically active "MNGF" of the mesenchymal limb tissue (Pollack et al., 1981; 1985; Kaminski, personal communication). Chemical characterization of the mesenchymal factor(s) has been deferred in favor of definitively establishing the developmental significance and extent of the motor neuron-target tissue relationship. The information thus far can be formulated into a model that summarizes the current understanding of how neural development is influenced by the motor neuron-target interactions.

Haptotaxis, as originally defined by Carter (1967), is the movement of a cell from a less adherent surface to a more adherent surface. Some investigators have compared substratum-associated growth factor activity to haptotaxis. However, a more accurate representation of the "MNGF" action implicated by these studies would be an amalgam of the concepts of chemotaxis, chemokinesis and haptotaxis. The directionality in the neurite response to target tissue in vitro and the substratum-localized neurite-promoting activity suggest that the "MNGF" may act in a haptochemotactic fashion. Data presented earlier indicate that the response of the motor neuron to the "MNGF" also involves a chemokinetic element which is consistent with the chemotactic responses of non-neuronal cell types that have a chemokinetic component (Snyderman and Goetzel, 1981). The combination of chemotactic and chemokinetic components of the neural response can account for the enhanced, directed neurite growth elicited by the target tissue.

Evidence for a neuron-substratum adhesion role in controlling the direction of neurite extension led Katz et al. (1984) to propose the "stochastic walk" hypothesis. By definition, a stochastic phenomenon requires the influence of a random variable. In their model of neurite elongation, the random variable is neuron-to-substratum adhesion. When the filopodia of the growth cone make sufficient adhesive attachments to the substratum, the growth cone develops a tension that pulls the trailing neurite (Bray, 1987). The direction of neurite growth can be predicted from the probability that sufficient adhesive contacts will be made with the substratum. A novel aspect of this model for controlled neurite growth would incorporate the action of a target-derived neuronal growth factor. For instance, the target-derived, substratum localizable "MNGF" elicits directed growth of spinal explant neurites, accelerates nerve fiber growth rate and alters growth rate cycles. These processes seem to be based in the action of a substratum-localized growth factor that increases metabolic activity (chemokinesis) of spinal cord motor neurons. This rate regulating component can enhance greatly the efficiency of the guidance system. If the growth cone encounters a gradient of substratum-bound growth factor, its response purportedly will be enhanced by the metabolic activation effect of the factor. Thus, the directional component and the rate component represent two separate processes, both regulated by the growth factor, that together result in an enhanced migration of the growth cone in a favorable direction. The combination of these two processes incorporated into the stochastic walk model of axon elongation modify it as a "biased stochastic walk". And so when a nerve fiber grows in the correct direction, with respect to the target-derived signal, its speed is increased so as to enhance the guidance process.

One can envision the target tissue releasing the putative motor neuron growth factor that then diffuses and binds to appropriate extracellular matrix sites thus establishing the guidance signal set. The binding of the "MNGF" to a substratum greatly improves the efficacy of the factor by localizing it to the neuron-substratum interface, by maintaining a concentration gradient, and most importantly by stabilizing the spatial relationship of the neuron and the signal origin. The difficulty in finding and characterizing neuronal growth factors in vivo may stem from the inherent high efficiency of the factor binding system with the consequence that very low levels of the factor may be physiologically adequate. A resultant axon-growth factor-substratum interaction could implement adhesion. This membrane-substratum adhesion may be translated into the reorganization of structural and contractile elements at the level of the cytoskeleton and membrane of the growth cone, the outcome of which is directional axon extension. Concurrently, the growth factor may bring about a chemokinetic, metabolic activation to facilitate neurite elongation, the stabilization process and the maintenance of functional neuron activities.

Superimposed upon the morphological response of the neuron to target tissue is the substratum-independent action of the target in enhancing cholinergic expression. It is significant that the limb target tissue is capable of eliciting this functional response only when it is mesenchymal. Temporal aspects of the interaction are provided by the stage-specific developmental competency of the participating tissues. This stage-specificity ensures that innervation occurs at the proper time and that the motor neurons have undergone appropriate cholinergic maturation. Spatial aspects of the present model are provided by the location of the target tissue, as the source of the "MNGF", relative to the central nervous system and by extracellular matrix components capable of binding and localizing the target-originated factor. Factor directed substratum adhesion can contribute to spatial affinity by altering growth rate and providing a biased stochastic walk. The postulated motor neuron growth factor that regulates or mediates several aspects of motor neuron development may be essential for the formation and maintenance of appropriate functional connections.

The neuron-target interactions that have been the topic of this chapter do not necessarily account for synaptic specificity, but they do seem to be part of the total developmental process. Target-derived neuron growth factors may contribute to the events leading to specificity by assuring that correct cell associations are established in advance of synaptogenesis. The present model of larval frog tissues provides the means for investigating developmentally significant neuron-target interactions.

ACKNOWLEDGMENTS

The author acknowledges a long-term, productive collaboration with Emanuel D. Pollack throughout the course of these investigations. Thanks are also extended to Veronica Liebig for her active participation in many of the experiments, and to George Dombrowski, Jr. for expert assistance in both the biochemical and computer programming aspects.

REFERENCES

Ashwell KW, Watson CR (1983). The development of facial motoneurons in the mouse: Neuronal death and the innervation of the facial muscles. J Embryol Exp Morphol 77:117-141.
Bennett MR (1983). Development of neuromuscular synapses. Physiol Rev 63:915-1048.
Black IB (1983). "Cellular and Molecular Biology of Neuronal Development." New York: Plenum Press, pp ix-xiv.
Bray D (1979). Mechanical tension produced by nerve cells in tissue culture. J Cell Sci 37:391-410.
Bray D (1987). Growth cones: do they pull or are they pushed? Trends Neurosci 10:431-434.
Burt AM (1970). A procedure for the histochemical demonstration of choline acetyltransferase. J Histochem Cytochem 18:408-415.
Carter SB (1967). Haptotaxis and the mechanism of cell

motility. Nature 213:256-261.
Constantine-Paton M, Law MI (1978). Eye-specific termination bands in tecta of three-eyed frogs. Science 189:639-641.
Davies AM, Thoenen J, Barde YA (1986). Different factors from the central nervous system and periphery regulate the survival of sensory neurons. Nature 319:497-499.
Farel PB, Bemelmans SE (1985). Specificity of motoneuron projection patterns during development of the bullfrog tadpole (Rana catesbeiana). J Comp Neurol 238:128-134.
Fonnum F (1975). A rapid radiochemical method for the determination of choline acetyltransferase. J Neurochem 24:407-409.
Harris WA (1986). Homing behavior of axons in the embryonic vertebrate brain. Science 320:266-269.
Heaton MB, Paiva M (1986). The influence of target tissue age on neurite outgrowth from chick embryo trigeminal motor nucleus explants. Develop Biol 116:314-318.
Heaton MB, Wayne DB (1986). Specific responsiveness of chick trigeminal motor nucleus explants to target-conditioned media. J Comp Neurol 243:381-387.
Hill BT, Whatley S (1975). A simple rapid microassay for DNA. FEBS Lett 56:20-23.
Hollyday M (1983). Development of motor innervation of chick limbs. In Fallon JF, Caplan, AJ (eds): "Limb Development and Regeneration, Part A." New York: Alan R. Liss, pp 183-193.
Jacob M, Christ B, Jacob HJ (1979). The migration of myogenic cells from the somites into the leg region of avian embryos. An ultrastructural study. Anat Embryol 157:291-309.
Kása P, Mann SP, Hebb C (1970). Localization of choline acetyltransferase. Nature 226:812-816.
Kater SB, Letourneau PC (eds) (1985). "Biology of the Nerve Growth Cone." New York: Alan R. Liss.
Katz MJ, George EB, Gilbert LJ (1984). Axonal elongation as a stochastic walk. Cell Motil 4:351-370.
Keletti G, Lederer WH (1974). "Handbook of Micromethods for the Biological Sciences." New York: Reinhold, pp 87-88.
Laing NG (1984). Motor innervation of proximally rotated chick embryo wings. J Embryol Exp Morphol 83:213-233.

Lance-Jones C, Landmesser L (1981). Pathway selection by chick lumbosacral motoneurons during normal development. Proc Roy Soc Lond 214:1-8.

Landmesser L (1978). The development of motor projections in the chick hind limb. J Physiol 284:391-414.

Letourneau P (1975). Cell-to-substratum adhesion and guidance of axonal elongation. Develop Biol 44:77-91.

Letourneau P (1987). What happens when growth cones meet neurites: attraction or repulsion? Trends Neurosci 10:390-393.

Lewis J, Al-Ghaith L, Swanson G, Khan A (1983). The control of axon outgrowth in the developing chick wing. In Fallon JF, Caplan AJ (eds): "Limb Development and Regeneration, Part A." New York: Alan R. Liss, pp 195-205.

Lockerbie RO (1987). The neuronal growth cone: A review of its locomotory, navigational and target recognition capabilities. Neurosci 20:719-729.

Muhlach WL, Pollack ED (1978). Improved method for the in vitro study of amphibian neural development utilizing Sykes-Moore chambers. Tiss Cult Assoc Man 4:875-879.

Muhlach WL, Pollack ED (1982). Target tissue control of nerve fiber growth rate and periodicity in vitro. Develop Brain Res 4:361-364.

Muhlach WL, Pollack ED (1984). Localized uptake of 2-deoxyglucose by the lateral motor column of spinal cord explants as a function of target and substratum. Soc Neurosci Abstr 10:1056.

Muhlach WL, Pollack ED (1986). Target tissue-directed neurite elongation explained by a "biased stochastic walk". Soc Neurosci Abstr 12:503.

Nurcombe V, Bennett MR (1983). The growth of neurites from explants of brachial spinal cord exposed to different components of wing bud mesenchyme. J Comp Neurol 219:133-142.

Pfenninger KH, Maylie-Pfenninger M-F, Friedman LB, Simkowitz P (1984). Lectin labeling of sprouting neurons. III. Type-specific glycoconjugates on growth cones of different origin. Develop Biol 106:97-108.

Pollack ED (1980). Target-dependent survival of tadpole spinal cord neurites in tissue culture. Neurosci Lett 16:169-174.

Pollack ED, Koves J (1975). In vitro cultivation of larval frog spinal cord explants. Tiss Cult Assoc Man

1:193-197.
Pollack ED, Liebig V (1977). Differentiating limb tissue affects neurite growth in spinal cord cultures. Science 197:899-900.
Pollack ED, Muhlach WL (1981). Stage dependency in eliciting target-dependent enhanced neurite outgrowth from spinal cord explants in vitro. Develop Biol 86:259-263.
Pollack ED, Muhlach WL (1982). Target control of neuronal development during formation of the spinal reflex arc: an operant model. J Neurosci Res 8:343-355.
Pollack ED, Muhlach WL, Liebig V (1981). Neurotropic influence of mesenchymal limb target tissue on spinal cord neurite growth in vitro. J Comp Neurol 200:393-405.
Pollack ED, Muhlach WL, Liebig V (1985). Substratum-mediation of neuron-target growth interactions in vitro. Cell Diff 16 Suppl:87.
Ramón y Cajal S (1929). "Studies on Vertebrate Neurogenesis." Guth L (1960,transl, ed): Springfield, IL: Charles C. Thomas Publishing.
Ruoslahti E, Pierschbacher MD (1987). New perspectives in cell adhesion: RGD and integrins. Science 238:491-497.
Rutishauser U (1984). Developmental biology of a neural cell adhesion molecule. Nature 310:549-553.
Scott SA (1988). Skin sensory innervation patterns in embryonic chick hindlimbs deprived of motoneurons. Develop Biol 126:362-374.
Snyderman RG, Goetzel EJ (1981). Molecular and cellular mechanisms of leukocyte chemotaxis. Science 213:830-837.
Sokoloff L (1981). The deoxyglucose method: theory and practice. Eur Neurol 20:137-145.
Stent GS (1985). Thinking in one dimension: The impact of molecular biology on development. Cell 40:1-2.
Taylor AC (1943). Development of the innervation pattern in the limb bud of the frog. Anat Rec 87:379-409.
Taylor AC, Kollros JJ (1946). Stages in the normal development of Rana pipiens larvae. Anat Rec 94:7-24.
Tosney KW, Landmesser LT (1985). Specificity of early motoneuron growth cone outgrowth in the chick embryo. J Neurosci 5:2336-2344.

MECHANISMS OF NEUROMUSCULAR JUNCTION DEVELOPMENT STUDIED IN TISSUE CULTURE

H. Benjamin Peng, Qiming Chen, M. William Rochlin, Dingliang Zhu and Brian Kay

Department of Cell Biology and Anatomy (H.B.P., Q.C., M.W.R., D.Z.) and Department of Biology (B.K.), University of North Carolina, Chapel Hill, North Carolina 27599

INTRODUCTION

The cell-to-cell interaction which leads to synapse formation is an intriguing problem in developmental neurobiology. This process can be conveniently studied in tissue culture. When processes of motor neurons come into contact with muscle cells in culture, functional synapses are formed; they undergo the same maturation process as those in vivo. The nerve-muscle co-culture is the conventional system for studying synaptogenesis. However, it is possible to simplify the analysis of this process by studying the development of synaptic specializations in the absence of either the pre- or the post-synaptic partner in separate neuron and muscle cultures. In the last several years, we have utilized these model culture systems to understand the mechanisms of synaptic development. The cultures are prepared from spinal cords or myotomes of Xenopus embryos. In addition to being easy to prepare and maintain, these cultures can be readily compared with the myotomal muscle in vivo, which forms the tail musculature of the tadpole. In this chapter, we will summarize our findings on the development of the neuromuscular junction (NMJ) from the use of Xenopus cultures. Furthermore, the use of techniques of molecular biology to identify the endogenous molecules involved in the neuromuscular interaction will be discussed.

INDUCTION OF PRESYNAPTIC DEVELOPMENT BY BASIC POLYPEPTIDE-COATED LATEX BEADS

Burry et al. (1980, 1984) previously showed that clustering of synaptic vesicles can be induced by polycation-coated beads in cultures of cerebellar neurons. Recently we carried out these experiments on explant cultures of Xenopus spinal cord (Peng, 1987). As shown in Fig. 1, varicosities similar to the presynaptic terminal are formed at the neurite-bead contacts. Within these terminals, vesicles 50-60 nm in diameter are clustered, often in juxtaposition to the membrane in contact with the beads. In addition, dense-cored vesicles, 80-100 nm in diameter, and smooth endoplasmic reticulum are also present within these varicosities. The size of these varicosities is in proportion to the area of bead-muscle contact. When beads which approximate the size of the neurite (about 1 µm) are applied to the neurites, submicron en passant-type junctions are formed along the process. But, when the size of the beads is much larger than the diameter of the neurite, the junction acquires the appearance of a nerve terminal, encompassing a substantial area on the bead's surface. This suggests that the nerve has the capacity to accommodate the target size in the development of the presynaptic terminal. On the average, 50% of the bead-neurite contacts exhibited such presynaptic-type specializations. Unlike the neuromuscular junction, however, the cleft between the bead and the neuritic membrane lacks a basement membrane. This suggests that the basement membrane at the NMJ is contributed by the muscle cell. As we shall see in the following discussion, this conclusion is supported by studies on the bead-induced postsynaptic specializations.

Structural evidence has shown that synaptic vesicles within the presynaptic nerve terminal interact with a cytoskeletal lattice (Hirokawa, 1983; Peng, 1983). The regulation of this interaction, e.g. by phosphorylation of proteins integral to the vesicles, may play an important role in synaptic transmission (Bahler and Greengard, 1987). One can imagine that the interaction of the beads with the neurite may elicit the development of this cytoskeletal specialization, which immobilizes synaptic vesicles as they are transported down the neurite by the anterograde axonal transport mechanism.

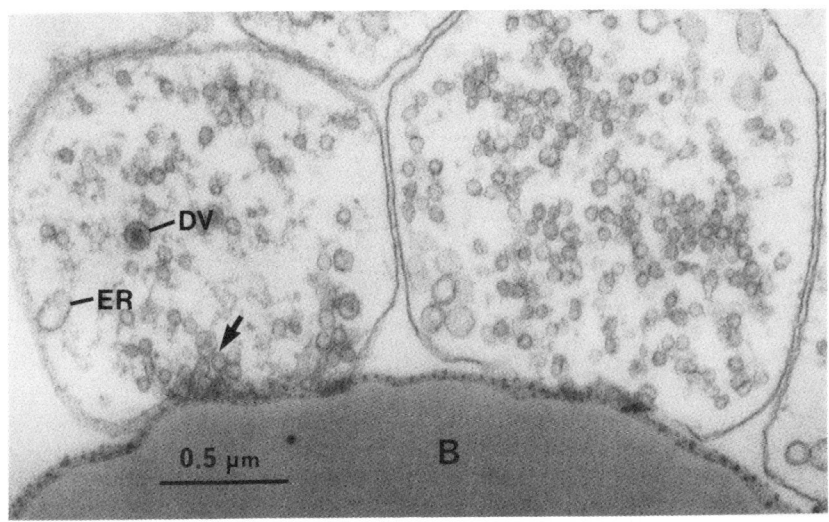

Figure 1. Presynaptic specializations induced by basic polypeptide-coated latex bead. B: bead; ER: smooth endoplasmic reticulum; DV: dense-core vesicle.

Thus, this bead-neurite co-culture should allow one to analyze the cellular machinery necessary for the assembly of the presynaptic terminal.

INDUCTION OF POSTSYNAPTIC DEVELOPMENT BY BASIC POLYPEPTIDE-COATED LATEX BEADS

In these studies, we cultured the myotomal muscle cells from Xenopus embryos. Latex beads coated with basic polypeptides such as polylysine or polyornithine were then applied to muscle cells to mimic the presynaptic input. An accumulation of acetylcholine receptors (AChRs) at the bead-muscle contacts occurs within a few hours after the bead application (Peng et al., 1981; Peng and Cheng, 1982). An example is shown in Fig. 2. These AChR clusters are discretely located at the bead-muscle contacts. The number of clusters is proportional to the number of bead-muscle contacts, and the size of the individual clusters also varies in proportion to the size of the beads used (Peng, 1986). In addition, acetylcholinesterase activity also develops at these bead-induced receptor clusters (Peng, 1987). Ultrastructural studies have revealed the development of an elaborate specialization at these sites, including infoldings of the membrane, a membrane-associated cytoplasmic density and a basement membrane (Peng and Cheng, 1982). All these structures are features of the postsynaptic membrane at the NMJ. Thus, the coated beads can mimic the nerve in inducing a local postsynaptic differentiation in the muscle cell.

Before innervation, AChRs are spontaneously

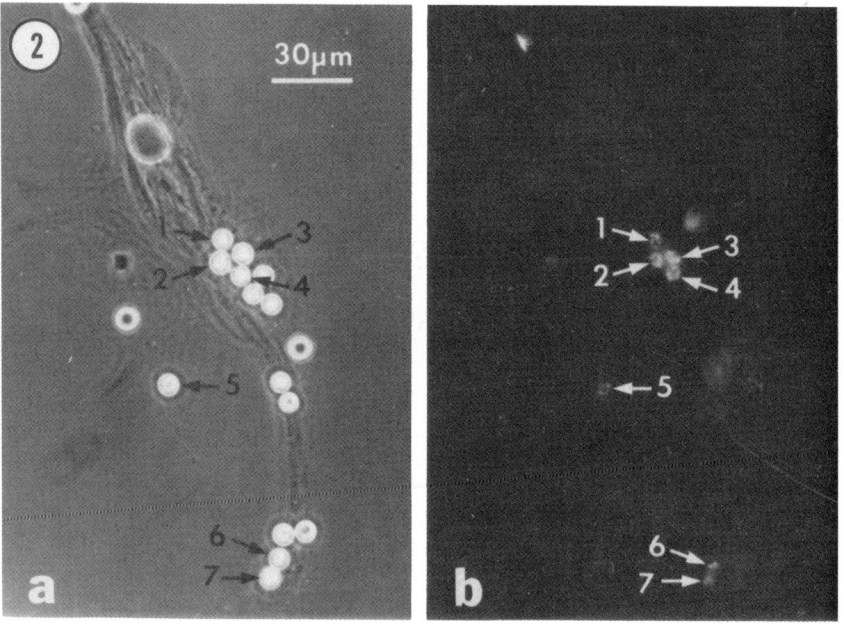

Figure 2. Formation of AChR clusters induced by polyornithine-coated latex beads. At the bead-muscle contacts (arrows in a), AChRs form discrete clusters as shown by fluorescence α-bungarotoxin labeling in b.

clustered in cultured muscle cells. During innervation, the nerve causes the dispersal of these preexisting AChR clusters in the extrajunctional area in addition to its effect of inducing a local clustering of AChRs. This is an example of the global effect of innervation. We found that this global effect of innervation also can be mimicked by the coated beads. As new clusters are assembled at the bead-muscle contacts, preexisting clusters away from the beads are gradually dispersed (Peng, 1986). Our data show that this process is not due to a depletion of the available AChR pool for the new cluster formation, but may be due to a direct effect of the bead stimulation. Thus, both the local and the global effect of innervation can be reproduced in this bead-muscle co-culture system.

ROLE OF ACHR DIFFUSION AND THE CYTOSKELETON IN THE FORMATION OF CLUSTERS

We have been using this model system for the past several years to understand the mechanism of AChR clustering. The formation of the clusters can result from either a lateral redistribution of AChRs preexisting on the cell surface or by a local insertion of AChRs from intracellular stores. Previous studies by Anderson and Cohen (1977) have shown that lateral translation of AChRs on the cell surface is involved in the nerve-induced clustering of AChRs. In our studies, we found that surface AChRs are drawn into cluster formation immediately following the addition of the beads. By first masking the surface AChRs with native α-bungarotoxin and then labeling the cells with fluorescently labeled toxin at various intervals, we were able to follow the incorporation of new receptors into the cell membrane. Our results have shown that there is no delay in the appearance of new receptors at the cell surface following the native toxin treatment. However, these new receptors begin to appear at the bead-muscle contacts after a four to eight hour delay. This suggests that there is no preferential insertion of new receptors at the site of cluster formation. Thus, in these cultured Xenopus muscle cells, the formation of clusters is brought about by a redistribution of AChRs which are already on the cell surface.

These results suggest that the lateral diffusion of AChRs within the plane of the membrane plays an important role in the clustering process. To further test this idea, we examined the effect of restricting the lateral mobility of AChRs in the formation of clusters. The tetravalent mannose-binding lectin, concanavalin A (Con A), binds to the subunits of AChRs and causes their immobilization as shown by fluorescence photobleaching studies. When Xenopus myotomal muscle cells were pulse-treated with Con A at a concentration of 50-100 µg/ml, the formation of clusters induced by the beads was suppressed. Its divalent analog, succinyl Con A, neither significantly reduces the lateral mobility of AChRs at similar concentrations nor does it block the clustering process. A reduction in the lateral mobility of AChRs also suppressed clustering induced by the nerve in Xenopus nerve-muscle co-cultures (Kodokoro et al., 1986). These results show that the lateral diffusion of AChRs in the membrane is an integral part of the mechanism of cluster formation.

As Edwards and Frisch (1976) first proposed, the AChR clustering may be explained by a diffusion-mediated trapping process. This model suggests that freely diffusing receptors are immobilized at the site of nerve-muscle contacts, or at the bead-muscle contacts in our system, by a localized molecular specialization which binds the AChRs. A candidate for the trapping mechanism is the membrane-associated cytoskeleton, since immunocytochemical studies have shown a close relationship between the AChR cluster and cytoskeletal proteins (Froehner, 1986). In our electron microscopical studies, we found that a meshwork of microfilaments is assembled at the bead-muscle contact sites before AChRs can be detected (Peng and Phelan, 1984). These data imply that this cytoskeletal specialization may be involved in the formation of the clusters. To understand the composition of this specialization, we have examined the appearance of three proteins at the bead-induced AChR clusters with immunofluorescence.

First, the appearance of the postsynaptic 43K protein was studied. This protein was first identified in the postsynaptic membrane of Torpedo electric organ, which is one of the richest sources of nicotinic synapses (Froehner, 1986). As shown in Fig. 3 c-d, the distribution of this protein in the postsynaptic membrane at the NMJ is identical to that of AChRs. Thus, it is a synaptic-specific protein. When cells treated with beads were labeled with antibodies against the 43K

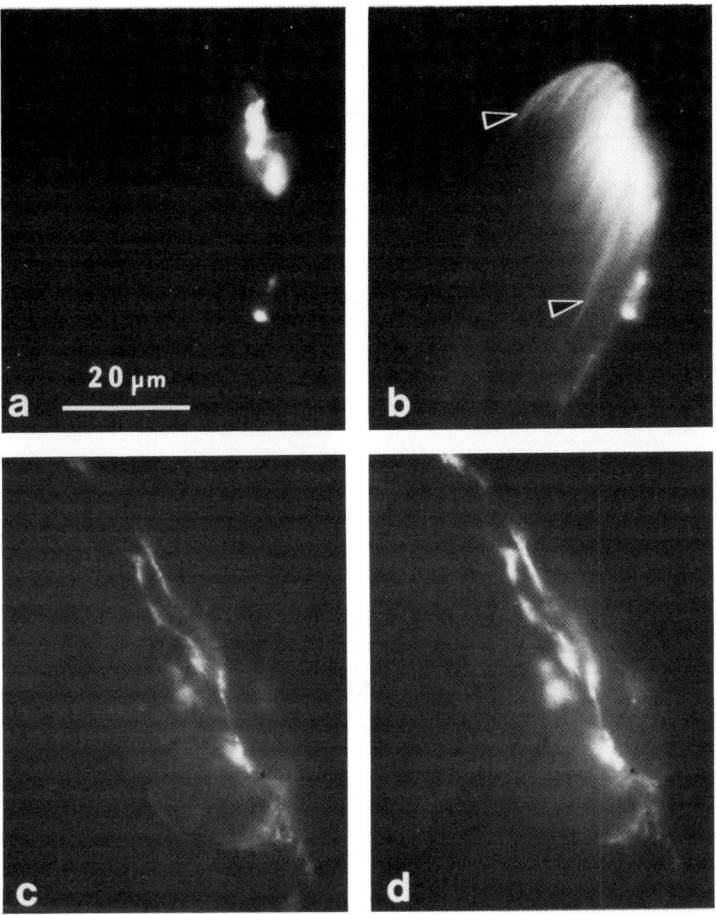

Figure 3. Co-localization of AChR clusters and the postsynaptic 43K and 58K proteins in myotomal muscle cells in vivo. Left: rhodamine image of α-bungarotoxin staining. Right: fluorescein image of antibody staining. (a-b) AChR cluster and 58K protein; (c-d) AChR cluster and 43K protein. Arrowheads in b point to invaginations of the myotendinous junction.

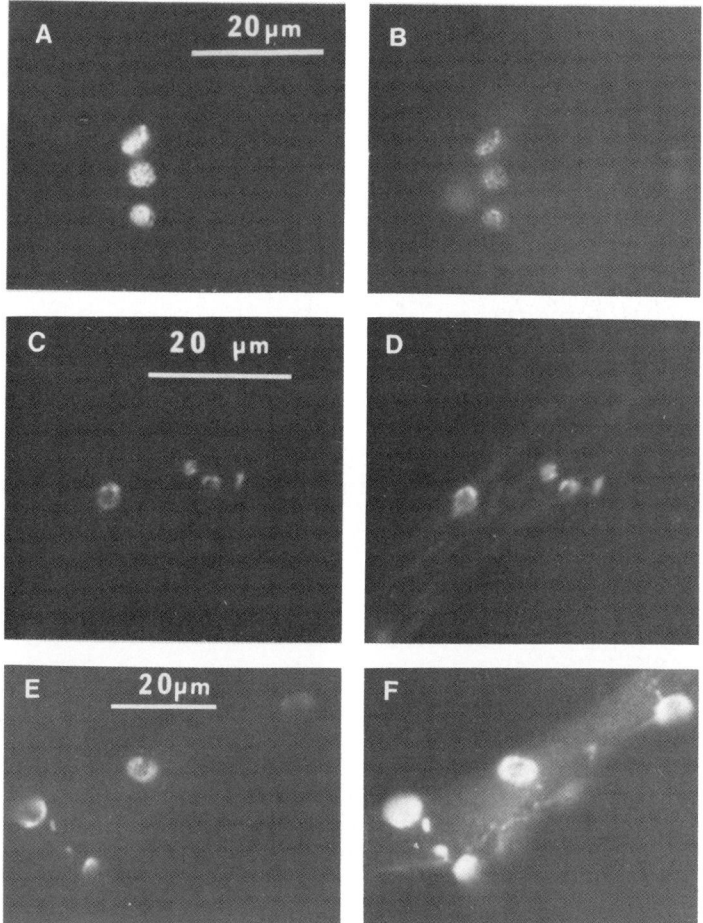

Figure 4. Association of bead-induced AChR clusters with 43K protein (A-B), 58K protein (C-D), or talin (E-F). For each pair, the AChR clusters are shown on the left and the antibody staining is shown on the right.

protein, it is clear that this protein is co-localized with the bead-induced AChR clusters (Fig. 4 A-B; also see Peng and Froehner, 1985). A second protein is the postsynaptic 58K protein, which was first identified

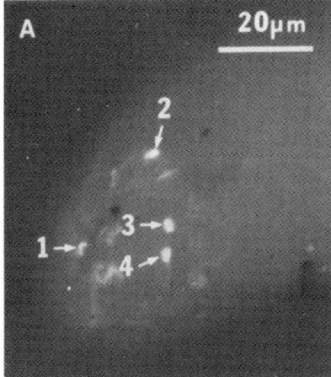 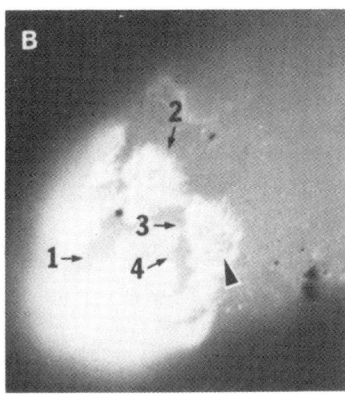

Figure 5. Localization of talin in the myotomal muscle cell in vivo. A: rhodamine α-bungarotoxin staining; B: FITC anti-talin antibody staining. Although talin is seen at the myotendinous junction (arrowhead in B), it is absent from the AChR-rich postsynaptic membrane (numbered positions in A and B).

also at the Torpedo electric organ postsynaptic membrane (Froehner et al., 1987). As shown in Fig. 3 a-b, antibody against this protein recognizes antigens both at AChR clusters and the extrasynaptic area adjacent to the postsynaptic membrane. Thus, this protein is shared by both the synaptic and the extrasynaptic membrane. At the bead-induced clusters, the presence of the 58K protein is also obvious (Fig. 4 C-D). A third cytoskeletal protein that we have examined is talin. This 215K protein mediates the interaction of actin filaments with plasma membrane receptors for extracellular matrix (Burridge, 1986). With antibodies against talin, we found that although this protein is present at the myotendinous junction, it is absent from the postsynaptic membrane of Xenopus muscle (Fig. 5). Interestingly, the bead-induced clusters are associated with talin (Fig. 4 E-F). These data show the versatility of the bead-induced clustering process in recruiting synaptic-specific, shared and extrasynaptic peripheral membrane proteins into the site of receptor concentration. Since

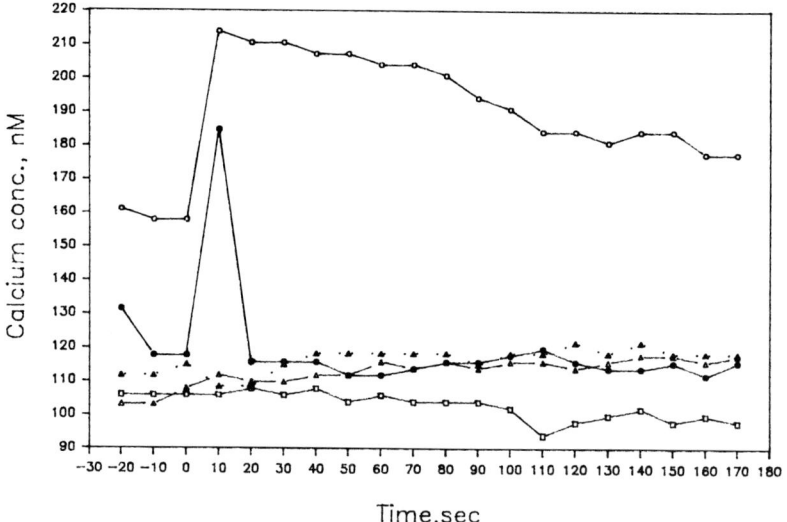

Figure 6. Changes in intracellular Ca^{2+} when muscle cells were treated with polyornithine-coated beads. The beads were added at time 0 and an immediate and transient rise in Ca^{2+} was observed (closed and open circles represent data from two different cells). Uncoated beads (open triangles) were ineffective in eliciting this Ca^{2+} transient, as were polyornithine-coated beads added in the presence of Ca^{2+}-free medium (squares) or 50 µM verapamil (solid triangles).

the beads induce a de novo assembly of AChR clusters, these data suggest that some of the proteins used in their formation may not be involved in their maintenance.

ROLE OF THE CALCIUM ION

The postsynaptic-type differentiation elicited by the beads should involve a local stimulation of the muscle. Since the cell membrane is in intimate contact with a highly charged substrate at the bead-muscle contact, it is conceivable that a change in the electric field strength across the membrane may occur at that locus. This would result in a change in the ion permeability. To test this hypothesis, we examined the role of Ca^{2+} influx on the bead-induced AChR clustering. By depriving the muscle cell of its extracellular Ca^{2+} supply with Ca^{2+}-free medium or with Ca^{2+} antagonists (including divalent cations Co^{2+}, Ni^{2+} or Mn^{2+}, or organic compounds such as verapamil or D-600), the formation of clusters induced by beads is reversibly suppressed (Peng, 1984). Recently, we have directly measured the change in intracellular Ca^{2+} accompanying the bead stimulation with fura-2 and digital video microscopy (Tsien et al., 1985). As shown in Fig. 6, a rapid transient rise in intracellular Ca^{2+} is observed at the time of the bead-muscle contact. This change is abolished by Ca^{2+}-free medium or by the calcium antagonist verapamil. Both treatments also suppressed the AChR clustering. Furthermore, uncoated beads, which do not cause AChR clustering, fail to elicit this Ca^{2+} transient. Thus, an increase in intracellular Ca^{2+} appears to be a necessary condition for the formation of AChR clustering. In the case of nerve-induced AChR clustering, it also has been shown that a deprivation of extracellular Ca^{2+} exerts an inhibitory effect (Henderson et al., 1984). This increase in intracellular Ca^{2+}, coupled with other second messenger systems, may be involved in the activation of the postsynaptic differentiation.

IDENTIFICATION OF THE TROPHIC MOLECULE

It is speculated that the nerve-muscle interaction which leads to synaptic differentiation is mediated by certain trophic molecules released by the motoneurons. Consistent with this hypothesis is the finding that extracts from brain, spinal cord or the synaptic basement membrane contain molecules which cause an increase in AChR clustering in cultured muscle cells (Usdin and Fischbach, 1986; Olek et al., 1983; Nitkin et al., 1987). Recently, we also have examined the effect of spinal cord extract from Xenopus larvae on the formation of AChR clusters in cultured Xenopus myotomal muscle cells. Spinal cords dissected from stage 50 Xenopus larvae were homogenized and centrifuged. The supernatant was then applied to the muscle culture. As shown in Fig. 7b, this crude spinal cord extract causes an obvious increase in AChR clustering after an overnight

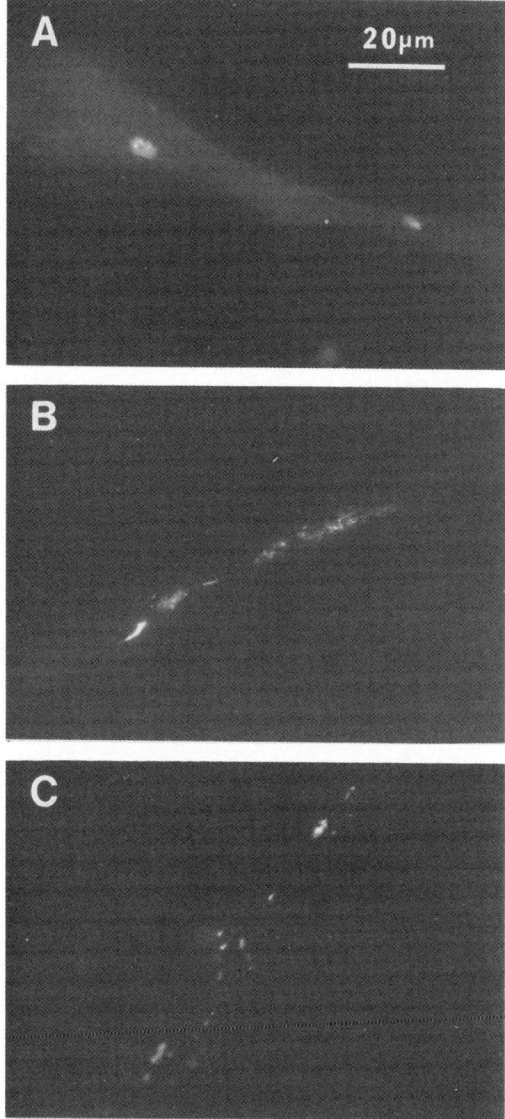

Figure 7. Effect of tissue extract on the formation of AChR clusters. The cells were treated with the extracts for 24 hr. and labeled with α-bungarotoxin. A: control (culture medium alone); B: 25 µg/ml spinal cord extract; C: 100 µg/ml muscle extract. The tissues were isolated from Xenopus tadpoles.

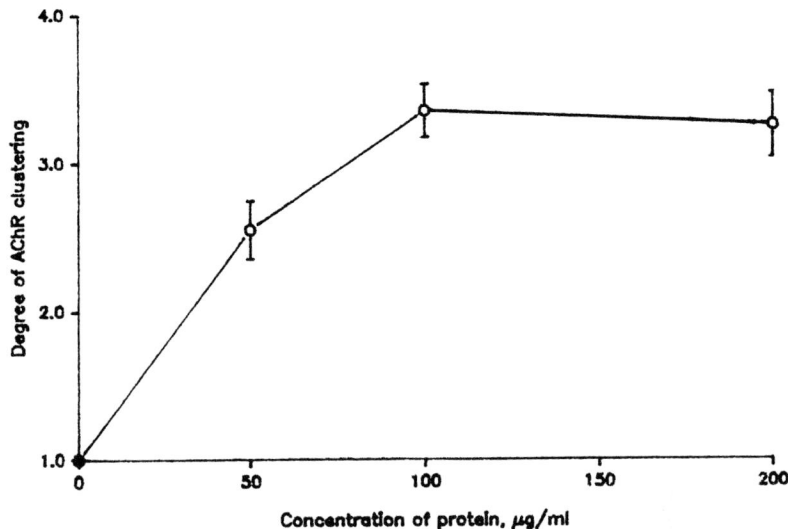

Figure 8. Quantitation of the AChR cluster-inducing activity in myotomal muscle extract. The number of AChR clusters per cell was measured and normalized with respect to the control value.

incubation. A three-fold increase in the number of AChR clusters per cell was observed at an extract protein concentration of 50 µg/ml. To examine whether AChR cluster-inducing activity also is present in the myotomal muscle, we made an extract from tails of stage 50 tadpoles whose spinal cords had been removed. As shown in Figs. 7c and 8, this muscle extract also causes a saturable increase in the AChR clustering in cultured cells. These results suggest that the muscle also is able to synthesize a trophic molecule for the postsynaptic differentiation. From our bead-muscle work, it is clear that the muscle cell is fully equipped with the machinery for this differentiation. Thus, the muscle may be in a totally autonomous status for synaptic development in the sense that it can synthesize its own molecules for both signaling and assembling the specializations. In this sense, the nerve may merely provide a substrate for the anchorage of these muscle-derived trophic molecules. This scheme also may explain

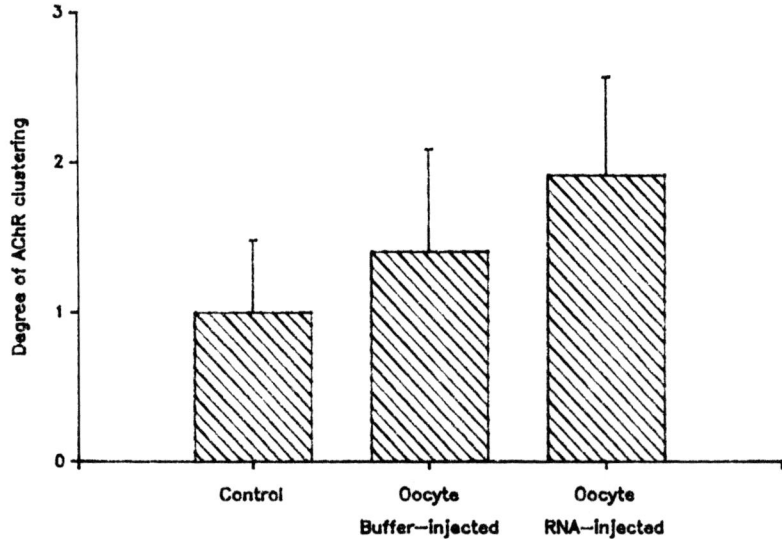

Figure 9. Effect of oocyte-conditioned medium on AChR clustering.

the induction of postsynaptic differentiation by the beads, since they may replace the nerve in offering such a substrate.

To further characterize these AChR cluster-inducing molecules, we examined whether mRNAs coding for these molecules are present within the tail musculature of Xenopus larvae. Poly (A)$^+$ RNAs were prepared from the tails. Judging from biochemical analyses, including in vitro translation and Northern blotting, our RNA preparations are enriched in muscle-specific messages, such as the Ca^{2+}-binding protein parvalbumin (Kay et al., 1987). We then injected these poly (A)$^+$ messages into Xenopus oocytes to effect their translation into proteins. The oocyte-conditioned medium is then assayed for its AChR cluster-inducing activity in myotomal muscle cell cultures. Our preliminary results (Fig. 9) demonstrate that cultures treated with the conditioned medium show a two-fold increase in AChR clustering over the untreated cultures. Even though medium conditioned by oocytes injected with buffer alone also caused a small increase in AChR clustering, the poly (A)$^+$-

injected oocytes caused an additional increase in cluster formation. These results suggest the presence of a secretory protein in the tail muscle which can stimulate the postsynaptic development. In the future, we plan to fractionate the muscle messages and have them expressed individually in oocytes. By performing bioassays on cultured muscle cells with individual fractions, we hope to identify the specific mRNA encoding the AChR cluster-inducing trophic factor(s). Similar approaches have been used to understand the expression of ionic channels from mRNAs isolated from the central nervous system.

CONCLUSION

Tissue culture offers a powerful system for understanding the development of the NMJ. In our approach, we have further simplified the culture system by studying the synaptic differentiation in separate neuron and muscle cultures. Basic polypeptides, when applied locally through the latex beads are recognized as signals for both the pre- and postsynaptic development in culture. This suggests that a single species of molecules may be involved in signaling these two types of development in vivo. Although the highly basic molecules used in our studies may not be present in vivo, it will be of great interest to find out whether the endogenous trophic molecules have, at the active locus, a sequence enriched in basic amino acids.

REFERENCES

Anderson MJ, Cohen MW (1977). Nerve-induced and spontaneous redistribution of acetylcholine receptors on cultured muscle cells. J Physiol (Lond) 268:757-773.
Bahler M, Greengard P (1987). Synapsin I bundles F-actin in a phosphorylation-dependent manner. Nature 326:704-707.
Burridge K (1986). Substrate adhesions in normal and transformed fibroblasts: organization and regulation of cytoskeletal, membrane and extracellular matrix components at focal contacts. Cancer Rev 4:18-78.
Burry RW (1980). Formation of apparent presynaptic elements in response to poly-basic compounds. Brain Res

184:85-98.

Burry RW, Kniss DA, Scribner LR (1984). Mechanisms of synapse formation and maturation. Current Topics Res Synapses 1:1-51.

Edwards C, Frisch HL (1976). A model for the localization of acetylcholine receptors at the muscle endplate. J Neurobiol 7:377-381.

Froehner SC (1986). The role of the postsynaptic cytoskeleton in AChR organization. Trends Neurosci 9:37-41.

Froehner SC, Murnane AA, Tobler M, Peng HB, Sealock R (1987). A postsynaptic 58K protein concentrated at acetylcholine receptor-rich sites in Torpedo electroplaques and skeletal muscle. J Cell Biol 104:1633-1646.

Henderson LP, Smith MA, Spitzer NC (1984). The absence of calcium blocks impulse-evoked release of acetylcholine but not de novo formation of functional neuromuscular synaptic contacts in culture. J Neurosci 4:3140-3150.

Hirokawa N (1983). Membrane specialization and cytoskeletal structures in the synapse and axon revealed by the quick-freeze deep-etch method. In Chang D, Tasaki I, Adelman WJ, Leuchtag HR (eds): "Structure and Function in Excitable Cells." New York: Plenum Press, pp 113-141.

Kay BK, Shah AJ, Halstead WE (1987). Expression of the Ca^{2+}-binding protein, parvalbumin, during embryonic development of the frog, Xenopus laevis. J Cell Biol 104:841-847.

Kidokoro Y, Brass B, Kuromi H (1986). Concanavalin A prevents acetylcholine receptor redistribution in Xenopus nerve-muscle cultures. J Neurosci 6:1941-1951.

Nitkin RM, Smith MA, Magill C, Fallon JR, Yao YM, Wallace BG, McMahan UJ (1987). Identification of agrin, a synaptic organizing protein from Torpedo electric organ. J Cell Biol 105:2471-2478.

Olek AJ, Pudimat PA, Daniels MP (1983). Direct observation of the rapid aggregation of acetylcholine receptors on identified cultured myotubes after exposure to embryonic brain extract. Cell 34:255-264.

Peng HB (1983). Cytoskeletal organization of the presynaptic nerve terminal and the acetylcholine receptor cluster in cell cultures. J Cell Biol 97:489-498.

Peng HB (1984). Participation of calcium and calmodulin in the formation of acetylcholine receptor clusters. J

Cell Biol 98:550-557.

Peng HB (1986). Elimination of preexistent acetylcholine receptor clusters induced by the formation of new clusters in the absence of nerve. J Neurosci 6:581-589.

Peng HB (1987). Development of the neuromuscular junction in tissue culture. CRC Crit Rev Anat Sci 1:91-131.

Peng HB, Cheng PC (1982). Formation of postsynaptic specializations induced by latex beads in cultured muscle cells. J Neurosci 2:1760-1774.

Peng HB, Cheng PC, Luther PW (1981). Formation of ACh receptor clusters induced by positively charged latex beads. Nature 292:831-834.

Peng HB, Froehner SC (1985). Association of the postsynaptic 43K protein with newly formed acetylcholine receptor clusters in cultured muscle cells. J Cell Biol 100:1698-1705.

Peng HB, Markey DR, Muhlach WL, Pollack ED (1987). Development of presynaptic specializations induced by basic polypeptide-coated latex beads in spinal cord cultures. Synapse 1:10-19.

Peng HB, Phelan KA (1984). Early cytoplasmic specialization at the presumptive acetylcholine receptor cluster: a meshwork of thin filaments. J Cell Biol 99:344-349.

Tsien RY, Rink TJ, Poenie M (1985). Measurement of cytosolic free Ca^{2+} in individual small cells using fluorescence microscopy with dual excitation wavelengths. Cell Calcium 6:145-157.

Usdin TB, Fischbach GD (1986). Purification and characterization of a polypeptide from chick brain that promotes the accumulation of acetylcholine receptors in chick myotubes. J Cell Biol 103:493-507.

HINDLIMB INNERVATION PATTERNS OF BULLFROG MOTOR AXONS DURING DEVELOPMENT AND REGENERATION

Matt T. Lee and Paul B. Farel[1]

Department of Physiology and Biophysics, University of Iowa, Iowa City, Iowa 52242 (M.T.L.) and Department of Physiology, University of North Carolina, Chapel Hill, North Carolina 27514 (P.B.F.)

INTRODUCTION

Although axonal regeneration following peripheral nerve injury shares some of the features of initial axon outgrowth during development, in many cases these two processes differ in terms of the specificity exhibited by the axons during synapse formation. In mammals (Bernstein and Guth, 1961; Tada et al., 1979; Brushart and Mesulam, 1980) and in the frog (Westerfield and Powell, 1983), the mechanisms that enable developing motor axons to establish appropriate connections with muscle are inoperative or ineffective when the axons are caused to regenerate during adulthood.

The failure of regenerating motor axons to reform normal patterns of synaptic connectivity could result from a loss during development of guidance factors produced by muscle (Slack et al., 1983) or embedded in peripheral nerve pathways (Landmesser, 1984). Alternatively, guidance cues may be present even in mature animals, but regenerating motor axons may lose the capacity to respond to these cues, because they either lack the necessary receptors or are confined by pre-existing channels of the distal nerve stump.

The experiments described in this chapter represent our initial efforts to understand why the ability of

---

[1]To whom correspondence should be addressed. Supported by NIH grants NS16030 and NS14899.

motoneurons to find their correct targets in development is not expressed during regeneration in the mature animal. We chose the bullfrog (Rana catesbeiana) for this work because its large size allows surgical manipulations to be performed even during the earliest stages at which motor axons begin to invade the hindlimb. As related in the next two sections, this has made it possible to ascertain the normal pattern of neuromuscular connectivity over the course of larval development and to determine the developmental period during which specific reinnervation of the hindlimb is lost. The remainder of the chapter investigates the possibility that regenerating motor axons are directed by structures in the distal stump.

SPECIFICITY OF NEUROMUSCULAR CONNECTIONS DURING DEVELOPMENT

In frogs (Cruce, 1974; Lamb, 1976), as in mammals (Romanes, 1964) and the chick (Landmesser, 1978), the location of the motoneuron somata in the lateral motor column (LMC) is related to the hindlimb muscles they innervate. Motoneurons in the dorsal part of the LMC innervate muscles in the posterior (ventral) portion of the limb, which are derived from the ventral premuscle mass. Motoneurons in the ventral part of the LMC supply muscles in the anterior (dorsal) portion of the limb, which arise from the dorsal premuscle mass. Furthermore, the position of motoneurons along the rostrocaudal axis of the LMC is related to the proximodistal location of the muscles they project to, with muscles in proximal limb regions innervated by rostral motoneurons.

To determine whether this pattern of connectivity is preceded by a less precise pattern in the early stages of neuromuscular development, retrograde labeling techniques were employed (Farel and Bemelmans, 1985a). Small amounts of horseradish peroxidase (HRP) were applied to one of three sites (dorsal thigh, ventral thigh, or ventral shank) in tadpoles from stages IV-XXIV (Taylor and Kollros, 1946) and in juvenile frogs. In each animal, the locations of labeled motoneurons were mapped along the dorsoventral and rostrocaudal axes of the LMC.

The results of this study showed that the distribution of labeled motoneurons along both axes was just as circumscribed in the youngest tadpoles, when the hindlimb is composed primarily of undifferentiated mesenchyme, as in any later stage or in juvenile frogs. Although these experiments spanned the period of naturally occurring cell death (Farel, 1987), there was, within the limits of resolution of the method used, no evidence for an early, diffuse pattern of neuromuscular connectivity in the bullfrog. These findings agree with those obtained for hindlimb motoneurons in the chick (Landmesser, 1978; Oppenheim, 1981; Hollyday, 1983) but disagree with the results of similar studies in the African clawed frog, Xenopus laevis (Lamb, 1976, 1977).

In Xenopus, neuromuscular connections appear to be less precise at stage 50 (Nieuwkoop and Faber, 1967), before the period of naturally occurring motoneuron cell death, than at stage 55, after cell death. It is possible that HRP may have spread inadvertently to adjacent regions of the smaller Xenopus hindlimbs at stage 50, causing the distribution of motoneurons innervating particular sites to appear larger at this stage. However, it is also conceivable that there are interspecies variations in the extent to which cell death is used to refine neuromuscular connections. If the latter possibility is true, the occurrence of inappropriate connections early in the development of a species may not be readily predictable from the phylogenetic position of that species.

SPECIFICITY OF NEUROMUSCULAR CONNECTIONS DURING REGENERATION

The specificity of hindlimb reinnervation exhibited by regenerating bullfrog motoneurons was assessed by retrograde labeling with HRP in the manner described above (Farel and Bemelmans, 1986). Motoneurons were axotomized by transecting the three ventral roots (VRs) that innervate the hindlimb in tadpoles at stages IV to XVII and in juvenile frogs. The motor axons were allowed to regenerate for five to seven weeks before HRP was applied to one of the three hindlimb regions used for the developmental studies. This time period proved to be sufficiently long for extensive reinnervation of the limb, as the number of motoneurons that could be labeled from the thigh was not significantly different from that in unoperated tadpoles. It was also sufficiently short that tadpoles rarely advanced more than one or two stages between VR transection and sacrifice.

Figure 1 illustrates several examples of the localization of labeled motoneurons obtained after regeneration. In tadpoles operated upon at early stages of development, HRP applied to the dorsal (Fig. 1, top) or ventral thigh (Fig. 1, middle) labeled motoneurons in the ventral or dorsal half of the LMC, respectively. This pattern of labeling is the same as that seen in unoperated animals, indicating that the regenerating motor axons had reinnervated the hindlimb with an almost normal level of neuromuscular specificity at these stages. In contrast, motoneurons labeled by HRP application to restricted hindlimb sites in more advanced tadpoles were distributed widely throughout the LMC (Fig. 1, bottom), suggesting that they had reinnervated the muscles of the limb nonspecifically.

The graphs in Fig. 2 show combined data on motoneuron localization from 47 tadpoles and five juvenile frogs after hindlimb reinnervation. Along both the rostrocaudal (Fig. 2, left) and dorsoventral axes of the LMC (Fig. 2, right), the percentage of motoneurons located in that part of the LMC appropriate for their peripheral termination was within normal values until stages VII/VIII. When motoneurons were axotomized after stage VIII, the frequency with which they reinnervated appropriate limb regions was significantly lower than normal.

Because motoneurons in the course of migration to the LMC can be identified as late as stage XIV in the bullfrog (Farel and Bemelmans, 1980; Liuzzi et al., 1983a), the possibility existed that the normal pattern of neuromuscular connectivity seen at early stages may have resulted from the initial axonogenesis of newly born motoneurons instead of (or in addition to) the regeneration of axotomized motoneurons. To determine the likelihood of this possibility, ^{3}H-thymidine (10 µCi at five-day intervals) was given to six tadpoles at stages VI-VIII during the seven-week period following VR transection. Excluding red blood cells and vascular endothelial cells, very few (mean ± s.e.m. = 18.8 ± 8.6; range = 7-27) tritium-labeled cells were found in the lumbar LMC on the operated side. However, it is

Figure 1. Motoneurons retrogradely labeled by HRP application to the hindlimb 5-6 weeks following ventral rhizotomy. Dorsal is toward the top of all micrographs. The midline is to the right in the top micrograph and to the left in the middle and bottom micrographs.
Top. Localization of labeled motoneurons to the ventral half of the lumbar LMC following HRP application to the dorsal thigh in a stage VI tadpole.
Middle. Localization of labeled motoneurons to the dorsal half of the lumbar LMC following HRP application to the ventral thigh in a stage V tadpole.
Bottom. Lack of localization of labeled motoneurons following HRP application to the ventral thigh in a stage XII tadpole. (From Farel and Bemelmans, 1986.)

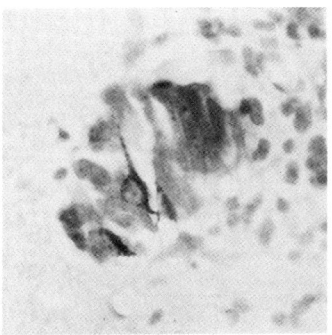
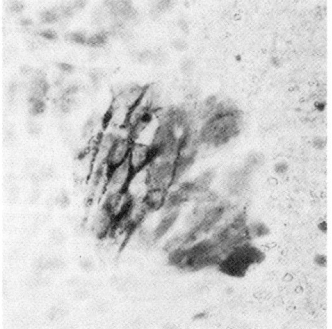
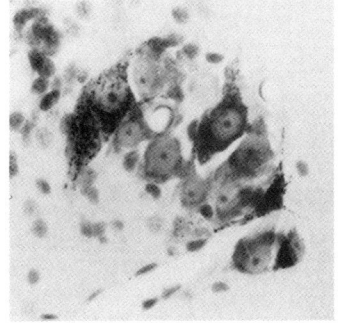

unlikely that even these few tritium-labeled cells were motoneurons, since they lacked the size and appearance of hindlimb motoneurons. Further, in five of these tadpoles HRP was applied to the hindlimb before sacrifice. In no instance was a profile labeled with both tritium and HRP. These results mean that newly born motoneurons did not contribute substantially to hindlimb reinnervation in these experiments.

Another possible source of reinnervating axons would be motoneurons that were born prior to ventral

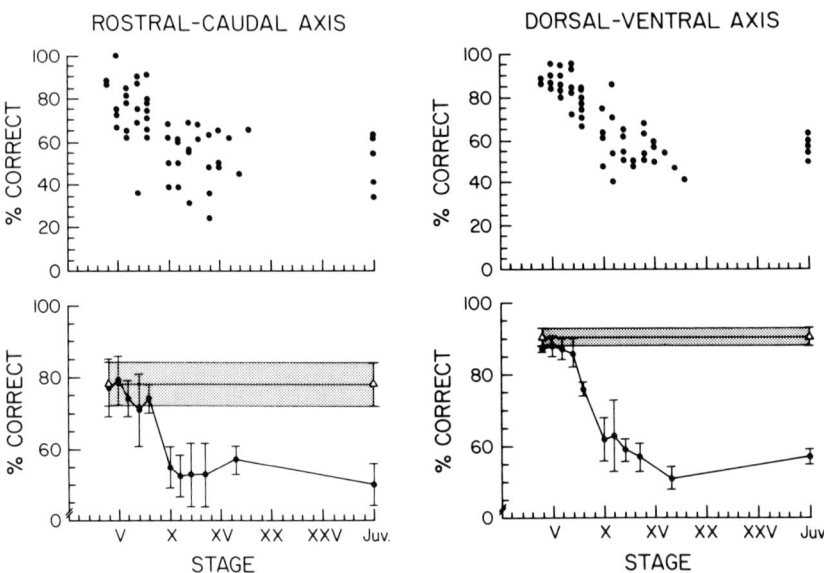

Figure 2. Localization along the rostro-caudal (left) and dorso-ventral (right) axes following hindlimb reinnervation. Ordinate (% correct) represents the percentage of motoneurons retrogradely labeled that are located within the expected half of the LMC. <u>Top</u>: Individual values obtained 5-7 weeks following ventral rhizotomy. <u>Bottom</u>: Mean values ± s.e.m. The shaded bar represents mean values (± 95% confidence interval) obtained in unoperated tadpoles. (From Farel and Bemelmans, 1986.)

rhizotomy but had not yet differentiated sufficiently to have axons in the severed ventral root. However, HRP placed on the ventral roots retrogradely labels virtually all motoneurons in the LMC (Farel, 1987) as well as those in the course of migration to the LMC (see above). These results eliminate the possibility that a significant number of motoneurons lacking axons in the ventral root existed at the time of transection.

We therefore conclude that reinnervation of the frog hindlimb following ventral root transection is due to the regeneration of severed axons, even at early stages of development.

The decline in regenerative specificity that occurs after stage VIII coincides with the period during which primary afferent fibers begin to invade the mantle zone of the spinal cord (Forehand and Farel, 1982; Liuzzi et al., 1983b) and reflex contractions of the hindlimb first can be elicited (Letinsky, 1974). The relationship of these events to regenerative specificity is unknown. However, the finding that regenerative specificity was unaffected when ventral root transection was combined with dorsal root ganglion removal (Farel and Bemelmans, 1985b) makes it unlikely that sensory fibers play a role in guiding regenerating motor axons.

GUIDANCE OF REGENERATING MOTOR AXONS BY THE DISTAL STUMP

Axons regenerating within peripheral nerves are found almost exclusively on the inside surface of Schwann tubes (Ramón y Cajal, 1928; Holmes and Young, 1942; Scherer and Easter, 1984; Scherer, 1986), which consist of the collagenous endoneurial sheaths and basal laminae of Schwann cells (Thomas, 1964). Schwann tubes retain their structure when the distal stump is denervated during Wallerian degeneration (Weddell, 1942), and it has been proposed that they exert a channeling influence on the axons that regenerate into them, each tube constraining its enclosed axons to grow only to the target located at the end of that tube (Glees, 1943). The nonspecific reinnervation that typically follows transection of a peripheral nerve or VR is thought to result from regenerating sprouts nonselectively entering the cut ends of tubes at the lesion site (Ramón y Cajal, 1928), although this idea has never been tested directly.

To ascertain whether regenerating bullfrog motor axons are guided by preformed channels, we examined the pathway choices made by the axons following transection of either the lumbar VRs or the spinal nerves (SNs) just proximal to the hindlimb plexus (Lee and Farel, 1988). These operations were performed on one side of juvenile frogs and tadpoles at stages XI-XVIII, that is, <u>after</u> the stages at which motoneurons can reestablish specific neuromuscular connectivity. In the case of VR transections, axons regrowing from each VR usually entered that root's own distal stump. Hence, if they were confined by structures in the stump, their ultimate destinations should have been appropriate for that root's normal field of innervation, even if they nonspecifically reinnervated particular muscles within that field.

Ventral root innervation fields were mapped by recording from the lumbar VRs (8,9, and 10) while stimulating each of 17 hindlimb nerves. The recordings were made after all spinal roots had been cut and the spinal cord had been removed from the preparation, eliminating the possibility of synaptic interactions between afferents and motoneurons. Therefore, the occurrence of spikes in a VR in response to stimulation of a limb nerve implies that VR contributed axons to the stimulated nerve.

Figure 3 illustrates the segmental innervation patterns for one hindlimb muscle nerve on both sides of an operated tadpole. In this example, stimulating the glutaeus magnus branch of the profundus anterior nerve on either side elicited antidromic impulses in VRs 9 and 10 but not in VR 8. Despite quantitative differences in the conduction velocities of the impulses on the two sides (a consistent finding in our preparations and in other studies; Sunderland, 1978), the qualitative pattern of innervation was the same on the two sides: motor axons regenerated into this nerve from segments 9 and 10 but not from segment 8, thereby reestablishing the normal innervation pattern of the nerve.

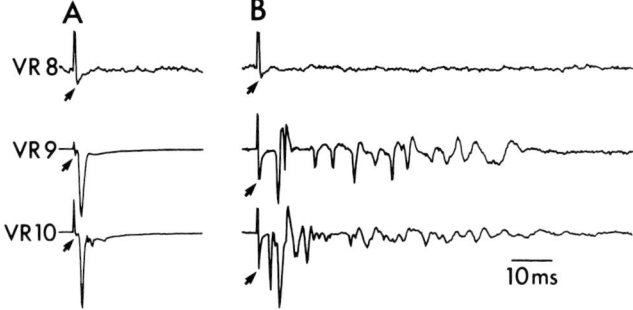

Figure 3. Recordings from the lumbar ventral roots on both sides of a tadpole, during stimulation of one of the hindlimb muscle nerves. On the intact (A) and regenerated (B) sides, antidromic action potentials were recorded in VRs 9 and 10, but not in VR 8, when the glutaeus magnus branch of the profundus anterior nerve was shocked. Each trace is an average of five sweeps. Arrows mark the stimulus artifacts. The recordings were obtained from a stage XIV tadpole, 57 days after VR transection. (From Lee and Farel, 1988.)

The segmental innervation patterns for all 17 hindlimb nerves are shown in Fig. 4 for limbs with a standard plexus (types C or D of Cruce, 1974), in which most of the axons are supplied to the plexus by SNs 9 and 10 in equal numbers. The graphs in this figure demonstrate that the hindlimb innervation fields of the regenerated axons closely resembled those that exist normally. This similarity even extended down to the level of particular branches of the major limb nerves. For example, the frequency with which VR 9 innervated the two branches supplying the gastrocnemius muscle was the same normally and after regeneration. A similar correspondence between normal and regenerated innervation patterns was obtained from limbs with an A-plexus type (not shown) in which SNs 8 and 9 provide most of the axons to the plexus. These results indicate that axons regenerating from a transected VR rarely, if ever, grew beyond the territory normally supplied by that VR.

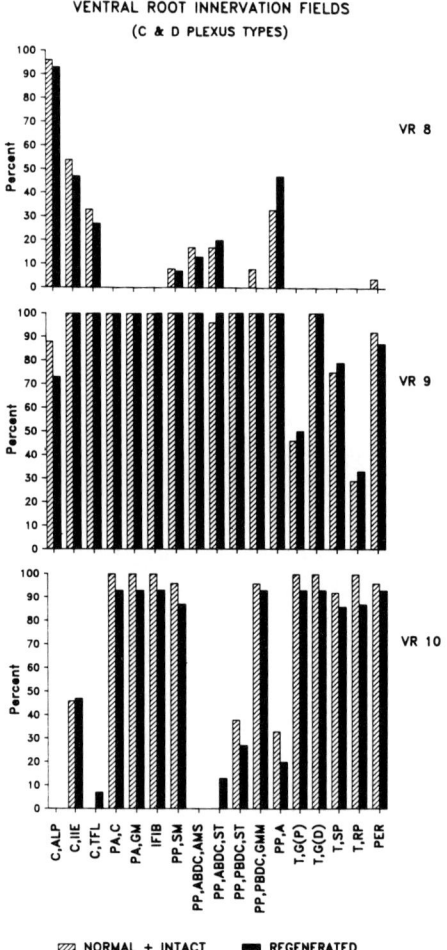

Figure 4. Segmental innervation of muscle nerves in hindlimbs with C- and D-plexus types, normally and following VR transection. The graphs show the percent of limbs in which each nerve was innervated by each VR. Normal + Intact: each nerve was sampled in 24 limbs (ten from normal, unoperated animals + 14 from intact, contralateral sides of operated animals). Regenerated: each nerve was sampled in 15 reinnervated limbs (except T,G(P), T,G(D), and T,SP, where n = 14). Abbreviations are based on the nomenclature of Gaupp (1896) and are defined in Table 1. From Lee and Farel (1988).

Table 1. Hindlimb nerves and abbreviations.

VR, ventral root
DR, dorsal root

Branches of the Crural Nerve:
    C,ALP, adductor longus and pectineus
    C,IIE, iliacus internus and externus
    C,TFL, tensor fasciae latae

Branches of the Profundus Anterior Nerve:
    PA,C, cruralis
    PA,GM, glutaeus magnus

IFIB, iliofibularis

Branches of the Profundus Posterior Nerve:
    PP,SM, semimembranosus
    PP,ABDC,AMS, anterior branch of descendens communis (innerv, adductor magnus and sartorius)
    PP,ABDC,ST, anterior branch of descendens communis (innerv. ventral head of semitendinosus)
    PP,PBDC,ST, posterior branch of descendens communis (innerv. dorsal head of semitendinosus)
    PP,PBDC,GMM, posterior branch of descendens communis (innerv. gracilis major and minor)
    PP,A, adductorius branch (innerv. adductor magnus, quadratus femoris, and obturator externus)
    MFCN, medial femoral cutaneous nerve

Branches of the Tibial Nerve:
    T,G(P), proximal branch to gastrocnemius
    T,G(D), distal branch to gastrocnemius
    T,SP, subaponeuroticus proprius branch (innerv. various muscles in the foot)
    T,RP, ramus profundus (innerv. muscles in the toes)

PER, peroneal nerve (innerv. muscles in the toes)

It may seem paradoxical that normal VR innervation fields were reestablished at stages when motoneurons do not specifically reinnervate their appropriate muscles. Since the axons in each VR project to a variety of muscles in different regions of the limb, it is possible for axons regenerating from a particular VR to make major projection errors at the level of individual muscles while remaining within the normal innervation field of that VR. Hence, non-specific target reinnervation can be compatible with the maintenance of normal segmental innervation patterns.

The return of normal segmental innervation fields during regeneration is consistent with the hypothesis that the axons were channeled to their destinations by pre-existing structures within each distal nerve stump. Alternatively, such innervation patterns might have reflected an ability on the part of the axons to recognize segmentally appropriate growth pathways. To distinguish between these alternatives, the three lumbar SNs were transected on one side at the point where they converged to form the hindlimb plexus in five tadpoles. This operation provided the regenerating axons with roughly equal access to the denervated stumps of all three spinal segments while leaving them free to respond to possible guidance cues in the hindlimb. Six weeks later, the innervation fields of motor axons from VRs 8 and 10 were determined for six hindlimb muscle nerves (Fig. 5). Motor axons regenerating from SN 8 were found only in the crural nerve branches, reestablishing the normal innervation pattern for that spinal segment. However, axons from SN 10 were found in all six limb nerves, including two which were never innervated by that segment normally. Thus, SN 10's axons did not maintain their normal segmental boundaries during regeneration. These findings therefore suggest that, at least for some regenerating motor axons, the reappearance of a normal hindlimb innervation pattern following VR transection did not result from an active selection of growth pathways on the basis of segmental cues. The reestablishment of normal segmental innervation patterns by fibers of SN 8 but not those of SN 10 is probably the result of the plexus geometry, which gives fibers of SN 10 greater access to pathways normally occupied by fibers of SN 8 than vice versa.

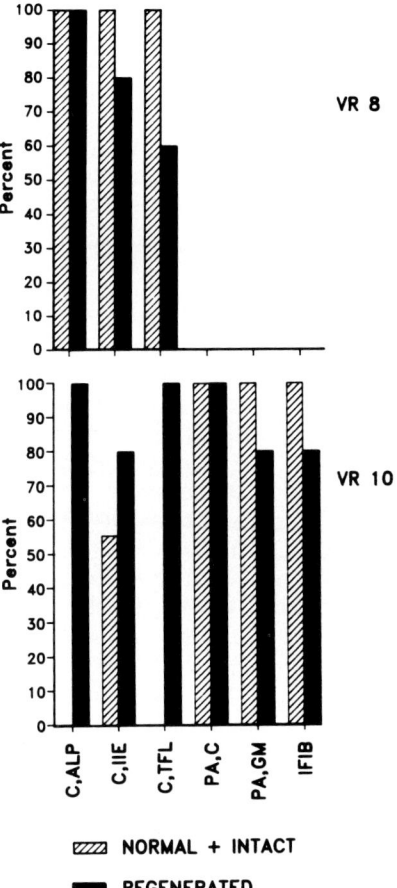

Figure 5. Segmental innervation of muscle nerves, normally and following spinal nerve transection. Normal + Intact: each nerve was sampled in nine limbs (four from normal, unoperated animals + five from intact, contralateral sides of operated animals). Regenerated: each nerve was sampled in five reinnervated limbs. In all limbs, the plexus was of the C- or D-type. Abbreviations are based on the nomenclature of Gaupp (1896) and are defined in Table 1. (From Lee and Farel, 1988.)

Spinal nerve transections sever both sensory and motor axons, thereby denervating cutaneous as well as muscle nerves. Following regeneration, motor axons grew into the medial femoral cutaneous nerve (a purely sensory pathway in normal limbs), as evidenced by the presence of antidromic spikes in the VRs or labeled motoneurons in the LMC when this nerve was stimulated or labeled with HRP. Hence regenerating motor axons did not appear to distinguish between sensory and motor pathways under these circumstances.

DISCUSSION

Our results support the hypothesis that bullfrog motor axons, when regenerating in frogs and advanced tadpoles, are constrained by structures they encounter as they penetrate the distal nerve stump. In these experiments, the axons did not discriminate among pathways on the basis of the muscles to which they led, the segmental labels they may have possessed, or the fact that they normally excluded motor axons in favor of sensory axons. However, we cannot rule out the possibility that these axons could make such distinctions under other conditions. The observation that regenerating motor axons in mature frogs can selectively reinnervate twitch vs. tonic fibers in the same muscle (Elizalde et al., 1983) suggests that these axons are capable of some selectivity in synapse formation. Moreover, regenerating preganglionic axons in the mammalian autonomic nervous system exhibit segmental selectivity during innervation of superior cervical ganglion neurons (Langley, 1897; Njå and Purves, 1977) and transplanted intercostal muscles (Wigston and Sanes, 1985). Finally, experiments in which regenerating axons were given a choice between two potential distal stumps using implanted, "Y"-shaped chambers have revealed preferences for native versus foreign nerve trunks (Politis, 1985) and motor versus sensory nerve pathways (Brushart and Seiler, 1987).

One candidate for the structures that constrain regenerating axons are the Schwann (endoneurial) tubes. However, the reported ability of regenerating axons to deviate from the paths of Schwann tubes (Ramón y Cajal, 1928; Bennett et al., 1973; Holder et al., 1984; Krarup and Gilliatt, 1985) argues against the idea that the axons are truly confined by them. Instead, the guidance of axons regenerating in the peripheral nervous system might be provided to some extent by both Schwann tubes and the perineurium, a sheath composed of several layers of flattened cells connected by tight junctions (Thomas and Olsson, 1975).

Two lines of evidence suggest that surviving perineurial sheaths may play a role in guiding regenerating axons. First, when a muscle is partially denervated, nodal sprouts from intact motor axons can leave the endoneurial tube of their parent axon to extend along a vacated nerve branch within the same perineurial sheath (Slack et al., 1979; Angaut-Petit et al., 1982). Second, unlike the endoneurium, in mature nerves the perineurium is relatively impervious even to diffusible substances due to the tight junctions between its cells (Sunderland, 1978). The diffusion barrier of the perineurium is not fully formed in immature animals (Hansson et al., 1971; Kristensson and Olsson, 1971), which may underlie the preferential reinnervation of motor nerves by regenerating motor axons in immature rats (Brushart, 1987) and the specific hindlimb regeneration seen in young tadpoles (Farel and Bemelmans, 1986). Determination of the contribution of the perineurium and other structures to the guidance of regenerating motor axons will require an analysis of the development and branching patterns of these structures in the peripheral nerves.

REFERENCES

Angaut-Petit D, Mallart A, Faille L (1982). Role of denervated sheaths and end-plates in muscle reinnervation by collateral sprouting in mouse. Biol Cell 46:277-289.
Bennett MR, McLachlan EM, Taylor RS (1973). The formation of synapses in reinnervated mammalian striated muscle. J Physiol 233:481-500.
Bernstein JJ, Guth L (1961). Nonselectivity in establishment of neuromuscular connections following nerve regeneration in rat. Exp Neurol 4:262-275.
Brushart TM (1987). Preferential reinnervation of motor nerves by regenerating motor axons. Soc Neurosci Abstr 13:1041.

Brushart TM, Mesulam M-M (1980). Alteration in connections between muscle and anterior horn motoneurons after peripheral nerve repair. Science 208:603-605.

Brushart TME, Seiler WA (1987). Selective reinnervation of distal motor stumps by peripheral motor axons. Exp Neurol 97:289-300.

Cruce WLR (1974). The anatomical organization of hindlimb motoneurons in the lumbar spinal cord of the frog, Rana catesbeiana. J Comp Neurol 153:59-76.

Elizalde A, Huerta M, Stefani E (1983). Selective reinnervation of twitch and tonic muscle fibres of the frog. J Physiol 340:513-524.

Farel PB (1987). Motoneuron number in the lumbar lateral motor column of larval and adult bullfrogs. J Comp Neurol 261:266-276.

Farel PB, Bemelmans SE (1980). Retrograde labeling of migrating spinal motoneurons in bullfrog larvae. Neurosci Lett 18:133-136.

Farel PB, Bemelmans SE (1985a). Specificity of motoneuron projection patterns during development of the bullfrog tadpole (Rana catesbeiana). J Comp Neurol 238:128-134.

Farel PB, Bemelmans SE (1985b). Specific regeneration of developing spinal motoneurons in the absence of peripheral sensory fibers. Soc Neurosci Abstr 11:975.

Farel PB, Bemelmans SE (1986). Restoration of neuromuscular specificity following ventral rhizotomy in the bullfrog tadpole, Rana catesbeiana. J Comp Neurol 254:125-132.

Forehand CJ, Farel PB (1982). Spinal cord development in anuran larvae. I. Primary and secondary neurons. J Comp Neurol 209:386-394.

Gaupp E (1896). "A. Ecker's und R. Wiedersheim's Anatomie des Frosches." Vieweg: Braunschweig.

Glees P (1943). Observations on the structure of the connective tissue sheaths of cutaneous nerves. J Anat 77:153-159.

Hansson G, Kristensson K, Olsson Y, Sjöstrand J (1971). Embryonal and postnatal development of mast cells in rat peripheral nerve. Acta Neuropathol 17:139-149.

Holder N, Tonga DA, Jasani P (1984). Directed regrowth of axons from a misrouted nerve to their correct muscles in the limb of the adult newt. Proc Roy Soc B 222:477-489.

Hollyday M. (1983). Development of motor innervation of

chick limbs. In Fallon JF, Caplan AI (eds): "Limb Development and Regeneration, Part A." New York: Alan R. Liss, pp 183-193.

Holmes W, Young JZ (1942). Nerve regeneration after immediate and delayed suture. J Anat 77:63-96.

Krarup C, Gilliatt RW (1985). Some effects of prolonged constriction on nerve regeneration in the rabbit. J Comp Neurol 68:1-14.

Kristensson K, Olsson Y (1971). The perineurium as a diffusion barrier to protein tracers: differences between mature and immature animals. Acta Neuropathol 17:127-138.

Lamb AH (1976). The projection patterns of the ventral horn to the hind limb during development. Develop Biol 54:82-99.

Lamb AH (1977). Neuronal death in the development of the somatotopic projections of the ventral horn in Xenopus. Brain Res 134:145-150.

Landmesser L (1978). The development of motor projection patterns in the chick hind limb. J Physiol 284:393-414.

Landmesser L (1984). The development of specific motor pathways in the chick embryo. Trends Neurosci 7:336-339.

Langley JN (1897). On the regeneration of pre-ganglionic and post-ganglionic visceral nerve fibres. J Physiol 22:215-230.

Lee MT, Farel PB (1988). Guidance of regenerating motor axons in larval and juvenile bullfrogs. J Neurosci (in press).

Letinsky MS (1974). The development of nerve-muscle junctions in Rana catesbeiana tadpoles. Develop Biol 40:129-153.

Liuzzi FJ, Beattie MS, Bresnahan JC (1983a). Dorsal root afferents contact migrating motoneurons in the developing frog spinal cord. Brain Res 262:299-302.

Liuzzi FJ, Beattie MS, Bresnahan JC (1983b). The development of the relationship between dorsal root afferents and motoneurons in the larval bullfrog spinal cord. Brain Res Bull 14:377-392.

Nieuwkoop PD, Faber J (eds) (1967). "Normal Table of Xenopus laevis (Daudin)." Amsterdam: North-Holland.

Njå A, Purves D (1977). Reinnervation of guinea pig superior cervical ganglion cells by preganglionic fibres arising from different levels of the spinal cord. J Physiol 272:633-651.

Oppenheim RW (1981). Cell death of motoneurons in the chick embryo spinal cord. V. Evidence on the role of cell death and neuromuscular function in the formation of specific peripheral connections. J Neurosci 1:141-151.

Politis MJ (1985). Specificity in mammalian peripheral nerve regeneration at the level of the nerve trunk. Brain Res 328:271-276.

Ramón y Cajal S (1928). "Degeneration and Regeneration of the Nervous System, Vol. 1." May RM (transl) London: Oxford University Press.

Romanes GJ (1964). The motor pools of the spinal cord. Prog Brain Res 11:93-119.

Scherer SS (1986). Reinnervation of the extraocular muscles in goldfish is nonselective. J Neurosci 6:764-773.

Scherer SS, Easter SS (1984). Degenerative and regenerative changes in the trochlear nerve of goldfish. J Neurocytol 13:519-565.

Slack JR, Hopkins WG, Pockett S (1983) Evidence for a motor nerve growth factor. Muscle Nerve 6:243-252.

Slack Jr, Hopkins WG, Williams MN (1979). Nerve sheaths and motoneurone collateral sprouting. Nature 202:506-507.

Sunderland S (1978). "Nerves and Nerve Injuries." New York: Churchill Livingstone.

Tada K, Oshita S, Yonenobu K, Ono K, Satoh K, Shimizu N (1970). Experimental study of spinal nerve repair after plexus brachialis injury in newborn rats: a horseradish peroxidase study. Exp Neurol 65:301-314.

Taylor AC, Kollros JJ (1946). Stages in the normal development of Rana pipiens larvae. Anat Rec 94:7-24.

Thomas PK (1964). Changes in the endoneurial sheaths of peripheral myelinated nerve fibres during Wallerian degeneration. J Anat 98:175-182.

Thomas PK, Olsson Y (1975). Microscopic anatomy and function of the connective tissue components of peripheral nerve. In Dyck PJ, Thomas PK, Lambert EH (eds): "Peripheral Neuropathy." Philadelphia: W.B. Saunders, pp 168-189.

Weddell G (1942). Axonal regeneration in cutaneous nerve plexuses. J Anat 77:49-62.

Westerfield M, Powell SL (1983). Selective reinnervation of limb muscles by regenerating frog motor axons. Develop Brain Res 10:301-304.

Wigston DJ, Sanes JR (1985). Selective reinnervation of intercostal muscles transplanted from different segmental levels to a common site. J Neurosci 5:1208-1221.

THE DEVELOPMENT OF SPINAL GANGLIA

Harold D. Bibb

Department of Zoology, University of Rhode Island, Kingston, Rhode Island 02881

INTRODUCTION

Following Shorey's (1909) initial use of larval Bufo americanus and Rana pipiens to investigate the effects of limb bud removal on the development of the ventral horn and spinal ganglia, a number of workers have used spinal ganglia, particularly the lumbar dorsal root ganglia that provide sensory innervation to the hindlimb, for research in developmental neurobiology. There are good reasons for this. After neural crest cells have aggregated in small groups to form rudiments that will become the spinal ganglia, neurogenetic processes are neatly localized within these discrete units; and because they are discrete units they are quite convenient for experimental manipulations. In detailing the advantages of using anuran larvae in the study of neurogenesis, Taylor (1943) pointed out the benefits of the presence of an essentially embryonic limb in a larval animal and observed that this permitted more localized and precise operations than could be performed on the younger stages of other vertebrates. Thus both the lumbar dorsal root ganglia and their target field are accessible for experimental alteration in anuran larvae.

In this chapter, the normal development of spinal ganglia will be reviewed with special emphasis on those that send sensory fibers to the hindlimb. Because the responses of the population of neurons within the ganglia to alterations of the limb target field and neuronotrophic effects of limb target tissues on neuritic outgrowth are discussed, a description of limb development also has been included. The Nieuwkoop and Faber (1956) staging system has been used throughout for Xenopus laevis, and the Taylor and Kollros (1946) staging system has been used for all Rana species.

NORMAL DEVELOPMENT OF SPINAL GANGLIA

After His' (1868) description of the origin of spinal ganglia from a narrow strip of ectoderm (Zwischentrang) present between the medullary plate and epidermal ectoderm, Harrison (1904, 1924) provided early experimental evidence for the neural crest origin of these structures in the frog. These results were supported by Raven (1931, 1936, 1937) who carried out xenoplastic transplantations of neural crest between Ambystoma mexicanum and either Triturus taeniatus or T. alpestris, and by Dushane's (1938) extirpation experiments on Ambystoma. (For reviews see Detwiler, 1936; Hörstadius, 1950; Pannese, 1974.)

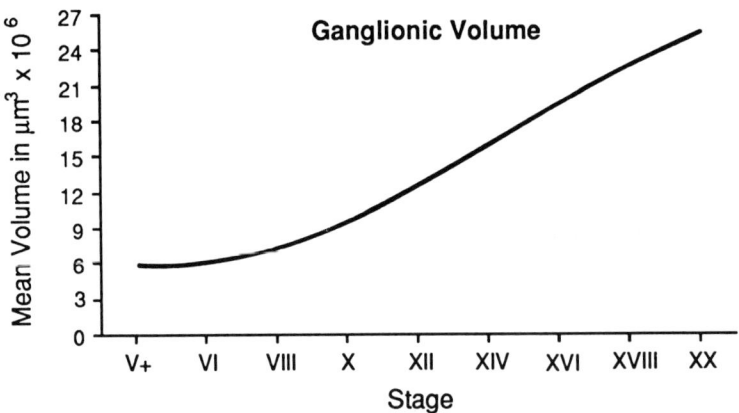

Figure 1. The volume of dorsal root ganglion 9 in Rana pipiens plotted against developmental stage. (Redrawn from Bibb, 1977.)

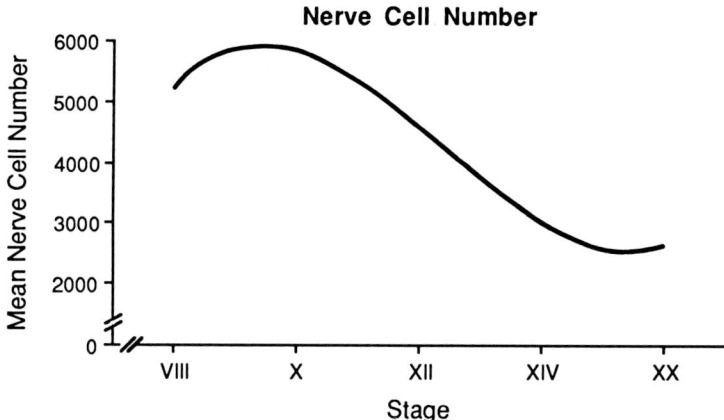

Figure 2. Nerve cell numbers in Rana pipiens dorsal root ganglion 9 plotted against developmental stage. (Redrawn from Bibb, 1977.)

Detwiler's (1937) drawings and reconstructions show the separation of the neural crest from the closing neural tube and the subsequent location of the crest dorsal to the tube in Ambystoma. As some of the neural crest migrates laterally and ventrally between the myotomes and the spinal cord, some cells aggregate into discrete segmentally arranged groups that form rudiments of the spinal ganglia. The metameric arrangement of the ganglia has been shown to be influenced by the somites (Lehmann, 1927; Detwiler, 1934). This work has been carefully reviewed by Detwiler (1936) and recently by Keynes and Stern (1986).

In Xenopus, the separation of the neural crest begins anteriorly with the closure of the neural tube at the same level at stage 22 (Nieuwkoop and Faber stage, Kollros, 1956). As neural tube formation proceeds in an anterior to posterior direction, the separation of the crest is not completed prior to stage 31, and the aggregation of crest cells as ganglionic rudiments is occurring at stages 37-38. At stage 39 each ganglion is small and made up of only six to ten cells; and by stage 44 some twenty to thirty small cells are present with conspicuous dorsal roots. In the adult frog, ten segmentally arranged ganglia are present on each side of the animal. As a result of the loss of the most anterior ganglion, two methods of numbering the ganglia have emerged. In Haslam's translation of Ecker's "Anatomy of the Frog" (1889), to which substantial original contributions had been made by R. Wiedersheim (see Ecker's preface to the second part), spinal nerves and their associated ganglia are numbered one through ten in an anterior to posterior sequence. However, in Gaupp's (1896) presentation of "Ecker's und Wiedersheim's Anatomie des Frosches", the loss of the first spinal nerve is taken into account, and the spinal nerves are numbered two through eleven. It is this second method of numbering that has been adopted for use here.

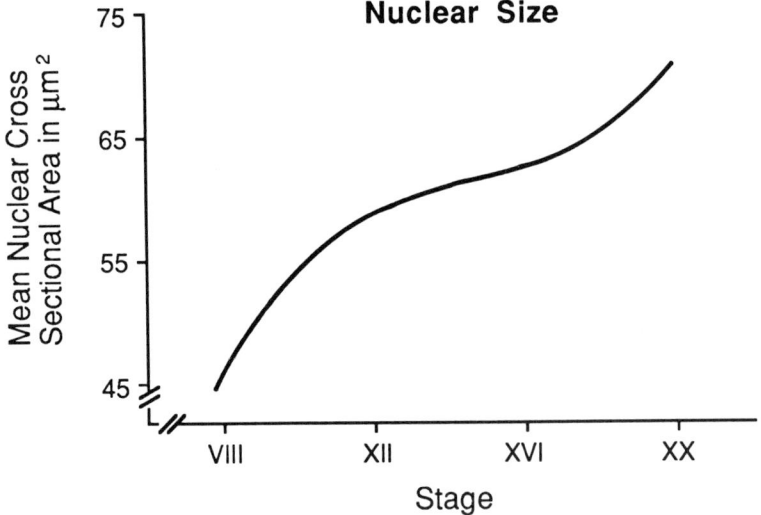

Figure 3. Nuclear sizes of nerve cells in dorsal root ganglion 9 in Rana pipiens plotted against developmental stage. (Redrawn from Bibb, 1977.)

The number of cells in the spinal ganglia and the size of the ganglia continue to increase as development proceeds. Prestige (1965) has provided careful descriptions of the changes in morphology of ganglion cells in Xenopus from stage 50, when the hindlimb bud is first constricted at its base and is approximately equivalent to that of a stage III Rana pipiens larva, to stage 59, after the forelimb has emerged and extends to the base of the hindlimb. In this same article, Prestige reports changes in the number of nerve cells present in ganglia 8, 9, and 10 between stage 50 and stage 65, when the tail is almost completely resorbed and is only about one-tenth the length of the body. During this period, the sum of the neurons present in ganglia 8, 9, and 10 on each side of the animal increases from approximately 1,500 at stage 50 to a peak of 9,000 to 10,000 cells at stages 57-59, before declining to approximately 8,500 neurons at stage 65.

Although a net decrease in neuronal numbers follows stage 59, degenerating cells are present in the ganglia as early as stage 53. The number of degenerating cells increases substantially following stage 53 and does not decrease until after stage 59.

Direct comparisons between Xenopus and Rana are not possible for much of the larval period because the data for nerve cell numbers in Xenopus are the sum of the neurons present in ganglia 8, 9, and 10 (Prestige, 1965), while those for R. pipiens (Bibb, 1977) and R. berlandieri (Bibb, 1978) are for ganglion 9 alone. In general, however, similar patterns emerge. A complete cell count of a single ninth ganglion from a stage VI R. pipiens larva showed the presence of 23 large cells and 2,190 small cells (Taylor, 1943). Based on the presence of fine fibers in the spinal nerve, Taylor argued that many of the small cells were in fact neurons. By stage VIII, slightly more than 5,000 nerve cells are present in ganglion 9 in R. pipiens, and the number in R. berlandieri is just over 3,000 at the same stage. These numbers reach a peak of approximately 8,700 nerve cells at stage X in R. pipiens and of slightly more than 6,500 at stage XII in R. berlandieri. Following the mid-larval peak in nerve cell numbers, these values decline to fewer than 3,000 neurons in ganglion 9 in R. pipiens at stage XX, and to approximately 2,500 nerve cells in the ninth ganglion of R. berlandieri at stage XVI. The pattern of this change in neuronal numbers is shown in Fig. 2. Degenerating nerve cells are present in the ninth ganglion at least from stage V⁺ forward throughout larval development in R. pipiens and R. berlandieri.

The overall size of the spinal ganglia increases throughout larval development (see Fig. 1 for the ninth ganglion in R. pipiens) as does cell size, as indicated by nuclear cross-sectional area (Kollros and McMurray, 1955). These changes are represented in Fig. 3.

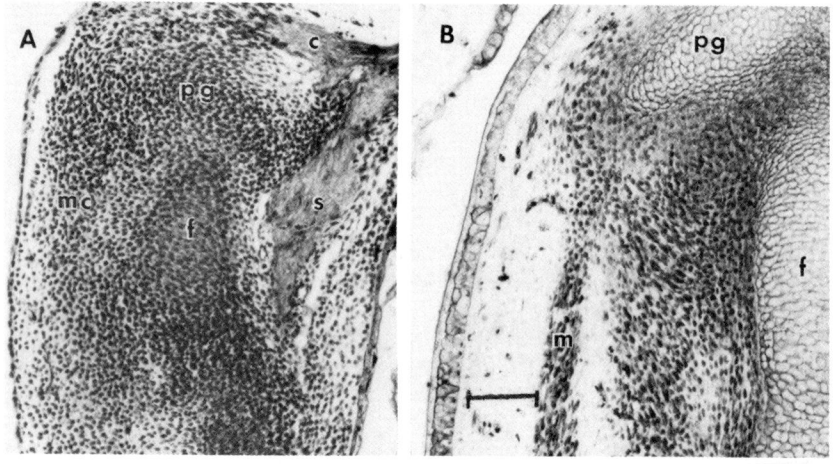

Figure 4. Longitudinal sections through the proximal area of Rana pipiens hindlimb buds. A: Stage VI⁻. The bifurcated main nerve trunk is present as the cruralis (c) and sciatic (s) branches. Chondrogenesis has just begun in the femur (f) but not in the pelvic girdle (pg). Rudiments of muscle are present as mesenchymal condensations (mc). B: Stage VIII. Chondrogenesis is well underway in the femur and the pelvic girdle. Myogenesis has begun in rudiments of individual thigh muscles (m). Bar = 80 µm.

HINDLIMB DEVELOPMENT

Because hindlimb tissues provide targets for the neurons of spinal ganglia 8, 9, and 10 and because the number of cells in a neuronal population is so clearly affected by the target (see following sections) it is appropriate to consider the development of the limb and the changes that occur within it. The following description is based largely on the work of Taylor (1943) with R. pipiens, Letinsky (1974) with R. catesbeiana and Newth (1956) with Xenopus laevis. Contributions from other workers are noted as appropriate.

In Xenopus the hindlimb bud is first visible externally at stage 46, and the rudiment is present as a mesenchyme-filled bud just prior to stage I in R. pipiens. At stages I and II the mesenchyme is more dense immediately beneath the epidermis than elsewhere in the rudiment. However, by stage III a medial condensation of mesenchyme is apparent in the rudiment in R. pipiens but is not present in R. catesbeiana. Also at stage III in R. pipiens, the main nerve trunk, which was present at the base of the limb bud at stage II, has bifurcated into the cruralis and sciatic divisions. This bifurcation occurs in Xenopus at stage 52 (Kollros, 1956) following nerve entry into the bud at stage 49 (Hughes and Tschumi, 1958), and in R. catesbeiana at stage IV following nerve entry into the limb bud at stage II.

Although condensations of the mesenchyme in stage IV R. pipiens hindlimb buds have formed the anlagen of the femur, and the tibia and fibula, these rudiments are much more distinctly outlined at stage V. Taylor (1943) indicates that these structures appear to have differentiated from the medial mesenchymal condensation that was first present at stage III. Mesenchymal primordia of these structures are first present at stage V in R. catesbeiana and at stage 51 in Xenopus. Chondrogenesis begins in the femur at stage VI in R. pipiens (Dunlap, 1966) and at stage 53 in Xenopus (Fig. 4).

Mesenchymal tissue that will give rise to the musculature of the hindlimb is present as two mesenchymal condensations in the bud at stage VI in R. pipiens (Dunlap, 1966). One of these is located dorso-laterally

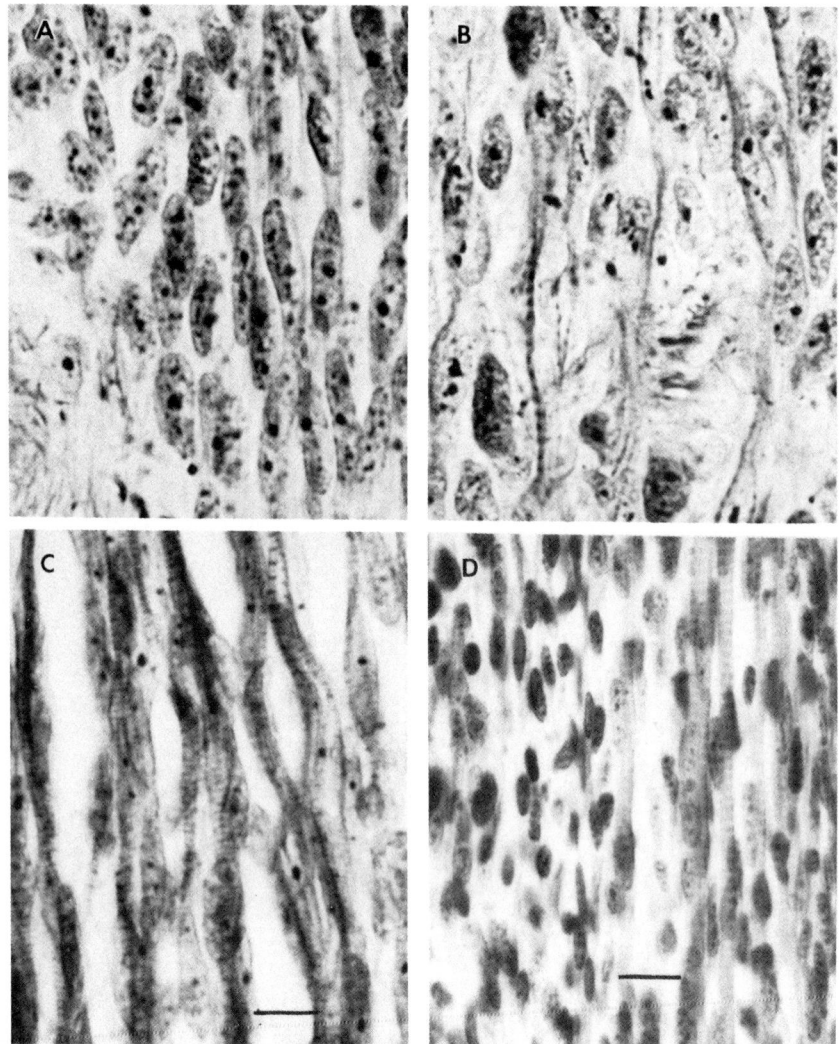

Figure 5. Myogenesis in <u>Rana pipiens</u> hindlimb. A: Stage VI, thigh. Alignment of myoblasts and incipient myotube formation. B: Stage VIII, thigh. Small myotubes present with cross-striations. C: Stage X, thigh. Many more myotubes are present containing larger numbers of nuclei, and cross-striations are more apparent. D: Stage XIII, shank. Groups of multinucleated muscle fibers are present in bundles. A-C: bar = 5 µm. D: bar = 15 µm.

in the limb rudiment and the other ventro-medially. Subdivision of the dorsolateral mass into the rudiments of individual muscles has begun at stage VI in R. pipiens. Development of both the skeletal components and the musculature of the limb bud proceeds in a proximal to distal direction, and the histogenesis of muscle fibers has begun in the thigh at stage 53 in Xenopus. In R. catesbeiana, myoblasts and cross-striated multinucleated myotubes are present in the most proximal region of the thigh at stage VII. Dunlap (1966) has reported the presence of cross-striated fibers in R. pipiens also at stage VII, while Taylor (1943) has indicated that cross-striations appear in the thigh as early as stage VI (Fig. 5).

Particularly toward the base of the rudiment, the epidermal covering of the limb bud in R. pipiens has been relatively well-differentiated from the first appearance of the structure, and at stage IV the deeper layer of the epidermis has become pseudostratified in the dorsal and lateral areas near the base.

As the mesenchymal components become incorporated into condensations that will differentiate as the muscular and skeletal elements of the limb, the quantity of mesenchymal tissue in the developing limb declines. Pollack and Richmond (1981) have shown that there is a rapid decline in the percentage of the limb as mesenchyme following stage IV in R. pipiens, and that after stage XI mesenchyme is essentially absent.

Accompanying the differentiation of muscular and skeletal components is the continued growth of nerves within the bud. The main mixed trunks of the thigh and shank are present at stage IV in R. pipiens, and the cruralis and sciatic branches run the length of the bud in R. catesbeiana at stage V. Two cutaneous branches, the ramus cutaneous femoris lateralis and the ramus cutaneous lateralis, are present in the tissue immediately beneath the epidermal layer of the stage IV limb bud in R. pipiens, and all cutaneous branches are present in the dermis at stage V. Sensory branches to the tendons and ligaments of the knee and ankle joints also are well-established at this time. At stage VI when, with the possible exception of the foot, the innervation pattern is complete, most cutaneous branches have reached the skin and given off collateral branches in R. pipiens. Although the innervation pattern is complete at stage VI in R. pipiens and R. catesbeiana, reflexive movement of the hindlimb does not occur until stage IX in R. pipiens, stage IX-X in R. catesbeiana, and stage 54 in Xenopus (Hughes and Tschumi, 1958). The development of muscle spindles appears to occur even later. Butler (1979) describes the first appearance of these structures in the iliofibularis muscle at stage XVIII in R. pipiens. (Further discussions on the innervation patterns of the developing limbs can be found in the chapters by Muhlach, by Lee and Farel and by Smith and Frank.)

RESPONSES TO PERIPHERAL CHANGE

Since the early demonstrations that the removal of the forelimb bud from Bombinator larvae resulted in the formation of a smaller than normal brachial plexus and a reduction in the size of the ventral horn of the spinal cord (Braus, 1906) and that limb bud removal in a variety of species including Bufo americanus and R. pipiens was followed by a reduction in the size of the ventral horn and limb-associated spinal ganglia (Shorey, 1909), it has been evident that the development of a neural center is influenced by its peripheral target. Contributions from a number of workers who have studied various neuronal populations in several species have substantially advanced our understanding of target effects on developing neural centers (reviewed in Piatt, 1948; Hughes, 1968; Kollros, 1968; Hamburger, 1976; Oppenheim, 1981; Purves and Lichtman, 1985). Here, however, we direct our attention to the responses of spinal ganglia to alterations of the peripheral target in the frog.

In a study of the development of the lumbar dorsal root ganglia in larval Xenopus, Prestige (1967) found that the removal of the developing hindlimb led to a reduction in the number of nerve cells in the affected ganglia. When the limb was removed at stages 53-55 and development was allowed to proceed for two weeks or longer, ganglia supplying the reduced target area contained less than 50% of the normal number of neurons. Amputation of the limb at stage 61 resulted in a more gradual reduction in nerve cell number; but two months after limb excision, neuronal numbers in ganglia on the side from which the limb had been removed contained approximately 50% of the normal number. Counts of degenerating nerve cells in affected and control ganglia showed that there were two periods during which large numbers of degenerating cells were present in the affected ganglia following amputation at stages 53-55. The first period of degeneration began one to two days following limb removal and continued for three to seven days, and the second period occurred during the third post-operative week. During other periods, however, the number of degenerating neurons in affected ganglia was frequently less than the number present in controls. However, the difference in the number of nerve cells present in control and affected ganglia was maintained or increased. This observation, and the pattern of degeneration in larvae from which the limb had been removed at other stages, suggested that amputation led not only to a greater than normal loss of neurons through degeneration, but also affected the production of neurons in these ganglia.

In studies designed to examine the effects of increasing the target area, two (8 and 10) of the three (8, 9, and 10) ganglia that provide the bulk of the sensory innervation to the hindlimb were removed from stage V R. pipiens in order to increase the size of the target available to the remaining ganglion (Bibb, 1977). At stage XX, the ninth ganglia with enlarged peripheral targets had attained volumes nearly twice as great as control ninth ganglia. Determinations of nuclear cross-sectional area as an index of neuron size (Kollros and McMurray, 1955) indicated that while nerve cells in these hypertrophic ganglia might increase in size relative to those in controls up through stage XII, this effect is transient and not present at stage XX.

Counts of nerve cells in control and hypertrophic ganglia showed that the size of the neuronal population in ganglia for which the target size had been increased was larger than that in control ninth ganglia at stage VIII and at subsequent stages through stage XX. At stage XX there are over 80% more nerve cells in hypertrophic than in control ganglia. In both control and hypertrophic ganglia the number of neurons reaches a peak at stage X and declines by 53% (approximately 3,000 neurons) in control ganglia by stage XX, and declines by 42% (approximately 3,700 neurons) in hypertrophic ganglia.

In order to determine if differences in proliferation might contribute to the hyperplasia of ganglia with enlarged peripheral targets, total counts of colchicine-accumulated mitotic figures were made at stages V^+, VI and alternate stages thereafter until stage XX. The numbers of mitotic figures in ganglia associated with expanded targets were significantly greater at every stage than those in control ganglia (Fig. 6). As discussed earlier (Bibb, 1977), it is not possible to assess the developmental fates of unlabeled mitotic products generated through the additional proliferation in ganglia with enlarged targets. Thus, the increased

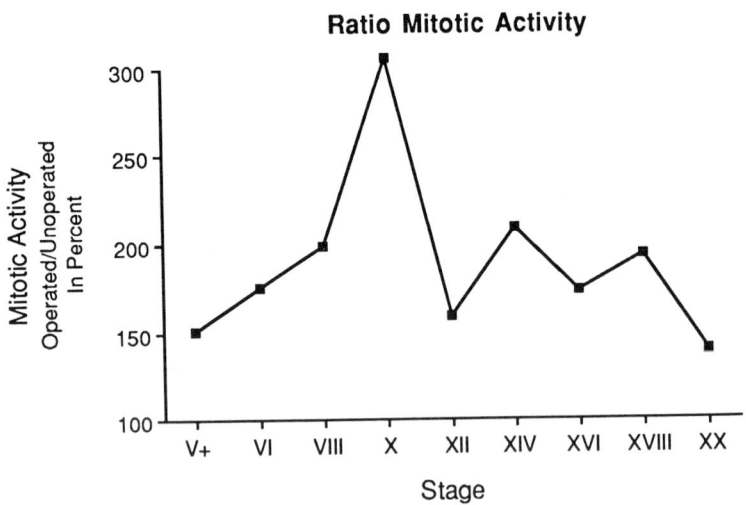

Figure 6. Mitotic activity in control and hypertrophic ganglia expressed as a ratio and plotted against developmental stage. (Redrawn from Bibb, 1977.)

numbers of neurons in hypertrophic ganglia cannot be definitively attributed to the increased proliferative activity. However, this possibility does merit further consideration in that there is enhanced mitotic activity as the ganglia become hyperplastic.

In another study aimed at determining the role of neuronal degeneration in the production of the hyperplastic condition, the technique described above was used to produce hypertrophy in the ninth ganglion of R. berlandieri larvae (Bibb, 1978). The number of nerve cells present in the ninth ganglia for which the peripheral target size had been increased was over 80% greater than that in the control ganglia at stage XVI. R. berlandieri shows peak numbers of neurons in control and hyperplastic ganglia slightly later in development (stage XII) than R. pipiens, but both show a pattern of peak numbers of neurons at mid-larval stages, followed by the loss of substantial numbers of neurons.

Because the hyperplastic condition was established between the time of target expansion at stage V and stage XII, degenerating neurons were counted in ganglia associated with increased peripheral areas and in control ganglia at closely grouped stages through the midlarval period and at stage XVI. Ninth ganglia with enlarged target sizes contained fewer, although not significantly so, degenerating neurons than control ganglia at each stage examined through stage X. At stages XII and XVI, however, neuronal degeneration was greater in hyperplastic ganglia than in controls. As only three animals were used at each stage, it is possible that a larger sample size would show significant differences in the neuronal degeneration that occurs while the hyperplastic condition is developing between stages V^+ and X.

Davis and Constantine-Paton (1983a,b) used an adaptation of the technique described above to study hyperplasia of the eleventh spinal ganglion (the tenth ganglion according to Haslam's translation of Ecker and Wiedersheim) and to determine the central and peripheral connectivity patterns that accompanied the hyperplasia. Interestingly, they found hyperplastic responses in the eleventh ganglion only in male larvae and male juveniles, and that unlike the responses of other dorsal root ganglia, peripheral enlargement via the removal of various combinations of ganglia that shared some portion of the same peripheral target frequently elicited a hyperplastic response from the eleventh ganglia both ipsilateral and contralateral to the enlarged periphery. Additionally, the hyperplastic response, sometimes more than 500% of normal, was often very great.

In their discussion, Davis and Constantine-Paton (1983a) were unable to account for the hyperplastic response in ganglion 11 solely on the basis of the rescue of neurons that normally would have died. Due to the magnitude of hyperplasia in affected ganglia, the speed of response, and the developmental stage of the animals in which the response could be elicited, they suggested that the availability of the expanded target might cause the recruitment of undifferentiated cells into mature sensory neurons, or that the enlarged target might stimulate an increase in the low proliferation rate of the ganglion.

Based on studies carried out on amniote species, the view has emerged that populations of neurons respond to target size only by increasing or decreasing the amount of cell death (reviewed in Oppenheim, 1981). However, each of the above-cited studies on the dorsal root ganglia in the frog provides some evidence that the production of neurons also may be affected (and see Kollros, this volume, on the same issue in the optic tectum). It is possible that this point will be clarified with the completion of studies on ganglionic labeling following target enlargement. Some additional support for the possible involvement of neuronal production in response to the target comes from a study of rat dorsal root ganglia (Devor et al., 1985) in which the change in neuronal number following sciatic nerve section was due more to adjustments in the addition of new neurons than from cell death.

GROWTH FACTORS AND ANURAN DORSAL ROOT GANGLIA

In introducing their report on the effects of Nerve Growth Factor (NGF) on the nervous system of Xenopus larvae, Levi-Montalcini and Aloe (1985) observed that little is known about the response of amphibian nervous systems to NGF. This observation could be extended to include neuronotrophic factors as a group (also see Muhlach, this volume). Levi-Montalcini and Aloe showed that daily injections of Xenopus larvae with 2-4 µgm NGF for a seven day period produced a substantial increase in the volume of dorsal root ganglia that could be attributed to a striking increase in both the size and number of cells.

Pollack's group had reported earlier that either NGF or target tissue elicits neuritic outgrowth from R. pipiens lumbar dorsal root ganglia in vitro. The target tissues used were spinal cord (Pollack et al., 1980) or tissues from the developing hindlimb (Pollack et al., 1979). When neither NGF nor target tissues were cultured with dorsal root ganglia (Pollack and Muhlach, 1982), neurite extension did not occur (Fig. 7). Further, the dorsal root ganglia are differentially responsive to target tissue in a stage-specific manner such that a maximum response is obtained in the presence of stage XI limb tissue in which little mesenchyme is present and muscle differentiation is well underway (Pollack and Muhlach, 1982). This observation is of particular interest in the context of Butler's (1979) study on the development of muscle spindles in the iliofibularis muscle. Although he does not find fully formed muscle spindles until stage XVIII, he argues that they may begin to develop as early as stage X.

It is perhaps important to remember that sensory fibers from the dorsal root ganglia reach the limb bud much earlier than stage XI, and that much of this early innervation is cutaneous. It is perhaps also significant that the skin covering the limb rudiment is relatively well-developed from the first appearance of the bud. Thus, trophic effects of the skin may be expressed earlier than those from differentiating muscle, and may be important in the early growth of sensory fibers within the limb bud.

Trophic factors from the skin also may be different from muscle-derived factor(s). Reports by Barde et al. (1980) and Davies et al. (1986) indicate that sensory neurons in the chick dorsal root ganglia and the mesencephalic trigeminal nucleus respond to more than a single neuronotrophic factor. This is not surprising since dorsal root ganglia have targets in the spinal cord and

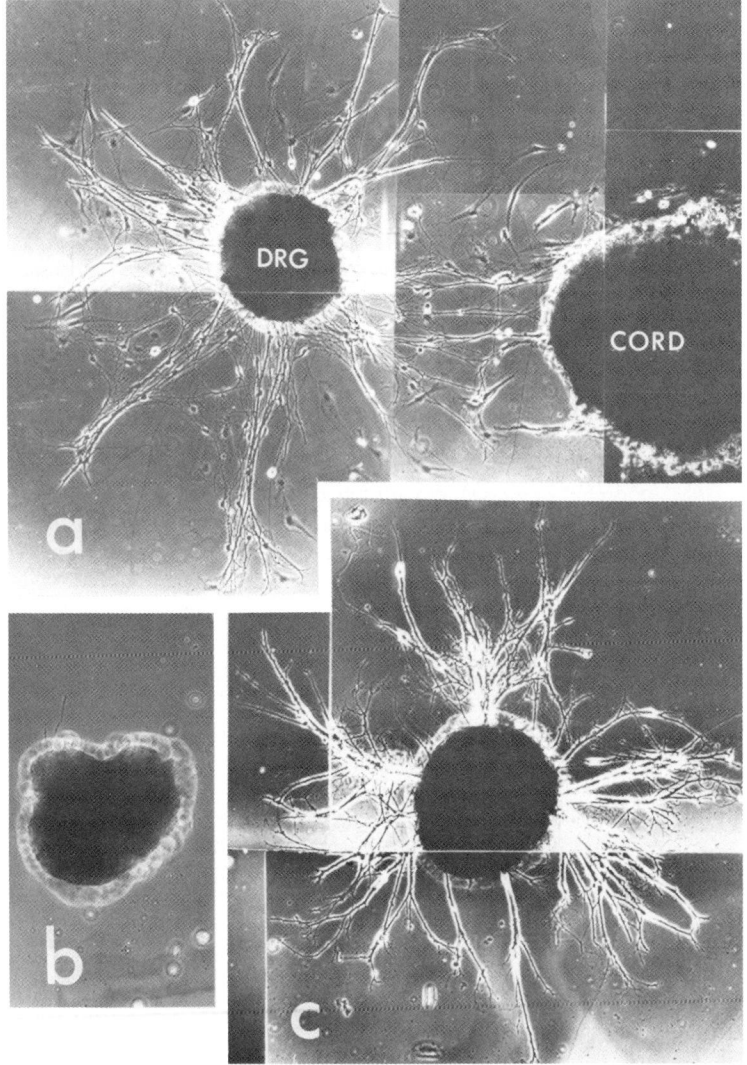

Figure 7. Cultures of stage XI Rana pipiens dorsal root ganglia (DRG) under varying conditions. a: Stage XI DRG with spinal cord explant. Cord-ganglion distance = 0.53 mm. b: Control ganglion grown in the absence of NGF and target tissue. Note absence of neuritic outgrowth. c: DRG treated with 5 biological units NGF. (From Pollack and Muhlach, 1982, courtesy of the authors.)

multiple targets in the developing limb. (Neuron-directed growth factors have been reviewed in Edgar, 1985; Lindsay et al., 1985; Levi-Montalcini, 1987).

CONCLUSIONS

In those anuran dorsal root ganglia for which data are available, developmental patterns are similar. The ganglia increase in size throughout the larval period, and the population of nerve cells within the ganglia increases until mid-larval stages and is then reduced substantially through neuronal degeneration.

In the normal development of the lumbar ganglia, neuronal degeneration is occurring during the same period that the nerve cell population is increasing in size and continues through the period of net nerve cell loss.

The ganglia respond to decreases in the size of the target field by becoming hypoplastic and to increases in the peripheral target by becoming hyperplastic. Mechanisms in addition to shifts in the normal pattern of nerve cell loss may be involved in these responses.

Neuronotrophic factors elicit neuritic outgrowth from anuran dorsal root ganglia, and it is possible that a variety of these factors ultimately may be shown to affect the neuronal populations of these ganglia.

ACKNOWLEDGMENTS

I am pleased to have the opportunity to express my appreciation for having had the good fortune to work with Professor Jerry J. Kollros and to benefit from his guidance. It also is a pleasure to acknowledge the contributions of Yongping Wang, Karen Montgomery and Abdul Elshaar in the work leading to the preparation of this chapter.

REFERENCES

Barde Y-A, Edgar D, Thoenen H (1980). Sensory neurons

in culture: changing requirements for survival factors during embryonic development. Proc Natl Acad Sci USA 77:1199-1203.

Bibb HD (1977). The production of ganglionic hypertrophy in Rana pipiens larvae. J Exp Zool 200:262-276.

Bibb HD (1978). Neuronal death in the development of normal and hyperplastic spinal ganglia. J Exp Zool 206:65-72.

Braus H (1906). Vordere Extremität und Operculum bei Bombinator larven. Ein Beitrag zur Kenntnis morphogener Correlation und Regulation. Morph Jahr 35:509-590.

Butler R (1979). The first appearance of muscle spindles in the iliofibularis muscle of the frog during metamorphosis. J Exp Zool 209:337-343.

Davies A, Thoenen H, Barde Y-A (1986). Different factors from the central nervous system and periphery regulate the survival of sensory neurons. Nature 319:497-499.

Davis MR, Constantine-Paton M (1983a). Hyperplasia in the spinal sensory system of the frog. I. Plasticity in the most caudal dorsal root ganglion. J Comp Neurol 221:444-452.

Davis MR, Constantine-Paton M (1983b). Hyperplasia in the spinal sensory system of the frog. II. Central and peripheral connectivity patterns. J Comp Neurol 221:453-465.

Detwiler SR (1934). An experimental study of spinal nerve segmentation in Ambystoma with reference to the plurisegmental contribution to the brachial plexus. J Exp Zool 67:395-441.

Detwiler SR (1936). "Neuroembryology." New York: Hafner.

Detwiler SR (1937). Observations upon the migration of neural crest cells, and upon the development of the spinal ganglia and vertebral arches in Ambystoma. Am J Anat 61:63-94.

Devor M, Govrin-Lippman R, Frank I, Raber P (1985). Proliferation of primary sensory neurons in adult rat dorsal root ganglion and the kinetics of retrograde cell loss after sciatic nerve section. Somatosensory Res 3:139-167.

Dunlap DG (1966). The development of the musculature of the hindlimb of the frog, Rana pipiens. J Morphol 119:241-258.

DuShane GP (1938). Neural fold derivatives in the

Amphibia: pigment cells, spinal ganglia and Rohon-Beard cells. J Exp Zool 78:485-503.
Ecker E (1889). "Anatomy of the Frog." Oxford: Clarendon Press.
Edgar D (1985). Nerve growth factors and molecules of the extracellular matrix in neuronal development. In Hopkins CR, Hughes RC (eds): "Growth Factors: Structure and Function." Cambridge: The Company of Biologists, pp 107-113.
Gaupp E (1896). "Ecker's und Wiedersheim's Anatomie des Frosches." Braunschweig: Vieweg und Sohn.
Harrison RG (1904). Neue Versuche und Beobachtungen über die Entwicklung der peripheren Nerven der Wirbeltiere. Bonn: Ges Natur Heilkunde, pp 55-62.
Harrison RG (1924). Neuroblast versus sheath cell in the development of peripheral nerves. J Comp Neurol 37:123-205.
Hamburger V (1976). The developmental history of the motor neuron. Neurosci Res Prog Bull 15 Suppl:1-37.
His W (1868). "Untersuchungen über die erste Analge des Wirbeltierleibes. Die Erste Entwicklung des Huhnchens im Ei." Leipzig: FCW Vogal.
Hörstadius S (1950). "The Neural Crest." London: Oxford University Press.
Hughes A (1968). "Aspects of Neural Ontogeny." London: Logos Press.
Hughes A, Tschumi PA (1958). The factors controlling the development of the dorsal root ganglia and ventral horn in Xenopus laevis (Daudin). J Anat (Lond) 92:498-527.
Keynes RJ, Stern CD (1986). Somites and neural development. In Bellairs R, Ede DA, Lash J (eds): "Somites in Developing Embryos." New York: Plenum, pp 289-299.
Kollros JJ (1956). The further development of the spinal cord, ganglia and nerves. In Nieuwkoop PD, Faber J (eds): "Normal Table of Xenopus laevis (Daudin)." Amsterdam: North-Holland, pp 63-73.
Kollros JJ (1968). Order and control of neurogenesis (as exemplified by the lateral motor column). Develop Biol Suppl 2:274-305.
Kollros JJ, McMurray V (1955). The mesencephalic V nucleus in anurans. I. Normal development in Rana pipiens. J Comp Neurol 102:47-64.
Lehmann FE (1927). Further studies on the morphogenetic role of the somites in the development of the nervous

system of amphibians. J Exp Zool 49:93-131.
Letinsky MS (1974). The development of nerve-muscle junctions in Rana catesbeiana tadpoles. Develop Biol 40:129-153.
Levi-Montalcini R (1987). The nerve growth factor: thirty-five years later. EMBO J 5:1145-1154.
Levi-Montalcini R, Aloe L (1985). Differentiating effects of murine nerve growth factor in the peripheral and central nervous system of Xenopus laevis tadpoles. Proc Natl Acad Sci USA 82:7111-7115.
Lindsay RM, Barde Y-A, Davies AM, Rohrer H (1985). Differences and similarities in the neurotrophic growth factor requirements of sensory neurons derived from neural crest and neural placode. In Hopkins CR, Hughes RC (eds): "Growth Factors: Structure and Function." Cambridge: The Company of Biologists, pp 115-129.
Newth DR (1956). The development of skeleton and musculature of pelvic girdle and hindlimbs. In Nieuwkoop PD, Faber J (eds): "Normal Table of Xenopus laevis (Daudin)." Amsterdam: North-Holland.
Nieuwkoop PD, Faber J eds (1956). "Normal Table of Xenopus laevis (Daudin)." Amsterdam: North-Holland.
Oppenheim RW (1981). Neuronal cell death and some related regressive phenomena during neurogenesis: a selective historical review and progress report. In Cowan WM (ed): "Studies in Developmental Neurobiology." New York: Oxford University Press, pp 74-133.
Pannese E (1974). The histogenesis of spinal ganglia. Adv Anat Embryol Cell Biol 47: Fasc 5. pp 1-97.
Piatt J (1948). Form and causality in neurogenesis. Biol Rev 23:1-45.
Pollack ED, Liebig V, Muhlach WL (1979). Limb target and nerve growth factor influence on nerve fiber growth from frog tadpole sensory ganglia in tissue culture. J Cell Biol 83:135a.
Pollack ED, Liebig V, Reed CR (1980). Stage-dependent growth influences on frog tadpole dorsal root ganglion neurites exerted by spinal cord explants in vitro. Soc Neurosci Abstr 6:377.
Pollack ED, Muhlach WL (1982). Target control of neuronal development during formation of the spinal reflex arc: an operant model. J Neurosci Res 8:343-355.
Pollack ED, Richmond M (1981). Analysis of mesenchyme in the developing hind limb of Rana pipiens larvae

with implications for neural development. J Morphol 169:253-257.

Prestige MC (1965). Cell turnover in the spinal ganglia of Xenopus laevis tadpoles. J Embryol Exp Morphol 13:63-72.

Prestige MC (1967). The control of cell number in the lumbar spinal ganglia during the development of Xenopus laevis tadpoles. J Embryol Exp Morphol 17:453-471.

Purves D, Lichtman JW (1985). "Principles of Neural Development." Sunderland, MA: Sinauer.

Raven CP (1931). Zur Entwicklung der Ganglienleiste. I. Die Kinematic der Ganglienleisten Entwicklung bei der Urodelen. Roux Archiv 129:179-198.

Raven CP (1936). Zur Entwicklung der Ganglienleiste. V. über die Differenzierung des Rumpfganglienleistenmaterials. Roux Archiv 134:122-145.

Raven CP (1937). Experiments on the origin of the sheath cells and sympathetic neuroblasts in Amphibia. J Comp Neurol 67:220-240.

Shorey ML (1909). The effect of the destruction of peripheral areas on the differentiation of neuroblasts. J Exp Zool 7:25-63.

Taylor AC (1943). Development of the innervation pattern in the limb bud of the frog. Anat Rec 87:379-413.

Taylor AC, Kollros JJ (1946). Stages in the normal development of Rana pipiens larvae. Anat Rec 94:7-24.

SPECIFICATION OF SPINAL SENSORY NEURONS DURING DEVELOPMENT

Carolyn Smith and Eric Frank

Department of Neurobiology, Anatomy and Cell Biology, University of Pittsburgh School of Medicine, Pittsburgh, Pennsylvania 15261

INTRODUCTION

The connections of primary sensory neurons are remarkably specific. The sensory neurons supplying each peripheral target project to particular areas in the spinal cord and have synaptic connections with specific subsets of the neurons in those areas (reviewed by Brown, 1981). The connections of the sensory neurons that supply muscle spindles provide a good example of this specificity. Spindle afferents project into the intermediate gray matter and ventral horn where they form synaptic connections with motoneurons. Each afferent arborizes in the vicinity of motoneurons supplying several different muscles but only establishes synaptic connections with some of these motoneurons. In general, afferents from a given muscle project to motoneurons supplying the same, or "homonymous", muscle and its synergists but not to motoneurons supplying antagonist muscles (Eccles et al., 1957). Cutaneous afferents, which project to the dorsal horn, must also have highly specific connections because individual dorsal horn neurons receive input from sensory neurons representing small areas on the body surface (Wall, 1973; Brown and Fuchs, 1975).

One hypothesis proposed to explain the development of these highly specific connections is that sensory neurons receive instructive signals from their peripheral targets, which they innervate first (Ramón y Cajal, 1911; Windle and Baxter, 1936), that specify their central targets (Weiss, 1936, 1942; Sperry and Miner, 1949; Miner, 1956). According to this hypothesis, developing sensory neurons initially may be pluripotent. An alternative possibility is that sensory neurons acquire affinities for particular peripheral and central targets before they form axons; their fates would be predetermined (Miner, 1956).

These hypotheses make different predictions about how sensory neurons might behave if forced to innervate a novel peripheral target. The first suggests that sensory neurons will make central connections appropriate to their novel target, while the second suggests that these connections might be inappropriate. These predictions have been tested in a series of experiments on frogs. The basic strategy in each of these studies was to force sensory neurons to innervate novel peripheral targets by surgical manipulations on tadpoles and then to examine the central connections of these sensory neurons in the adult frog. In this chapter, we discuss the relevance of the findings to the problem of when and how the connections of sensory neurons are specified. To provide a framework for this discussion, we begin with a brief summary of the organization of sensory projections in adult frogs and a description of the time course of their development.

ORGANIZATION OF SENSORY PROJECTIONS IN ADULT FROGS

Our description is based on anatomical studies of Rana catesbeiana and Rana pipiens (Joseph and Whitlock, 1968; Frank and Westerfield 1982a; Székely et al., 1982; Jhaveri and Frank, 1982; Liuzzi et al., 1985; Smith and Frank, 1988a). The sensory neurons of concern are those in dorsal root ganglia (DRGs) that supply the trunk and the limbs. In the terminology of Ecker (1889) which we have adopted, the ganglion associated with the brachial nerve is DRG 2. The forelimb is usually innervated exclusively by sensory neurons in DRG 2 but, occasionally, is also innervated by some sensory neurons in DRG 3. The trunk is innervated by DRGs 3 through 6 and the hindlimb by DRGs 7, 8 and 9.

The areas of the spinal cord in which sensory

fibers from these ganglia arborize are illustrated in Fig. 1. Fibers from the brachial ganglion project to the rostral half of the spinal cord while fibers from the lumbosacral ganglia project to the caudal half. Thoracic sensory neurons arborize at thoracic levels of the spinal cord and, for neurons in DRG 3, in an area rostral to dorsal root 2. Thoracic ganglia are composed predominantly of cutaneous sensory neurons which project to the dorsal horn. The brachial and lumbosacral ganglia contain, in addition to cutaneous afferents, many afferents from muscle spindles. These spindle afferents project more ventrally in the gray matter and make direct synaptic connections with motoneurons (Frank and Westerfield, 1982a). Thoracic ganglia probably contain few, if any, spindle afferents because spindles are not present in the axial muscles of frogs (Ceccherelli, 1904).

The central connections of spindle afferents from forelimb muscles of R. catesbeiana have been examined by horseradish peroxidase (HRP) labeling and by intracellular recording methods (Frank and Westerfield, 1982a; Jhaveri and Frank, 1983; Lichtman and Frank, 1984; Lichtman et al., 1984). The sensory neurons that have

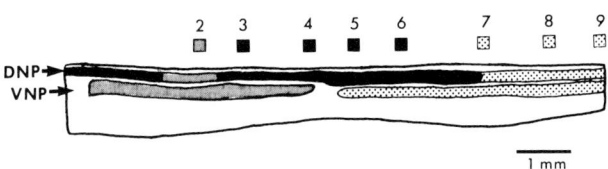

Figure 1. Drawing of a parasagittal section of the spinal cord illustrating the terminal fields of sensory fibers from brachial, thoracic and lumbosacral dorsal roots. The level of entry of the roots and the type of shading used to illustrate their terminal fields are indicated by the boxes above the drawing. The dorsal neuropil (DNP) is composed of cutaneous afferents and the ventral neuropil (VNP) of muscle afferents. Projections from thoracic and limb afferents overlap in the DNP.

been examined in the most detail are those that supply the medial head of the triceps muscle. Medial triceps afferents arborize in a region of the spinal cord containing the motoneurons supplying several different forelimb muscles, including the triceps muscles. Each afferent has synaptic connections with nearly 100% of the motoneurons supplying the medial head of the triceps muscle and with about half of the motoneurons supplying the other two heads. They rarely provide any input at all to subscapularis or pectoralis motoneurons, even though these motoneurons are located in the same region of the brachial spinal cord.

DEVELOPMENT OF SENSORY NEURONS

By the time tadpoles hatch from their eggs, the dorsal root ganglia have already formed, and some sensory neurons have differentiated (Nieuwkoop and Faber, 1956). However, the generation of sensory neurons continues during the larval period. Counts of sensory neurons in lumbosacral DRGs of Xenopus laevis (Prestige, 1965) and R. pipiens (Bibb, 1978) show that the numbers reach a peak at about the time the digits of the hindlimb form (stage 55 in Xenopus, as defined by Nieuwkoop and Faber, 1956, and stage XII in R. pipiens, as defined by Taylor and Kollros, 1946). The numbers then decline to the adult level at about stage 60 (Xenopus) or stage XVI (R. pipiens). Tritiated thymidine labeling studies in Rana showed that most sensory neurons have been generated by stage XVIII (Davis and Constantine-Paton, 1983; Mendelson and Frank, 1987). Thoracic sensory neurons also are generated during the first half of the larval period. Only about 50% of the sensory neurons in DRG 4 have been generated at stage VII in R. catesbeiana (Smith, 1988, in prep.). In Xenopus, the number of thoracic sensory neurons rises until stage 54 and declines to the adult level at stage 59.

Although sensory neurons are still being generated during the first half of the larval period, some neurons differentiate and form peripheral and central projections. The early-developing neurons in thoracic ganglia innervate skin of the trunk and project to thoracic levels of the spinal cord and to the brain stem, like the thoracic sensory neurons in adult frogs (Smith and

Frank, 1988a). For example, at stage III (Fig. 2), DRG 3 neurons project to the dorsal horn at thoracic levels and in the area near the obex, as do DRG 3 neurons in the adult. The organization of their projections does not change during the larval period. Some sensory neurons in brachial and lumbosacral ganglia form peripheral and central projections at stage III-IV, when the limbs consist only of small buds. These neurons arborize in the dorsal horn. Projections to the intermediate gray matter, the termination site of muscle spindle afferents, begin to form around stage VII (Forehand and Farel, 1982; Liuzzi et al., 1985; Smith and Frank, 1988a). By stage XIV, brachial and lumbosacral sensory

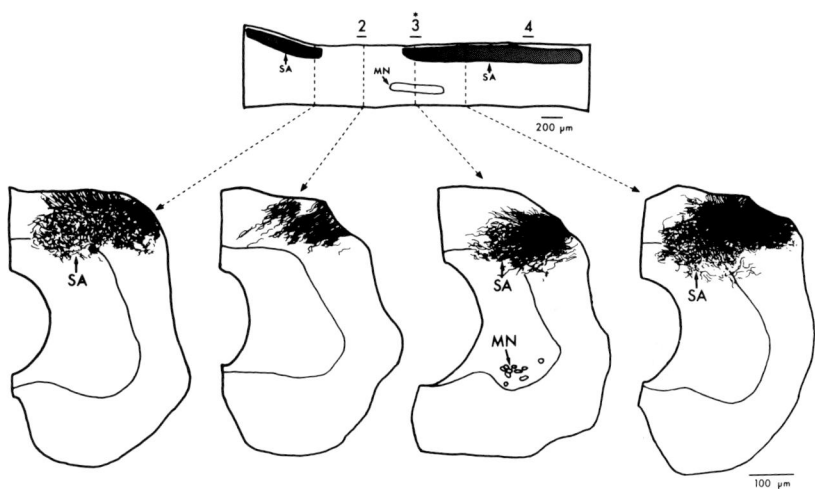

Figure 2. Central projections from DRG 3 neurons in a stage III-IV tadpole. Sensory and motor neurons were labeled by exposing the dorsal and ventral roots to HRP. The drawings at the bottom show HRP-labeled sensory fibers and motoneuron cell bodies in transverse sections from the spinal cords. A parasagittal view of the projections is shown at the top. DRG fibers pass through the level of dorsal root 2 in the dorsal funiculus but do not arborize at this level. SA: sensory arborizations; MN: motoneurons. (From Smith and Frank, 1988a.)

neurons have formed dense plexuses in both the dorsal horn and intermediate gray matter.

Tadpoles respond to tactile stimulation of the trunk even at early larval stages, indicating that the sensory neurons that innervate the trunk skin have functional synaptic connections in the central nervous system. Responses can be elicited by stimulating the limbs beginning around stage X (Letinsky, 1975; Frank and Westerfield, unpubl. observations). Sensory neurons do not have direct connections with motoneurons at this stage, although some ventrally-projecting sensory fibers from lumbosacral ganglia extend into the vicinity of motoneurons (Liuzzi et al., 1985). Contacts between sensory fibers and motoneurons are observed at stage XIII-XIV in the lumbosacral region (Liuzzi et al., 1985) and at stage XVI-XVII in the brachial region (Jackson and Frank, 1987). Electrical stimulation of forelimb muscle afferents evokes small monosynaptic EPSPs in some brachial motoneurons at stage XVI-XVII (Frank and Westerfield, 1983). The amplitudes of the monosynaptic EPSP's produced by stimulating individual muscle nerves increase during the period between stage XVII and XXII which suggests that synaptic connections continue to develop during this period.

Sensory neurons could form synaptic connections exclusively with appropriate types of spinal neurons from the very beginning. However, a highly specific pattern of connections could also be created by pruning an initially diffuse set of connections. Frank and Westerfield (1983) examined projections from medial triceps muscle afferents onto motoneurons in R. catesbeiana tadpoles to determine whether the initial connections of these sensory neurons are specific or diffuse. As is illustrated in Fig. 3, triceps afferents project more strongly to triceps motoneurons than to adjacent non-triceps motoneurons in tadpoles, just as they do in adult frogs. For example, at stage XVIII, which is only one stage after connections between triceps afferents and motoneurons can first be detected electrophysiologically, EPSP's evoked by triceps afferents in triceps motoneurons are five to 10 times larger than in subscapularis and pectoralis motoneurons. This ratio is nearly identical to that found in the adult.

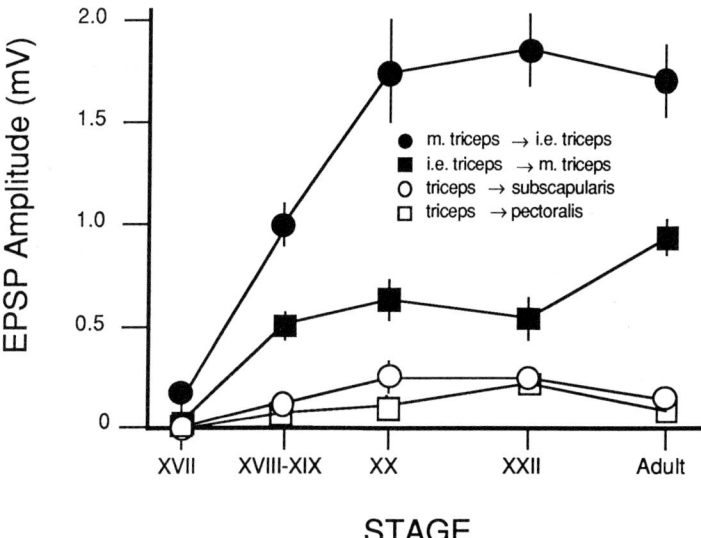

Figure 3. Development of monosynaptic connections between muscle afferents and motoneurons. EPSPs produced in motoneurons by stimulating triceps muscle afferents were measured from intracellular records. They were judged to be monosynaptic if they had central latencies of 3 ms or less (see Frank and Westerfield, 1983, for details). Monosynaptic EPSPs are first detectable at stage XVII. At all stages, EPSPs evoked in triceps motoneurons are larger than those produced in non-triceps motoneurons. (After Frank and Westerfield, 1983.)

This early specificity suggests that sensory neurons have affinities for particular spinal neurons at the time they form their central connections. When does specification occur? One possibility is that sensory neurons are specified before axon outgrowth and that they selectively innervate both their peripheral and central targets. Alternatively, sensory neurons may be pluripotent initially and become specified after they innervate their peripheral targets. This problem has been addressed by examining the connections of sensory neurons that were provided with novel peripheral targets during their development.

CONSEQUENCES OF SKIN ROTATION

A number of different types of surgical manipulations have been done in an attempt to force developing sensory neurons to innervate foreign targets. In one series of studies, a strip of skin was removed from the trunk of R. pipiens tadpoles and replaced with its dorsoventral axis reversed so that skin from the back and belly was interchanged. After the tadpoles metamorphosed, the reflexes evoked by touching the graft were examined. Normal frogs respond to tactile stimulation by wiping the point stimulated. However, when the skin was rotated at stage XIV or earlier, the responses elicited by stimulating the graft were often misdirected; when the back was touched, the frog wiped its belly and vice versa (Miner, 1956; Jacobson and Baker, 1969). Thus, some of the sensory neurons innervating the graft must have formed central connections appropriate to the type of skin they innervated. This finding was interpreted as evidence that the central connections of cutaneous sensory neurons are actually determined by biochemical properties of the skin they innervated (Miner, 1956).

Wiping reflexes can be elicited first at about stage XX in both normal and skin-rotated frogs (Jacobson and Baker, 1969). Interestingly, the first wipe reflexes in skin-rotated frogs are often normal. Misdirected reflexes are, at first, elicited from a small region in the center of the graft. This region then expands gradually to include most of the graft. On the basis of these observations, Gaze (1970) suggested that the formation of misdirected reflexes may involve two steps: (1) specification of the sensory neurons by the foreign skin (before stage XV) and (2) expression of this specificity in the formation of connections during metamorphosis.

If all sensory neurons innervating the graft formed central connections appropriate to the type of skin they innervated, then frogs with rotated skin would produce only misdirected reflexes. However, most produce normal reflexes on some trials. A possible explanation is that sensory neurons which had already formed connections when the skin was rotated retained their original central connections despite being forced to innervate foreign skin. By stage XV, most thoracic sensory neurons already may have formed connections, and this may be the reason that frogs develop only normal reflexes when the skin is rotated after this stage. Sklar and Hunt (1973) reasoned that if sensory neurons can become stably specified during early larval stages, then frogs should develop both normal and misdirected reflexes when the skin is rotated at an early stage and then returned to its original position. Contrary to this prediction, they found that frogs developed only normal reflexes following skin rotation at stage V or X and re-rotation at stage XIII. However, since the percentage of neurons that innervate the skin during this period might be small, this finding is not a compelling reason to abandon the idea that some neurons can be stably specified by the periphery at early stages.

An alternative explanation of the misdirected reflexes in skin-rotated frogs is that sensory neurons have a special affinity for a particular type of skin and that some are able to innervate the correct type of skin even when it has been moved to the novel location. For example, prespecified belly-skin neurons may grow around the side of the body to reach belly-skin that has been moved to the back. Studies by Bloom and Tompkins (1976) and Heidemann (1977) suggest that selective reinnervation by this mechanism is responsible for the belly-directed reflexes elicited by stimulating the back in skin-rotated frogs. However, Baker et al. (1977) argue that this cannot be the complete explanation because back skin that has been grafted to the belly is only innervated by nerves that supply the belly, and yet the responses elicited by stimulating it are directed to the back.

Another way in which prespecified sensory neurons could reach the correct type of skin in skin-rotated frogs is by sending their axons into the opposite cutaneous nerve from normal. Baker et al. (1978) examined the locations of the cell bodies of sensory neurons projecting into the dorsal and ventral cutaneous nerves in normal and skin-rotated frogs to see whether the topographic organization of the ganglia provides evidence that selective innervation occurs by this mechanism. The results were equivocal. In both normal and skin-rotated frogs, about 10% more neurons in the dorsal half of the ganglion innervated dorsal skin than ventral skin while the reverse was true of neurons in the ventral part of the ganglion. This observation can be explained by a mechanism involving either peripheral specification or prespecification by assuming that, during development, neurons in the dorsal and ventral halves of the ganglion project predominantly into the corresponding peripheral nerves. If sensory neurons are specified by their targets, then they would form appropriate central connections regardless of which type of skin they innervated. If they were prespecified, neurons that innervated the incorrect type of skin might die so that only those that innervated the correct type would form central connections.

The effects of skin rotation on the central projections of thoracic sensory neurons have also been examined. Székely et al. (1982) used cobalt labeling to compare projections to the spinal cord from subdivisions of thoracic nerves in normal and skin-rotated frogs. As is illustrated in Fig. 4, the central projections from nerves supplying belly and back skin overlap extensively in normal frogs. In skin-rotated frogs, the central projections from the same nerves were not significantly different from normal. Thus, there is no direct evidence that skin rotation produces anatomical changes in the central connections of sensory neurons.

REFLEXES ELICITED FROM SUPERNUMERARY LIMBS

Thoracic sensory neurons can be forced to innervate a limb by removing the limb from one individual and grafting it to the back of another. Weiss (1936) examined the reflexes elicited by stretching muscles in the supernumerary limbs of frogs and salamanders. Stretch of a given muscle produced a reflex contraction in both that muscle and the homologous muscle in the host's normal limb. Weiss assumed that the sensory neurons that innervated muscles in the supernumerary limbs were not the ones that would normally supply those muscles. Since these sensory neurons mediated appropriate reflexes, he concluded that their functional properties were determined by the muscles, a process he termed "modulation".

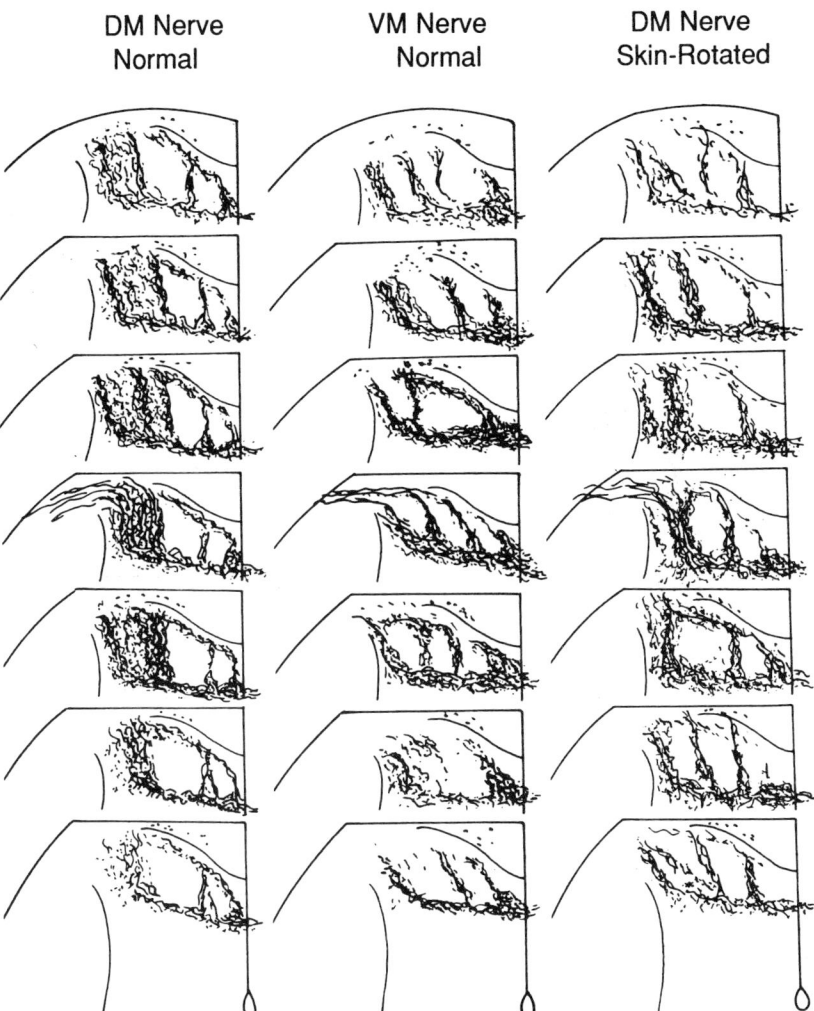

Figure 4. Central projections from cutaneous nerves in normal and skin-rotated frogs. Dorsomedial (DM) or ventromedial (VM) nerves were labeled with cobalt chloride and drawings were made of the stained sensory fibers in the dorsal horn at different rostrocaudal levels. Note that the projection from the DM nerve in the skin-rotated frog is not markedly different from the projection of either the DM or VM nerve in normal frogs. (After Székely et al., 1982.)

Subsequent studies have shown that muscles develop in supernumerary limbs only when the limbs are innervated by brachial or lumbosacral nerves (reviewed by Mendell and Hollyday, 1976). Since the supernumerary limbs studied by Weiss had well developed muscles and were mobile, they were probably innervated by spinal segments and ganglia that normally supply the limbs.

Although supernumerary limbs innervated exclusively by thoracic spinal nerves are immobile, they are sensitive to tactile stimulation: touching the limb evokes a response in the host's own hindlimb or forelimb (Miner, 1956; Mendell and Hollyday, 1976). Which limb responds depends on which nerves innervate the supernumerary limb. If it is innervated by caudal thoracic nerves, the host's hindlimb responds; whereas, if it is innervated by rostral thoracic nerves, the forelimb responds. Hollyday and Mendell (1975) used both behavioral observations and electrophysiological methods to assess the specificity of responses elicited by touching supernumerary hindlimbs in Xenopus. When the limb was grafted sufficiently early in development (before stage 55), the responses evoked by touching it were typical of those produced by limb afferents and, in some cases, unlike those produced by normal thoracic sensory neurons. These findings suggest that supernumerary hindlimbs induce thoracic sensory neurons to make connections they normally would not make.

CONNECTIONS OF THORACIC SENSORY NEURONS
FORCED TO INNERVATE FORELIMB MUSCLES

Thoracic ganglia in bullfrogs normally are composed predominantly of cutaneous sensory neurons that innervate skin of the trunk and project to the dorsal horn. The aim of the experiments described in this section was to find out whether thoracic sensory neurons in bullfrog tadpoles can innervate forelimb muscles and, if so, whether they form central connections typical of forelimb muscle afferents.

The three types of manipulations that have been used to force thoracic sensory neurons to innervate the forelimb are illustrated in Fig. 5. In the first (A), the ganglion that normally supplies the forelimb, DRG 2, was removed from tadpoles (Frank and Westerfield, 1982b). When DRG 2 was removed before stage X, the forelimb was innervated by neurons in DRG 3. In the second (B), DRGs 2 and 3 were removed and neurons in DRG 4 were forced to innervate the forelimb by redirecting the fourth spinal nerve (SN 4) into the path of the brachial nerve (Smith, 1986; Smith and Frank, 1988b). Alternatively, DRG 2 was removed and SN 3 was redirected. In the third (C), DRGs 2 and 3 were removed and two or three midthoracic DRGs (4, 5 and 6) were transplanted to the position previously occupied by DRG 2 (Smith and Frank, 1987).

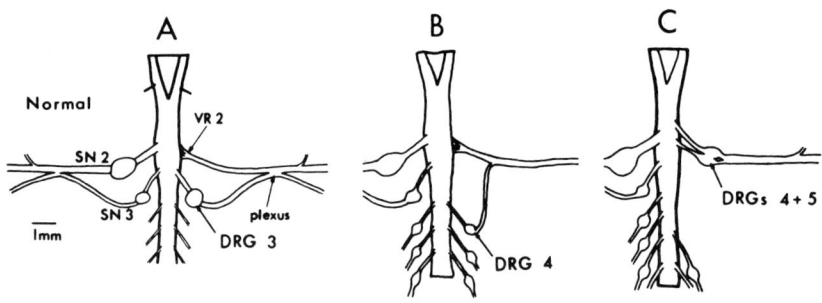

Figure 5. Schematic diagrams of the innervation of the forelimb in frogs following surgical manipulations at early larval stages. A: Removal of DRG 2. Spinal nerve (SN) 3 fuses with the brachial nerve. DRG 3 is enlarged and some sensory neurons in DRG 3 now innervate the forelimb. VR 2 = 2nd ventral root. B: DRGs 2 and 3 removed; SN 4 re-routed. Both DRGs 2 and 3 are absent. The forelimb is now innervated by sensory neurons in DRG 4. C: DRGs 2 and 3 removed; DRGs 4 and 5 transplanted to the brachial level. The transplanted sensory neurons innervate the forelimb and project into the brachial spinal cord. (A: after Frank and Westerfield, 1982b; B: after Smith and Frank, 1988b; C: after Smith and Frank, 1987.)

To determine whether these manipulations caused thoracic sensory neurons to innervate forelimb muscles, recordings were made from the dorsal roots containing their central processes, and muscle nerves were electrically stimulated. If the nerve contained sensory fibers, action potentials were observed in the dorsal root recording. When the surgical operations were done at stage X or earlier, thoracic sensory neurons often innervated muscles. Furthermore, recordings from muscle nerves showed that these neurons were sensitive to stretch, which suggests that they terminated on spindles. When the surgical manipulations were done at stages XI to XV, only a few thoracic sensory neurons innervated muscles. The ganglia also were much smaller than normal which suggests that the surgical operations caused the degeneration of many sensory neurons.

The central projections from thoracic ganglia that were forced to innervate the forelimb were examined by HRP labeling. When the surgical manipulations were done at stage X or earlier, the thoracic sensory neurons formed two distinct neuropils, one in the dorsal horn and the other in the intermediate gray matter, as is illustrated in Figs. 6 and 7. The dorsal neuropil is the termination site of cutaneous afferents in normal frogs, and the ventral neuropil is the termination site of muscle spindle afferents (Jhaveri and Frank, 1983). When the manipulations were done at later stages, fewer sensory neurons projected ventrally, in keeping with the observation that few of them innervated muscles.

Thoracic sensory neurons normally arborize at thoracic levels of the spinal cord and near the obex. Although their axons pass through the brachial region, they do not arborize at this level. However, when induced to innervate the forelimb, thoracic sensory neurons arborized in the brachial region, even when their cell bodies were still at the thoracic level. This expansion of the central projections could mean that the level of a sensory neuron's arborization is determined by its peripheral target. However, an alternative possibility is that sensory neurons were attracted by the partially deafferented spinal cord. To distinguish between these explanations, we compared the projections formed by DRG 4 neurons in frogs in which the fourth spinal nerve was either redirected into the forelimb or

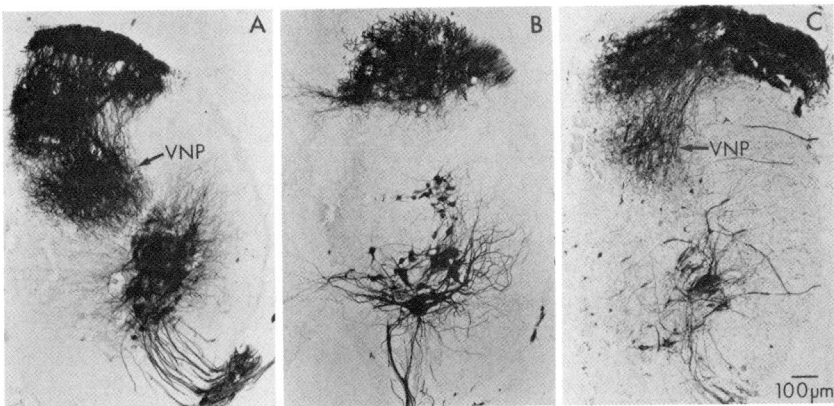

Figure 6. Central projections from normal and transplanted sensory neurons. A: Projections from DRG 2 in normal frog. B: Projections from DRG 4 in normal frog. C: Projections from DRGs 4 and 5 after transplantation to the brachial level at stage VIII. Sensory and motor neurons were labeled by exposing the brachial nerve or dorsal and ventral roots to HRP. Sections from the spinal cord were processed with diaminobenzidine. Note that transplanted thoracic sensory neurons form a ventral neuropil (VNP) whereas normal thoracic sensory neurons to not. (After Smith and Frank, 1987.)

left intact and in which both DRGs 2 and 3 were removed (Smith, 1986; Smith and Frank, 1988b). As can be seen in Fig. 7, DRG 4 neurons projected further rostrally and formed more ventrally-projecting branches when peripheral nerve 4 was redirected into the forelimb than when it was left intact. The fact that simply removing DRGs 2 and 3 caused DRG 4 neurons to project somewhat further rostrally than normal and to form some terminations characteristic of forelimb muscle afferents may be related to the electrophysiological observation that a few of them innervated the forelimb (Smith, unpubl. observations). The finding that the number of neurons projecting into the brachial level correlates with the number innervating the forelimb supports the suggestion that the levels at which sensory neurons arborize depend on their peripheral targets.

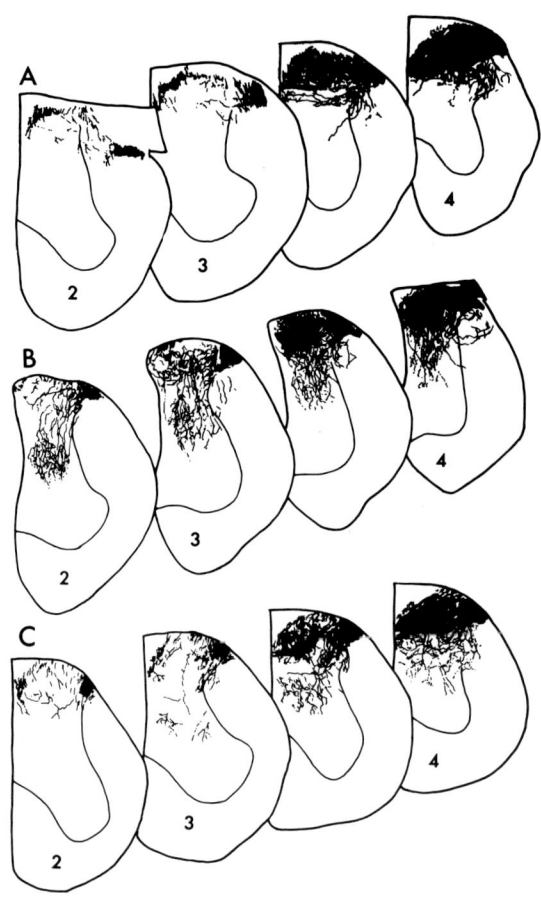

Figure 7. Influences of peripheral nerve re-routing and partial deafferentation of the spinal cord on the central projections from DRG 4 neurons. The central projections were stained by exposing the 4th dorsal root to HRP. Drawings were made of HRP-labeled sensory fibers in transverse sections from the spinal cord at the levels of the 2nd, 3rd, and 4th dorsal roots. A: Projections from DRG 4 neurons in a normal frog. B: Projections from DRG 4 neurons in a frog in which DRGs 2 and 3 were removed and spinal nerve 4 redirected into the forelimb. C: Projections from DRG 4 neurons in which DRGs 2 and 3 were removed without disrupting spinal nerve 4. (After Smith and Frank, 1988b.)

In normal frogs, sensory neurons supplying forelimb muscles have direct excitatory connections with the motoneurons supplying specific muscles. To determine whether thoracic sensory neurons that innervated forelimb muscles made synaptic connections with motoneurons and, if so, whether they selected motoneurons appropriate for the muscles they innervated, we measured the latencies and amplitudes of the responses produced in motoneurons by stimulating muscle nerves. The responses consisted of EPSPs that occurred at short central latencies, which suggests that they were produced monosynaptically. Furthermore, the pattern of connections between sensory neurons and motoneurons supplying different muscles was the same as in normal frogs. For example, medial triceps afferents projected more strongly to triceps motoneurons than to subscapularis or pectoralis motoneurons. The specificity of the projections of triceps afferents in individual animals can be conveniently expressed in terms of a specificity index defined as:

$$SI = 1 - \frac{\text{EPSP amplitude in non-triceps motoneurons}}{\text{EPSP amplitude in triceps motoneurons}}$$

This measure has the property that values near 1.0 indicate that projections onto triceps motoneurons are stronger that those onto non-triceps motoneurons while values near 0 indicate that projections onto both types of motoneurons are equally strong. As is illustrated in Fig. 8, the specificity indices for frogs whose forelimbs were innervated by thoracic sensory neurons are within the range found in normal frogs.

It seems unlikely that thoracic DRGs contain sensory neurons prespecified to innervate particular muscles in the forelimb and neurons in the brachial spinal cord. Therefore, the finding that thoracic sensory neurons made connections with the correct types of motoneurons when they innervated forelimb muscles suggests that they were instructed to form these connections by the periphery. Muscles may have distinctive labels that induce the sensory neurons that innervate them to acquire their own distinctive labels and, thus specify their central connections, as suggested by Weiss (1936). Since each muscle contains the axons of a unique set of motoneurons, sensory neurons that innervate a given muscle could also be uniquely specified by the motoneurons that supply that muscle (Honig, 1982).

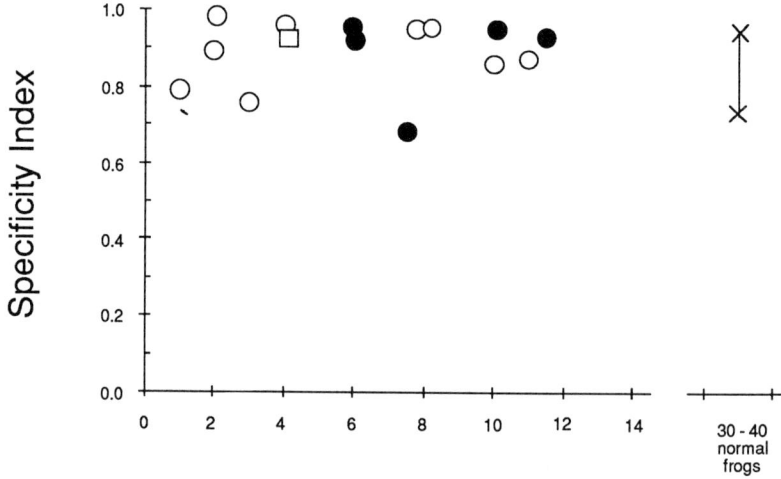

Figure 8. Specificity of the connections made by thoracic sensory neurons that innervated the medial triceps muscle plotted as a function of the number of sensory neurons that innervated this muscle. The specificity indices were calculated as described in the text. The number of medial triceps sensory neurons was estimated by recording from the cut peripheral end of the dorsal root while stimulating the medial triceps nerve at progressively increasing strengths (see Sah and Frank, 1984, for details). Each point represents an animal in which thoracic sensory neurons were forced to innervate the forelimb by one of the manipulations illustrated in Fig. 5 (A: open circles; B: squares; C: closed circles). The values for normal frogs are from Sah and Frank, 1984.

BIRTHDATES OF THORACIC SENSORY NEURONS THAT INNERVATE THE FORELIMB

In the experiments described in the preceding section, thoracic ganglia were forced to innervate the forelimb at stages when they contain both differentiated neurons and dividing cells. Which of these cells innervate the forelimb? This question was addressed by using ^{3}H-thymidine to determine the birthdates of sensory neurons in thoracic ganglia that were transplanted to the brachial level (Smith, 1988, in prep.). When tadpoles were injected with ^{3}H-thymidine from shortly after the time the ganglia were transplanted (stages VII-IX) until stage XVIII, between 65% and 85% of the sensory neurons in the transplanted ganglia were labeled. Thus, while some of the sensory neurons that innervated the forelimb may have innervated the trunk before they were transplanted, most were newly-generated sensory neurons. In thoracic ganglia from the unoperated side which were examined for comparison, approximately 50% of the neurons were labeled. Counts of the unlabeled sensory neurons in control and transplanted ganglia showed that many differentiated sensory neurons did not survive transplantation. These neurons may have died because they were deprived of trophic factors that they need for their survival and normally obtain from their peripheral targets (Levi-Montalcini and Angeletti, 1968; Hendry et al., 1974; Hamburger and Yip, 1984).

CAN MATURE SENSORY NEURONS BE RESPECIFIED?

Sensory neurons in adult animals can be forced to innervate foreign peripheral targets by redirecting their peripheral axons. However, they retain their original central connections even when these connections result in inappropriate reflexes (Sperry, 1941). The central connections of sensory neurons appear to be quite resistant to change even at stages shortly after their formation. For example, when muscle afferents were forced to innervate an antagonistic muscle in newborn kittens and then examined in the adult cat, they were found to project to motoneurons supplying their original muscle and its synergists (Eccles et al., 1962). Their projections to motoneurons supplying their new target muscle were little, if any, larger than normal. Similarly, muscle afferents forced to innervate a synergistic muscle projected more strongly to motoneurons supplying their original muscle than to those supplying the new one (Mendell and Scott, 1975).

In these experiments, sensory neurons may have been

respecified but incapable of expressing their new specificities because they were unable to break their original connections. The results might be different if sensory neurons were forced first to innervate a novel target and then allowed to reform their central connections. An experimental test of this suggestion is feasible in frogs because amphibian sensory neurons can re-establish specific synaptic connections in the spinal cord after transection of the dorsal root (Sah and Frank, 1984). We re-routed the medial triceps muscle nerve into the subscapularis muscle in juvenile frogs, and after allowing time for the sensory axons in this nerve to innervate their new target, we crushed the dorsal root so that the central projections from these sensory neurons would degenerate. Three months later, when central projections from the crushed dorsal root had re-formed, the pattern of connections between muscle afferents and motoneurons was investigated electrophysiologically. Although subscapularis muscle afferents normally project strongly to subscapularis motoneurons, the triceps sensory afferents that were forced to innervate the subscapularis muscle did not. Instead, they projected strongly to triceps motoneurons, as is typical of triceps afferents in normal frogs. While these observations are based on studies of only four animals, the results suggest that mature sensory neurons in frogs are not respecified by forcing them to innervate a different target.

CONCLUSIONS

The studies described in the preceding sections show that thoracic sensory neurons in tadpoles at early larval stages can innervate foreign targets and form central connections appropriate to those targets. Sensory neurons in adult frogs can innervate novel targets but seem to retain affinities for central neurons appropriate to their original targets. A straightforward explanation of these observations is that developing sensory neurons are specified by their peripheral targets, but that once specified, they retain their specificities even if forced to innervate a different target.

An alternative possibility is that sensory neurons are prespecified to select a particular peripheral target and form central connections appropriate to it. For this hypothesis to explain the finding that thoracic sensory neurons can innervate the limbs, it is also necessary to postulate that the dorsal root ganglia contain neurons prespecified to innervate targets they do not normally encounter. This suggestion seems reasonable since many sensory neurons die during normal development; the neurons that do not survive might be ones that failed to innervate appropriate targets.

An extreme form of this hypothesis is that each ganglion contains the full complement of sensory neurons needed to innervate every target in the body. However, numerical considerations suggest that this is unlikely to be the case. Even if the number of sensory neurons generated exceeded the number present in the adult by nearly three-fold, as is suggested by Prestige's studies (1965), the excess in each ganglion is not enough to include all the neurons needed to innervate the entire body. One way around this difficulty would be to postulate that each target at a given level of the body has a unique label, but that the same sets of labels are used at different levels. Some support for the idea that the same labels may be used at the brachial and lumbosacral levels is provided by behavioral observations on frogs with supernumerary limbs.

Perhaps a more prudent approach is to be open to both types of explanations. The connections of sensory neurons may be determined in part by properties that they acquire before axon formation and in part by their peripheral targets. For example, sensory neurons may be committed to innervating a particular <u>type</u> of target (eg. skin or muscle) but not a specific target. They may also be committed to projecting to a particular area in the spinal cord (e.g., dorsal horn or intermediate gray matter). However, their choices of which particular spinal neurons to innervate may depend on instructive signals they receive from their peripheral targets. This type of hypothesis is in keeping with the observation that cells are often committed to developing a particular phenotype at the time they withdraw from the mitotic cycle but also provides a mechanism for ensuring that sensory neurons form central connections appropriate to their targets.

REFERENCES

Baker RE, Corner MA, Veltman WAM (1978). Topography of cutaneous mechanoceptive neurones in dorsal root ganglia of skin-grafted frogs. J Physiol (Lond) 284:181-192.

Bibb HD (1978). Neuronal death in the development of normal and hypertrophic spinal ganglia. J Exp Zool 206:65-72.

Bloom EM, Tompkins R (1976). Selective reinnervation in skin rotation grafts in Rana pipiens. J Exp Zool 195:237-246.

Brown AG (1981). "Organization in the Spinal Cord." Berlin: Springer-Verlag.

Brown PB, Fuchs JL (1975). Somatotopic representation of hindlimb skin in cat dorsal horn. J Neurophysiol 38:1-9.

Ceccherelli G (1904). Sulle "terminazioni nervose a paniere" del Giacomini, nei muscoli dorsali degli Anfibi anuri adulti. Anat Anz 24:428-435.

Davis MR, Constantine-Paton M (1983). Hyperplasia in the spinal sensory system of the frog. I. Plasticity in the most caudal dorsal root ganglion. J Comp Neurol 221:453-465.

Eccles JC, Eccles RM, Lundberg A (1957). The convergence of monosynaptic excitatory afferents on to many different species of alpha motoneurons. J Physiol (Lond) 138:22-50.

Eccles JC, Eccles RM, Shealey CN, Willis WD (1962). Experiments utilizing monosynaptic excitatory action on motoneurons for testing hypothesis relating to specificity of neuronal connections. J Neurophysiol 24:559-580.

Ecker E (1889). "Anatomy of the Frog." Oxford: Clarendon Press.

Forehand CJ, Farel PB (1982). Spinal cord development in anuran larvae. I. Primary and secondary neurons. J Comp Neurol 209:386-394.

Frank E, Westerfield M (1982a). Synaptic organization of sensory and motor neurones innervating triceps brachii muscles in the bullfrog. J Physiol (Lond) 324:479-494.

Frank E, Westerfield M (1982b). The formation of appropriate central and peripheral connexions by foreign sensory neurones of the bullfrog. J Physiol (Lond) 324:495-505.

Frank E, Westerfield M (1983). Development of sensory-motor synapses in the spinal cord of the frog. J Physiol (Lond) 343:593-610.

Gaze RM (1970). "Formation of Nerve Connections." New York: Academic Press.

Hamburger V, Yip JW (1984). Reduction of experimentally induced neuronal death in spinal ganglia of the chick embryo by nerve growth factor. J Neurosci 1:60-71.

Heidemann WK (1977). Neurophysiological and behavioral evidence for selective reinnervation in skin-grafted Rana pipiens. Proc Natl Acad Sci USA 74:5749-5753.

Hendry IA, Stockel K, Thoenen H, Iversen LL (1974). The retrograde axonal transport of nerve growth factor. Brain Res 86:103-121.

Hollyday M, Mendell L (1975). Area specific reflexes from normal and supernumerary hindlimbs of Xenopus laevis. J Comp Neurol 162:205-220.

Honig MG (1982). The development of sensory projection patterns in embryonic chick hind limb. J Physiol (Lond) 330:175-202.

Jackson PC, Frank E (1987). Development of synaptic connections between muscle sensory afferents and motor neurons: anatomical evidence that postsynaptic dendrites grow into a pre-formed sensory neuropil. J Comp Neurol 255:538-547.

Jacobson M, Baker RE (1969). Development of neuronal connections with skin grafts in frogs: behavioral and electrophysiological studies. J Comp Neurol 137:121-142.

Jhaveri S, Frank E (1983). Central projections of the brachial nerve in bullfrogs: muscle and cutaneous afferents project to different regions of the spinal cord. J Comp Neurol 221:304-312.

Joseph BS, Whitlock DG (1968). Central projections of selected spinal dorsal roots in anuran amphibians. Anat Rec 160:279-288.

Letinsky MS (1974). The development of nerve-muscle junctions in Rana catesbeiana tadpoles. Develop Biol 40:129-153.

Levi-Montalcini R, Angeletti P (1968). Nerve growth factor. Physiol Rev 48:534-569.

Lichtman JW, Frank E (1984). Physiological evidence for specificity of synaptic connections between individual sensory and motor neurons in the brachial spinal cord of the bullfrog. J Neurosci 4:1745-1753.

Lichtman JW, Jhaveri S, Frank E (1984). Anatomical basis of specific connections between sensory axons and motor neurons in the bullfrog's brachial spinal cord. J Neurosci 4:1754-1763.

Liuzzi FJ, Beattie MS, Bresnahan JC (1985). The development of the relationship between dorsal root afferents and motoneurons in the larval bullfrog spinal cord. Brain Res Bull 14:377-392.

Mendell LM, Hollyday M (1976). Spinal reflexes in anurans with an altered periphery. In Llínas R, Precht W (eds): "Frog Neurobiology." Berlin: Springer-Verlag, pp 793-810.

Mendell LM, Scott JG (1975). The effect of peripheral nerve cross union on connections of single Ia fibers to motoneurons. Exp Brain Res 22:221-234.

Mendelson B, Frank E (1987). Sensory neurons that innervate a specific target are generated over a protracted developmental period. Soc Neurosci Abstr 13:1456.

Miner N (1956). Integumental specification of sensory fibers in the development of cutaneous local sign. J Comp Neurol 105:161-170.

Nieuwkoop PD, Faber PG (1956). "Normal tables of Xenopus laevis." Amsterdam: North-Holland.

Prestige MC (1965). Cell turnover in the spinal ganglia of Xenopus laevis tadpoles. J Embryol Exp Morphol 13:63-73.

Ramón y Cajal S (1911). "Histologie du Systeme Nerveuse de l'homme et des vertebres." Azoulay L (transl), 1972. Madrid: Instituto Ramón y Cajal.

Sah DWY, Frank E (1984). Regeneration of sensory-motor synapses in the spinal cord of the bullfrog. J Neurosci 4:2784-2791.

Sklar J, Hunt RK (1973). The acquisition of specificity in cutaneous sensory neurons: a reconsideration of the integumental specification hypothesis. Proc Natl Acad Sci USA 70:3684-3688.

Smith CL (1986). Sensory neurons with rerouted peripheral axons make appropriate central connections. Soc Neurosci Abstr 12:542.

Smith CL, Frank E (1987). Peripheral specification of sensory neurons transplanted to novel location along the neuraxis. J Neurosci 7:1537-1549.

Smith CL, Frank E (1988a). Specificity of sensory projections to the spinal cord during development in bullfrogs. J Comp Neurol (in press).

Smith CL, Frank E (1988b). Peripheral specification of sensory connections in the spinal cord. Brain Behav Evol (in press).
Sperry RW (1941). The effect of crossing nerves to antagonistic muscles in the hind limbs of the rat. J Comp Neurol 75:1-19.
Sperry RW, Miner N (1949). Formation within sensory nucleus V of synaptic associations mediating cutaneous localization. J Comp Neurol 90:403-423.
Székely G, Matesz K, Baker RE, Antal M (1982). The termination of cutaneous nerves in the dorsal horn of the spinal cord in normal and in skin-rotated frogs. Exp Brain Res 45:19-28.
Taylor AC, Kollros JJ (1946). Stages in the normal development of Rana pipiens larvae. Anat Rec 94:7-23.
Wall PD (1973). Dorsal horn electrophysiology. In Iggo A (ed): "Handbook of Sensory Physiology, vol. II." Berlin: Springer-Verlag, pp 253-270.
Weiss P (1936). Selectivity controlling the central-peripheral relations in the nervous system. Biol Rev 11:494-531.
Weiss P (1942). Lid closure reflex from eyes transplanted to atypical locations in Triturus torosus: evidence of a peripheral origin of sensory specificity. J Comp Neurol 77:131-169.
Windle WF, Baxter RE (1936). Development of reflex mechanisms in the spinal cord of albino rat embryos: Correlation between structure and function and comparisons with the cat and the chick. J Comp Neurol 63:189-209.

SECTION III

NEURONAL ORDER, DIFFERENTIATION, AND POPULATION ADJUSTMENTS

SECTION III. NEURONAL ORDER, DIFFERENTIATION AND POPULATION ADJUSTMENTS

The final four chapters highlight the developmental neurobiology of the frog through a focus on higher CNS neurons: their differentiation and numerical control, their relationship to afferent inputs, their formation into characteristic lamina in the brain and the structured sequence of events in neurogenesis.

Having considered thus far developmental events at lower levels of the neuraxis that might provide insight into general mechanisms of nervous system development, a return to the central nervous system is appropriate. Although an overwhelming task, there is considerable interest in the development of individual neurons and their eventual mediation of embryonic behavior. It has become possible to identify specific spinal and hindbrain neurons relative to their neurotransmitter properties and thereby follow individual neuron differentiation within the organism.

Other questions have been addressed through the use of the visual system and the cerebellum in the frog. In the case of the optic tectum there are two primary concerns. First is a return to the issue of neuron number regulation that has been particularly controversial in the case of the tectum. Second is a continuing focus on the manner by which development of the tectum lays down the cellular network that serves as the target for incoming retinal ganglion fibers. The issue of specificity is exemplified nowhere better than in the case of the retinotectal projection. Finally the genesis, migration and settling patterns of neurons are seen most remarkably in the cerebellum where neurodevelopment and metamorphic regulation become intertwined.

In its entirety, this volume is directed to the fact that the developing frog is a favorable model for delving into the primary processes of neural development: neuron generation, neuron migration, neuron differentiation, neuron growth and maturation, and neuron death. Through temporally restricted interactions and a rigorous sequence of events, the individual neurons become integrated into a unified, functional nervous system.

THE EARLY DEVELOPMENT OF NEURONS IN XENOPUS EMBRYOS REVEALED BY TRANSMITTER IMMUNOCYTOCHEMISTRY FOR SEROTONIN, GABA AND GLYCINE

Alan Roberts

Department of Zoology, University of Bristol, Bristol, BS8 1UG, England

INTRODUCTION

Immunocytochemistry offers exciting prospects of breakthroughs in our understanding of how neuronal growth cones navigate a correct course to their targets. However, before pathway selection can be studied we need to know what cell classes are present and how each class of cell develops to establish its normal dendritic arbor and axonal projection. Immunocytochemistry can help here as well. Antibodies are now available which recognize a number of neuronal transmitter substances. Among these, three have been applied to the developing nervous system of the amphibian Xenopus laevis. These antibodies reveal cells which may use serotonin, GABA or glycine as their transmitter at very early stages in their morphological differentiation. We can therefore, ask a series of questions about each specific cell class: When and where do the first immunoreactive cells of each class appear? At what stage of differentiation is transmitter first expressed? What is the pattern of early axonal outgrowth and growth cone behaviour? How does the population expand? In this chapter I will review the results from recent studies on the early development (up to hatching) of five classes of neuron in Xenopus embryos and then see whether any general conclusions can be drawn about the first steps in the morphological differentiation of spinal cord neurons.

SEROTONIN

Methods for revealing serotonin have been available for some time and have been used to study the development of raphespinal cells in the hindbrain of some representative vertebrates (fish: Ekström et al., 1985; Amphibian: Sims, 1977; bird: Wallace, 1975; Mammal: Lidov and Molliver, 1982; Wallace and Lauder, 1983). In Xenopus, van Mier et al. (1986) showed that serotonin-like immunoreactive (SER) cells first appeared in the

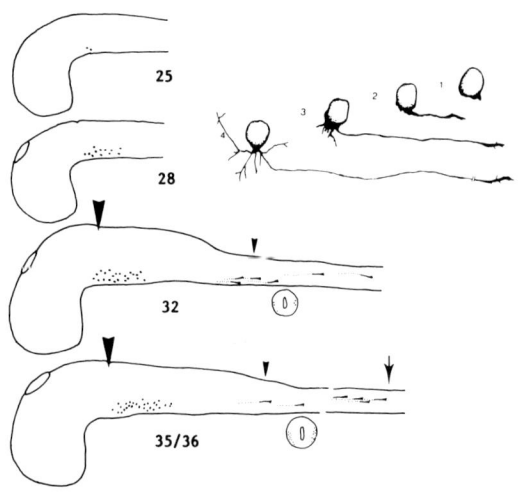

Figure 1. Development of hindbrain raphespinal neurons with serotonin-like immunoreactivity in Xenopus embryos, at the stages indicated, seen in lateral views of the brain and spinal cord. Hindbrain extends from large arrowhead to obex at small arrowhead. Arrow indicates level of anus. Scale: 200 µm. Caudally directed growth cone shows extent of projection into spinal cord. In these and all subsequent lateral views, somata are shown only on one side of the nervous system. (Redrawn from van Mier et al., 1986.) Inset: numbered steps in the development of hindbrain SER raphespinal neurons. (From van Mier et al., 1986.) Lateral view: caudal to the right.

rostral hindbrain at stage 25 (Nieuwkoop and Faber, 1956) about five hours after closure of the neural tube (Fig. 1). Fifteen hours later, at stage 32, a population of about 20 raphespinal neurons is present on each side of the hindbrain and SER axons extend into the spinal cord. By the time of hatching, stage 37/38, SER axons have reached the level of the anus and are distributed throughout the dorsoventral extent of the marginal zone of the mid-trunk spinal cord.

At the cellular level, serotonin-like immunoreactivity was first expressed in cells at the stage when their initial axonal growth cone was forming. It was clear in both axons and growth cones, and allowed a series of steps in the development of a SER raphespinal neuron to be defined (Fig. 1). This series of pictures also suggests that a single axon is produced and is directed caudally, before dendrites begin to grow.

GABA

Antibodies to the complexes formed by gamma-amino butyric acid (GABA) during glutaraldehyde fixation were first described by Storm-Mathisen et al. (1983). In the Xenopus embryo these antibodies have been used to follow the development of two classes of spinal cord neuron and one class of hindbrain neuron. These now will be considered in turn.

Kolmer-Agduhr (K-A) cells (Dale et al., 1987a) are spinal cerebrospinal fluid-contacting neurons with cilia and microvilli protruding into the spinal canal (neurocoel) and an ascending ipsilateral axon. They label strongly for GABA. Similar neurons are present in the spinal cords of all vertebrate groups (Agduhr, 1922; Kolmer, 1921; Vigh and Vigh-Teichmann, 1973) and show GABA-like immunoreactivity in rats (Barber et al., 1982). Their function is unknown. K-A cells are first labeled by the GABA antiserum at stage 25 in the rostral spinal cord (Fig. 2; Dale et al., 1987b). In subsequent stages, K-A cells are added more caudally, and also by in-fill between the more precocious cells. There is, therefore, a clear rostrocaudal developmental gradient. At the caudal end of the cell column labeled cells are seen, well separated from each other and with a single,

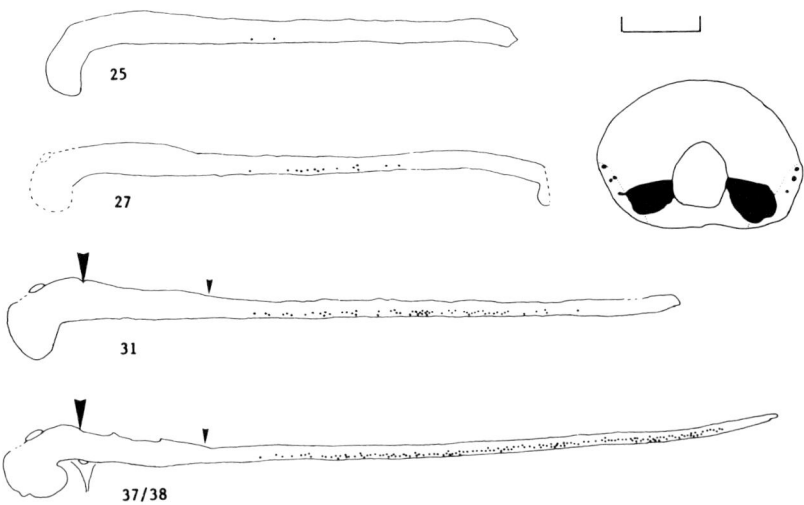

Figure 2. Development of spinal Kolmer-Agduhr (K-A) cells with GABA-like immunoreactivity at stages indicated. Conventions as in Fig. 1. Transverse section shows K-A cells in caudal spinal cord at stage 37/38, scale: 30 µm. Scale for side views: 400 µm. (Redrawn after Dale et al., 1987a,b.)

heavily labeled growth cone (Fig. 3). Since K-A cells have no dendrites, these must be axonal growth cones. Such growth cones which had extended less than 60 µm are always directed rostrally with a mean deviation from the longitudinal axis of 16.8° (S.D. 13.7°, n = 12). K-A cell growth cones can fasciculate with other labeled axons, but this is not necessary to establish their rostral direction of growth (see Fig. 3a).

Ascending interneurons are the second class of spinal neuron with GABA-like immunoreactivity (Roberts et al., 1987). By stage 37/38 these neurons form a longitudinal column of cells on either side, in the dorsal half of the spinal cord (Fig. 4). They have ascending axons, and dendrites in the dorsal half of the marginal zone. These neurons are first labeled at stage 26 in

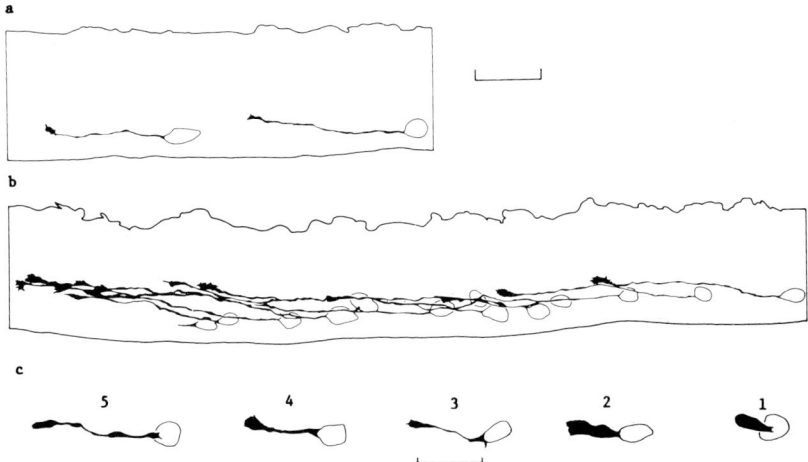

Figure 3. Axon outgrowth from Kolmer-Agduhr cells. Camera lucida drawing in lateral view: (a) wholemount spinal cord at stage 25 and (b) at stage 29/30; (c) series of cells showing stages in early axon outgrowth. Rostral to left. Scale: (a) and (b) 40 µm; (c) 30 µm. (Redrawn from Dale et al., 1987b.)

the caudal hindbrain. By stage 28 their axonal projection is clear as they lie in an ascending tract of labeled axons with ascending growth cones at its rostral end in the hindbrain (Fig. 4). The population of labeled ascending interneurons increases by addition of cells at the caudal end of the column and by in-fill. The initial outgrowth of the axon was not revealed clearly by the antibody labeling, but no caudally directed growth cones were seen and the tract formed by these cells was fairly compact (Fig. 4). The pattern of axon outgrowth is, therefore, reliable and rostral. Dendritic growth cones were also seen emerging from the somata of these neurons, forming an increasingly complex arbor in the dorsal half of the marginal zone.

The third class of cells with GABA-like immunoreactivity are mid-hindbrain reticulospinal neurons (Roberts et al., 1987). These neurons have a bilateral

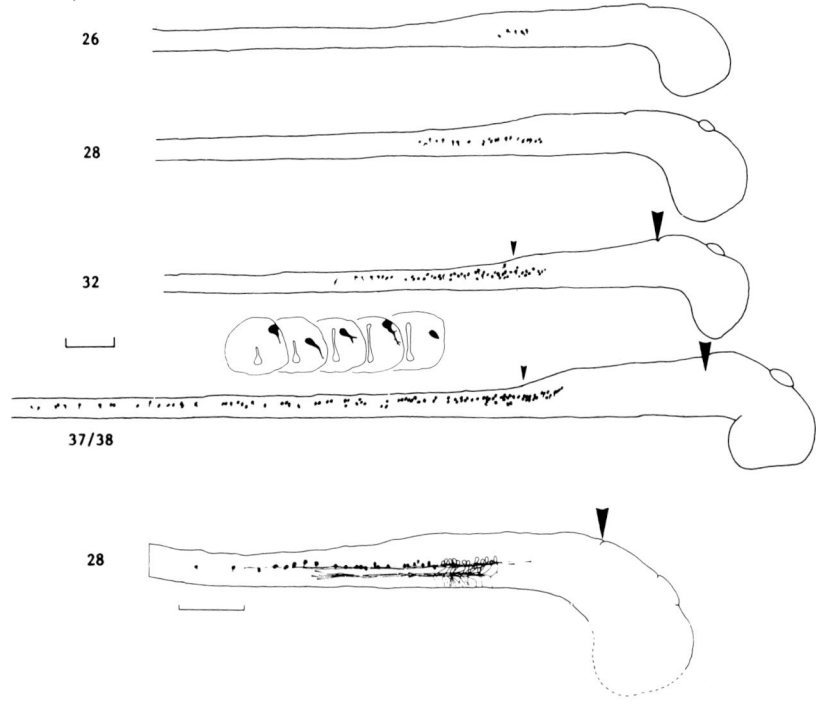

Figure 4. Development of "ascending" interneurons with GABA-like immunoreactivity at stages indicated. Transverse sections show location of somata at stage 37/38 (scale: 60 µm). Lowest drawing (scale: 150 µm) shows ascending somata (filled) and mid-hindbrain reticulospinal somata (clear) with their axons forming dorsal ascending tracts respectively. Scale for upper wholemounts: 200 µm. (Redrawn from Roberts et al., 1987.)

projection to the spinal cord. When first labeled at stage 25 or 26 (Fig. 5) each cell has a single ventral axon which crosses under the hindbrain. By stage 28 these crossed axons have turned caudally to form a clear descending tract in the ventral half of the spinal marginal zone (Fig. 4). However, from stage 28 onwards many of these cells show an ipsilateral descending axon and growth cone. The cells therefore project to both

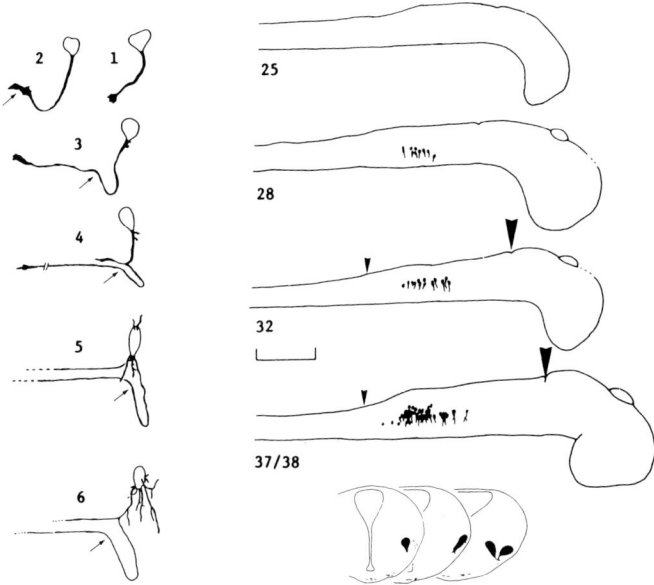

Figure 5. Development of mid-hindbrain reticulospinal neurons with GABA-like immunoreactivity at stages indicated. Transverse sections show location at stage 37/38 (scale: 74 µm). Diagrams (1) to (6) on the left are based on camera lucida drawings of lateral views. They show how descending contra- and ipsilateral axons and mainly dorsoventral dendrites develop (scale: 56 µm). Arrows show where contralateral axons reach the marginal zone on opposite side. (Partly redrawn from Roberts et al., 1987.)

sides of the spinal cord by growing a secondary ipsilateral axon which often forms as a branch from the first decussating axon (Fig. 5). Dendrites are extended from the initial segment of the axon and from the soma into the marginal zone. They tend to form after the axon is well developed.

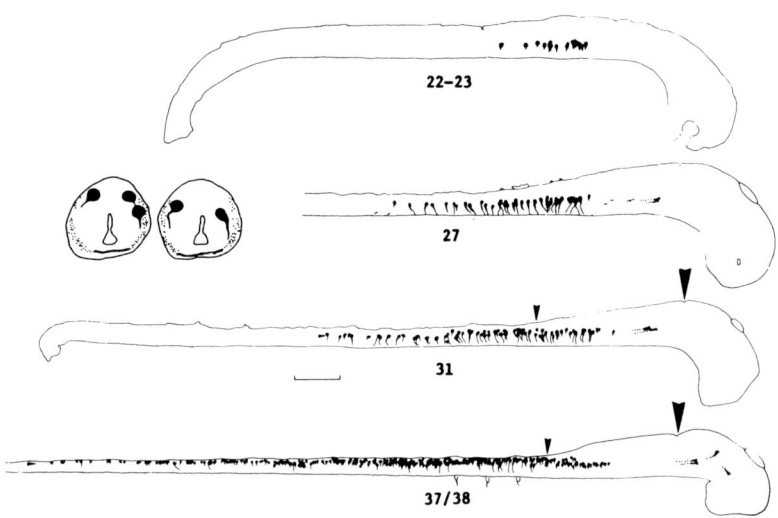

Figure 6. Development of "commissural" interneurons with glycine-like immunoreactivity at stage indicated. The most rostral and caudal labeled growth cones (out of scale) indicate the extent of GLY axonal projections. Transverse sections show locations of somata and GLY labeled axons in the spinal cord at stage 37/38 (scale: 60 µm). Scale: 200 µm.

GLYCINE

In the Xenopus embryo spinal cord a class of reciprocal inhibitory interneurons producing strychnine-sensitive inhibition have been identified anatomically (Dale, 1985). It has now been shown that these same "commissural" interneurons have glycine-like immunoreactivity (GLY) (Dale et al., 1986). The glycine antibody has therefore been used to follow the development of this class of spinal interneuron (Roberts et al., in preparation). "Commissural" interneurons first label for GLY at an earlier stage of development than the cells described above. They are present in the caudal hindbrain/cervical spinal cord as the neural tube is just closing at stage 22 to 23 (Fig. 6). Numbers then

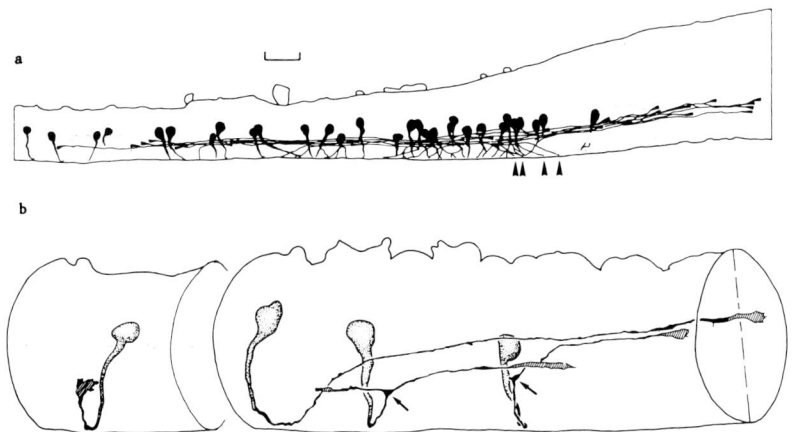

Figure 7. Axonal projections of "commissural" interneurons with GLY seen in lateral view. (a) All labeled cells and clear growth cones on one side at stage 27. Ventral decussating axons are clear. Arrowheads show caudally directed axons of rostral cells on other side of hindbrain (scale: 60 µm). (b) Cells illustrating stages in the development of contralateral projections: growth cones hatched, rostral to right (scale: 17 µm).

increase by caudal addition and by in-fill, as with the other spinal cell classes.

Early stages in differentiation can be seen most clearly at the caudal end of the cell column from stage 27 onwards. "Commissural" interneurons usually first show GLY when their axon has already grown ventrally and circumferentially to cross the floor-plate and reach the opposite side (Fig. 7). In the ventral marginal zone on the contralateral side the growth cones either turn rostrally or branch to descend and ascend. In each case their direction of growth changes, from ventral and circumferential to longitudinal. The axons of most cells initially grow rostrally. However, cells at the rostral end of the cell column, in the hindbrain, grow an axon first in a caudal direction (arrowheads in Fig. 7). Since all "commissural" interneurons revealed by intracellular marker injection had both caudal and rostral contralateral axons (Soffe et al., 1984; Dale, 1985) it is likely that secondary descending axons are formed later, rather in the way that the ipsilateral descending axon is formed in mid-hindbrain reticulospinal neurons. In a minority of cases a secondary axon forms ipsilateral to the soma. Dendrites of "commissural" interneurons grow from the initial segment of the axon laterally into the marginal zone. They are not very clear in wholemounts but are beginning to form as soon as the axonal growth cone has reached the opposite side.

CONCLUSIONS

Transmitter immunocytochemistry has allowed early stages in the differentiation of a number of different neuron classes to be seen in wholemount preparations of the developing Xenopus nervous system. Large numbers of cells have been studied for each cell class and at each developmental stage. These observations can be related to those obtained on the early stages of spinal neuron development using reduced silver and Golgi staining (Ramón y Cajal, 1890; Barron, 1944; Hughes, 1959; Wentworth, 1984), TEM reconstruction (Holley and Silver, 1987) and horseradish peroxidase injection into blastomeres (Jacobson and Huang, 1985). A number of general features emerge from these studies.

Initial Axon Growth

Firstly, initial axon growth is in a specific direction for each class of neuron. Of the evidence reviewed here the Kolmer-Agduhr cells provide the clearest example (Dale et al., 1987b). The single growth cones seen emerging from K-A somata were all rostrally directed (see Fig. 3). In other cell classes where growth cones were not labeled so close to the soma there was no evidence for any "misdirected" other axons in the process of retraction. This all points to the orientation of axonal outgrowth being determined before the growth cone is produced.

Secondly, within the marginal zones of the spinal cord and hindbrain initial axon outgrowth is limited for the cells I have described to one of three orientations: ascending longitudinal (Kolmer-Agduhr cells, ascending interneurons), descending longitudinal (raphespinal neurons), and ventral circumferential (commissural interneurons, mid-hindbrain reticulospinal neurons). Of cells described previously in Xenopus, Rohon-Beard neurons have ascending and descending initial projections (Jacobson and Huang, 1985), and motor neurons have descending central projections (Hughes, 1959). There are, therefore, no examples of initial axon outgrowth in a dorsal or strongly oblique orientation. This limited range of orientations implies a very limited number of controlling factors.

Thirdly, each of the cell classes confined to the CNS and described above in Xenopus has a single axon which forms before the dendrites appear (cf. Barron, 1944). The single axon may branch at a distance from the soma, but the soma only seems to "allow" one axon (cf. Dotti and Banker, 1987). In contrast, primary sensory Rohon-Beard neurons with peripheral neurites and lying in the dorsal spinal cord do not follow this rule and have a bipolar soma with ascending and descending axons (Jacobson and Huang, 1985).

Fourthly, each neuron is a pioneer and has initial outgrowth in an appropriate direction without contact with its peers. This was particularly clear for commissural interneurons and Kolmer-Agduhr cells where, at the caudal end of the cell column, individual neurons could be seen as having grown an axon before contacting labeled peers. The same conclusion was reached by Holley and Silver (1987) after serial reconstruction of neurons in the chick spinal cord. In the vertebrate CNS there seems to be little evidence that the first cells to differentiate within a class are different from those which appear later. The whole concept of pioneers whose specialized properties or random growth establishes pathways to be followed by later cells does not appear to have been substantiated (cf. Harrison, 1910; Weiss, 1950). Even after contacting their peers, the growing CNS axons in the Xenopus embryo spinal cord do not seem to show a very strong tendency to form tight fascicles either when growing longitudinally in the marginal zone, or when growing circumferentially in the floor-plate. They can fasciculate but also defasciculate. In the marginal zone growth is broadly longitudinal and may be facilitated by the tendency for growing along other axons, but this process is not slavish as might be expected of axons whose only mode of navigation was fasciculation with their peers.

Expression of Transmitter

In cultured motoneurons of Xenopus and chick (Young and Poo, 1983; Hume et al., 1983) acetylcholine may be released from growth cones. Antibodies labeling 'serotonin', 'GABA' and 'glycine' now suggest that these transmitters are also present in the growth cones of various classes of neuron in the CNS. In all cases, transmitter labeling was present by the time the growth cone had extended less than 100 µm from the soma. For the cerebrospinal fluid-contacting Kolmer-Agduhr cells, labeling for GABA was present as the initial axonal growth cone emerged from the soma. This evidence suggests, furthermore, that process growth and transmitter expression are initiated more or less synchronously. Since specific transmitter uptake systems (Lamborghini and Iles, 1985) and receptors (Bixby and Spitzer, 1984) appear at similar stages of development, it is possible that all these features may be co-induced by the same developmental switch (Dale et al., 1987b).

The transmitter antibodies suggest that transmitter molecules are located throughout the cell and its processes. By revealing the whole cell, and the whole population of each class of cell, we have been able to follow the development of both individual morphology and the whole population. The rostrocaudal developmental gradient has been graphically displayed. For the spinal cell classes, we have seen that each population first appears in a rostral position and is then increased by two processes: caudal addition and in-fill between earlier differentiating cells. This is similar to the pattern described for sensory Rohon-Beard cells by Lamborghini (1980).

PROSPECT

I have reviewed the pattern of development of five

classes of neuron in the spinal cord and hindbrain of the Xenopus embryo on the basis of evidence from cell labeling using antibodies to complexes formed by putative transmitter molecules. These techniques open the door to similar studies in other groups to test the generality of the conclusions from Xenopus. They offer opportunities for experimental manipulation and give new insights into the anatomy of the spinal cord. These now need to be investigated in an effort to relate each developing population of neurons to a role in generating the developing behaviour of these simple vertebrates (Roberts et al., 1986).

REFERENCES

Agduhr E (1922). Über ein zentrales Sinnesorgan bei den Vertebraten. Z Anat Entwickl 66:223-360.

Barber RP, Vaughn JE, Roberts E (1982). The cytoarchitecture of GABAergic neurons in rat spinal cord. Brain Res 238:305-328.

Barron DH (1944). The early development of the sensory and internuncial cells in the spinal cord of the sheep. J Comp Neurol 81:193-225.

Bixby JL, Spitzer NC (1984). The appearance and development of neurotransmitter sensitivity in Xenopus embryonic spinal neurones in vitro. J Physiol (Lond) 353:143-155.

Dale N (1985). Reciprocal inhibitory interneurons in the Xenopus embryo spinal cord. J Physiol (Lond) 363:61-70.

Dale N, Ottersen OP, Roberts A, Storm-Mathisen J (1986). Inhibitory neurones of a motor pattern generator in Xenopus revealed by antibodies to glycine. Nature 324:255-257,

Dale N, Roberts A, Ottersen OP, Storm-Mathisen J (1987a). The morphology and distribution of "Kolmer-Agduhr" cells, a class of cerebrospinal fluid-contacting neurons revealed in the frog embryo spinal cord by GABA immunocytochemistry. Proc Roy Soc B 232:193-203.

Dale N, Roberts A, Ottersen OP, Storm-Mathisen J (1987b). The development of a population of spinal cord neurons and their axonal projections revealed by GABA immunocytochemistry. Proc Roy Soc B 232:205-215.

Dotti CG, Banker GA (1987). Experimentally induced

alteration in the polarity of developing neurons. Nature 330:254-256.

Ekström P, Nyberg L, van Veen T (1985). Ontogenetic development of serotonergic neurons in the brain of a teleost, the three-spined stickleback. An immunohistochemical analysis. Develop Brain Res 17:209-224.

Harrison RG (1910). The outgrowth of the nerve fibre as a mode of protoplasmic movement. J Exp Zool 9:787-848.

Holley JA, Silver J (1987). Growth pattern of pioneering chick spinal cord axons. Develop Biol 123:375-388.

Hughes A (1959). Studies in embryonic and larval development in Amphibia. II. The spinal motor root. J Embryol Exp Morphol 7:128-145.

Hume RI, Role LW, Fischbach GD (1983). Acetylcholine release from growth cones detected with patches of acetylcholine receptor-rich membranes. Nature 305:632-634.

Jacobson M, Huang S (1985). Neurite outgrowth traced by means of horseradish peroxidase inherited from neuronal ancestral cells in frog embryos. Develop Biol 110:102-113.

Kolmer W (1921). Das "Sagitallorgan" der Wirbeltiere. Z Anatl Entwickl 60:652-717.

Lamborghini JE (1980). Rohon-Beard cells and other large neurons in Xenopus embryos originate during gastrulation. J Comp Neurol 189:323-333.

Lamborghini JE, Iles A (1985). Development of a high affinity GABA uptake system in embryonic amphibian spinal neurons. Develop Biol 112:167-176.

Lidov HGW, Molliver ME (1982). Immunohistochemical study of the development of serotonergic neurons in the rat CNS. Brain Res Bull 9:559-604.

Nieuwkoop PD, Faber J (1956). "Normal Tables of Xenopus laevis (Daudin)." Amsterdam: North-Holland.

Ramón y Cajal S (1890). A quelle époque apparaissent les expansions des cellules nerveuse de la moëlle épinière du poulet? Anat Anz 5:609-613, 631-639.

Roberts A, Dale N, Ottersen OP, Storm-Mathisen J (1987). The early development of interneurons with GABA immunoreactivity in the central nervous system of Xenopus laevis embryos. J Comp Neurol 261:435-449.

Roberts A, Soffe SR, Dale N (1986). Spinal interneurons and swimming in frog embryos. In Grillner S, Stein PGS, Stuart DG, Forssberg H, Herman RM (eds):

"Neurobiology of Vertebrate Locomotion." London: Macmillan, pp 279-306.

Sims TJ (1977). The development of monoamine-containing neurons in the brain and spinal cord of the salamander, Ambystoma mexicanum. J Comp Neurol 173:319-336.

Soffe SR, Clarke , Roberts A (1984). Activity of commissural interneurones in spinal cord of Xenopus embryos. J Neurophysiol 51:1257-1267.

Storm-Mathisen J, Leknes AK, Bore AT, Vaaland JL, Edminson P, Haug FS, Ottersen OP (1983). First visualisation of glutamate and GABA in neurones by immunocytochemistry. Nature 301:517-520.

van Mier P, Joosten HWJ, van Rheden R, ten Donkelaar HJ (1986). The development of serotonergic raphespinal projections in Xenopus laevis. Int J Develop Neurosci 4:465-476.

Vigh B, Vigh-Teichmann I (1973). Comparative ultrastructure of the cerebrospinal fluid-contacting neurons. Int Rev Cytol 35:189-251.

Wallace JA (1985). An immunocytochemical study of the development of central serotonergic neurons in the chick embryo. J Comp Neurol 236:443-453.

Wallace JA, Lauder JM (1983). Development of the serotonergic system in the rat embryo: an immunocytochemical study. Brain Res Bull 10:459-479.

Weiss P (1950). Deplantation of fragments of nervous system in amphibians. I. Central reorganization and the formation of nerves. J Exp Zool 113:397-461.

Wentworth LE (1984). The development of the cervical spinal cord of the mouse embryo. II. A Golgi analysis of sensory, commissural and association cell differentiation. J Comp Neurol 222:96-115.

Young SH, Poo MM (1983). Spontaneous release of transmitter from growth cones of embryonic neurones. Nature 305:634-637.

TOWARD AN UNDERSTANDING OF TECTAL DEVELOPMENT IN FROGS

Jerry J. Kollros

Department of Biology, University of Iowa, Iowa City, Iowa 52242

INTRODUCTION

It has been known for some 80 years (Steinitz, 1906) that removal of one eye rudiment from a frog embryo or larva produces optic tecta of two quite different sizes by the time of metamorphosis. The tectum contralateral to the operation (since optic nerve decussation is essentially complete) is considerably smaller than the ipsilateral control tectum. Additional details were provided by Dürken (1913, 1930), and by Larsell (1929, 1931) in Hyla regilla. However, the mechanism responsible for these different tectal sizes was not elucidated. Later studies in fish implicated failure of the tectal cells to grow (Pflugfelder, 1952), or failure of the usual number of cells to differentiate (Leghissa, 1951). Meanwhile, it had been shown in the chick that, following early unilateral eye rudiment removal, the two tecta developed in identical fashion through the first 12 days of incubation, after which substantial degeneration and cell death was seen in the deprived tectum (Filogamo, 1950). In 1953, however, it was shown by Kollros that removal of the embryonic eye is followed, early in larval life (by stage V), by a reduction of cell proliferation in the tectum which lacked optic fiber input, and that the reduction in mitotic activity increased progressively with developmental stage to the period of metamorphic climax, such that the disparities in cell production rates were calculated to be adequate to account for the progressively increasing differences in cell numbers between the two tecta. This method of tectal size adjustment, i.e., by reduced mitotic activity as a result of reduced fiber input into the brain, appears to be unique to anurans. Even so, this method has apparently failed to gain the acceptance it deserves (Jacobson, 1978; Hamburger and Oppenheim, 1982; Purves and Lichtman, 1985). Even Currie and Cowan (1974), who record the same phenomenon, and seek to limit it to reduced glial cell production, exclude the possibility that neuronal production is involved. Further data (Kollros, 1982; Kollros and Thiesse, 1988; Kollros, unpubl.) in Hyla, Pseudacris, Rana and Xenopus, however, provide additional documentation of significant impact of unilateral enucleation upon contralateral mitotic rates; hence, the current dogma which denies or fails to recognize such effects requires immediate rectification. Also requiring rectification is the assumption (Currie and Cowan, 1974) that such differences in mitotic rate as do occur are accounted for entirely by smaller numbers of glial cells, an assumption stated positively by Cowan (1981), but only on the basis of the assumptions presented in the 1974 work with Currie (op. cit.), and also emphasized by Jacobson (1978). Just prior to the end of metamorphosis, when mitotic figures are scarce, differences in division rates between the two sides are no longer consistent.

The early embryonic tectum (Shumway stage 22 or earlier) is composed exclusively of cells, from ependyma to pial border. The first invasion of optic nerve fibers is visible at stage 23, in a small zone near the rostral pole of the tectum (Currie and Cowan, 1975), and it is here that the first cells leave the common core of deep layers to migrate into this superficial neuropil (Kollros, 1953). The coverage of the tectum by optic nerve fibers proceeds fairly rapidly at first, and then more slowly, so that more medial and more caudal regions are covered (Fig. 1); not until the very end of the larval period is such coverage of the tectum complete (Currie and Cowan, 1975). Meanwhile, the superficial neuropil has thickened, and cells from the deeper layers have invaded it, creating distinctive layers 7, 8, and 9. Somewhat later the deeper thin neuropil layers appear, layer 5 before layer 3. The layering is first apparent at the rostral pole of the tectum, extends caudad, and is best appreciated in parasagittal sections over stages

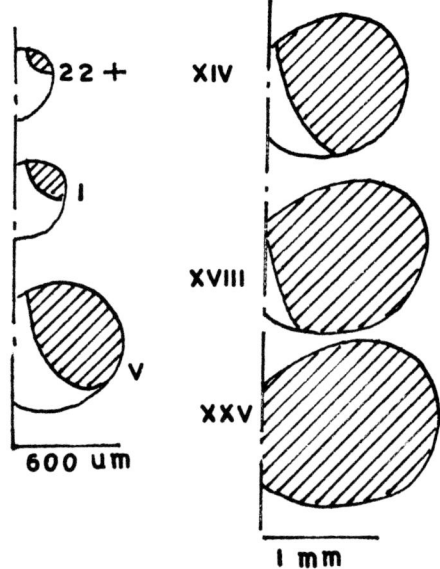

Figure 1. Progressive spread of optic nerve fibers over the developing tectum of Rana pipiens. Data of Currie and Cowan (1975) were used in constructing these representations.

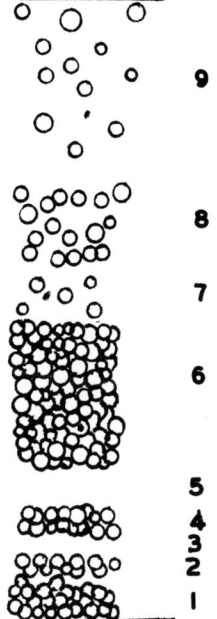

Figure 2. A short segment of the midtectum at metamorphic climax is represented to show the cellular layering. Layers 3 and 5 are fiber layers alone; some seven fiber layers interlace with the scattered cells of layers 7-8-9. The cells of layers 2, 4, and 6 are generally tightly packed, with overlapping nuclear profiles.

I through X^+. The cellular lamination of the tectum is shown in Fig. 2, although the complexities of fiber layering in layers 7-8-9 (see Lázár, 1984, for these details) are not included.

Tectal cell divisions, from early larval stages onward, are distributed throughout the tectum, but always with more divisions caudad than rostrad (Kollros, 1953, 1982; Kollros and Thiesse, 1988; Eichler, 1971; Straznicky and Gaze, 1972; Currie, 1974; Currie and Cowan, 1974). The autoradiographic study of Straznicky and Gaze (1972) led them to interpret tectal growth in Xenopus as a series of "wedges", with new cells being produced exclusively near the midline in a somewhat broader band caudad than craniad. Each newly formed "wedge" pushed the older tectal elements laterad and rostrad. Their Figure 30 is unequivocal in this matter; further, it suggests that less than one-sixth of the tectum is formed after stage 54. This interpretation of tectal growth was accepted by Currie and Cowan (1974), even though the plot of distribution of mitotic figures at stage XIV failed to conform to such a concept and presented a very broad medial "wedge". Other investigators have also accepted the "wedge" concept. Data are now available to refute it, or at least to require major modifications of it (e.g., Eichler, 1971; Kollros and Thiesse, 1988; Kollros, unpubl.).

Cell death is involved in the final determination of cell number in a variety of structures, including many cell groups in the nervous system (Glücksman, 1951; Jacobson, 1978; Purves and Lichtman, 1985). There has been, however, no mention of cell death by the host of researchers who have dealt with retinotectal relationships in postmetamorphic frogs, nor by the early investigators of tectal development in frogs, nor by Currie and Cowan (1974). Kollros (1953) reported that larval enucleation was followed by both reduction in mitotic activity and by cell death. Later (1982) he reported very limited numbers of pyknotic cells in both control and deprived tecta in stage III through V tadpoles, but concluded that a significant role of cell death in determining final tectal cell numbers in normal animals was very unlikely. Careful and extensive studies of later larval stages (Kollros and Thiesse, 1988; Kollros, unpubl.) require a revision of this view, and it can now be reported that pyknotic cell numbers increase during larval life almost to the start of metamorphic climax, fall thereafter, and are virtually absent by three weeks after the end of metamorphosis. Further, if an eye is removed from a larva, increased rates of cell death are invariably seen in the contralateral tectum within 24 hours. The frog, therefore, displays both cell death and reduced rates of cell production as methods of controlling tectal cell number following enucleation. The details of tectal cell formation and the impact of eye removal at different stages, in several frog species, follow.

MATERIALS AND METHODS

Procedures for the study of larval R. pipiens are given in Kollros and Thiesse (1988). They include fixation in Bouin's fluid, serial section at 10 µm, and staining with hematoxylin and light green. R. pipiens eggs were obtained from frogs purchased from Kons Scientific, Germantown, WI. Eggs of R. sylvatica were collected by Robyn Lilehei in Missouri and Minnesota. Xenopus eggs were purchased from Carolina Biological Supply Co., Burlington, NC. Hyla and Pseudacris were collected as eggs and tadpoles in Iowa City. These several species were treated in the same fashion as R. pipiens. In all cases, experimental animals were maintained singly in one liter of water at 20°C, fed commercial canned spinach, and operated upon under urethane anesthesia.

RESULTS

Mitotic Activity

Mitoses have been counted in every tectal section in several species of anurans. Fig. 3 displays the counts in single tecta of control animals or in the control tectum of animals following unilateral enucleation. The data on R. pipiens, with peak activity at stage X are from Kollros and Thiesse (1988). Comparable data on Hyla versicolor are also presented, with a slightly later peak of mitotic activity. This delay correlates well with fragmentary data on the other hylid,

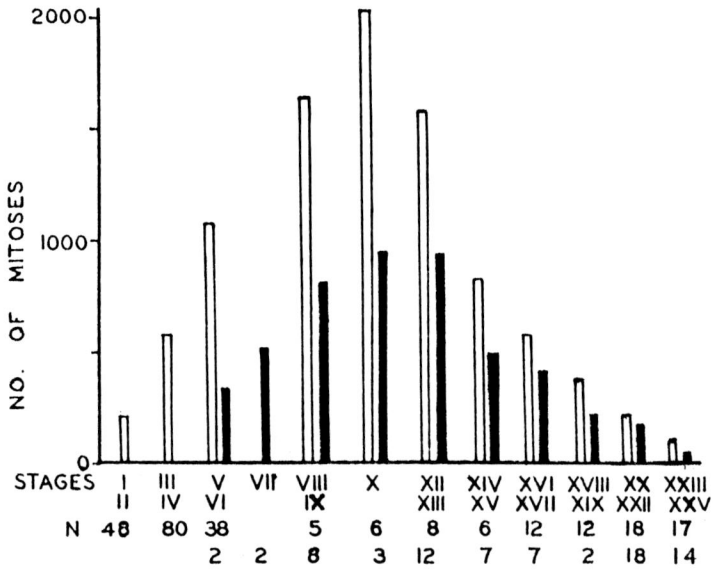

Figure 3. Mean numbers of mitoses in control tecta of R. pipiens (open bars and upper N values) and Hyla versicolor (solid bars and lower N values) larvae.

Pseudacris triseriata, also small and rapidly developing. The Rana data correlates well with information on Xenopus laevis (Table 1), with peak mitotic activity at stages comparable to those of peak activity in R. pipiens. In all of these species the numbers of mitotic figures near the end of metamorphosis are reduced to below 10% of the peak values, and just after metamorphosis mitotic figures are either entirely absent, or nearly so.

For R. pipiens it has been calculated that the figures seen at any instant of fixation represent less than 10% of the figures which might be accounted for in a 24 hour period. Thus in R. pipiens, if one animal were to be fixed every day of an average larval period, from stage I through XXV (stages of Taylor and Kollros, 1946), some 85,000 division figures would be seen;

TABLE 1. Mitoses in Control Xenopus Tecta

Stage	N	Range	Mean	±S.E.
47	1		136	
51	5	333-448	386	21
53	3	564-621	599	13
54[a]	1		646	
55[a]	3	481-729	574	58
56	9	255-563	355	63
57	2	239-455	347	
58	2	176-258	217	
59	1		113	
60	6	95-182	131	11
61	7	31-92	56	8
62	5	31-73	43	7
63	2	46-52	49	
64	7	25-72	42	6
65	5	32-48	39	3
66	8	12-71	48	7

[a]Stages with peak numbers, equivalent to stages IX to XI of Rana pipiens.

however, it is likely that close to 1,000,000 cells are produced during the larval period, substantially more than survive at stage XXV or in early postmetamorphic periods (see Cell Numbers below).

Whenever an eye rudiment is removed from an embryo of R. pipiens a reduced rate of mitotic activity is recorded in the contralateral tectum, but not until 15 or more days later, i.e., at stages III⁺ or IV. On the other hand, if enucleation is performed in larval stages V or later, the differences in rate ordinarily appear by three to five days after the operation. In all of these cases, the longer the time or stage interval between enucleation and fixation, the greater will be the disparity between sides in rates of mitotic activity. For example, early larval enucleation coupled with fixation in larval stages XVII or later produces differences of 50% or more. What requires emphasis is the fact that

TABLE 2. Reductions in Mitotic Activity (in %) 3 to 9 Days After Eye Removal at the Stages Indicated

	(R. pipiens)[a]					
Days Postop.	3	4	5	7	9	Mean
Stages						
XIII	3	7	31	27	34	20
XVI or XVII	5	20	37	49	37	30
XIX or XX	25	26	17	24	20	23
Mean	11	18	28	33	30	24

[a]Each figure represents one animal.

ingrowing optic nerve fibers spread only gradually over the tectum (Fig. 1), and the differences in mitotic activity can be seen only in those tectal regions which have been deprived of optic fiber input. Those regions of the tectum not yet covered by such fibers show essentially identical rates of cell divisions on the two sides. Thus, as an increasing fraction of the tectum becomes covered by retinal fibers, the degree of difference in division activity between sides becomes enhanced. Limiting the study to periods of three to nine days after unilateral enucleation, with an average between five and six days, about 10% difference develops at stage V. It is 20% by stage XIII and 30% by stage XVI, with decreasing values for series initiated later (Table 2) when mitotic activity is greatly reduced. In each of these, however, had samples been taken after nine days, the disparities between the two sides would have been still greater, except perhaps for the most advanced stages. Such differences are more accentuated rostrad than caudad throughout development, in correlation with the greater coverage of the tectum by retinal fibers, even though the numbers of dividing cells are always greater caudad. The results given above for R. pipiens are duplicated in other species, so far as degree of tectal involvement is concerned. For the small hylids, however, the reduction of mitotic activity correlates better with developmental age than with stage. By the end of the larval period in Pseudacris, for example, the maximum differences in mitotic rates are closer to 30% than the 50% seen in R. pipiens.

Ependymal Area

All of the early studies on the effects of early unilateral enucleation reported a reduction of tectal dimensions in all three planes, and a reduction in size (e.g., ependymal area) of the tectal ventricles (Kollros, 1953). The degree of reduction in ependymal surface area and of numbers of mitotic figures are virtually the same at early larval stages (Kollros, 1982), but later the drop in mitotic activity outpaces the reduction in ependymal surface. In contrast, when enucleations are performed in late larval stages (Kollros and Thiesse, 1988), the reduction in mitotic activity is rather rapid (Table 2), while the impact on ependymal area is relatively slow and of lesser magnitude. Incomplete data on Hyla and Xenopus reveal the same kind of responses as in Rana.

Cell Death

In large control tecta of advanced larval stages of R. pipiens there may be over 6,000 cells on each side in 10 µm transverse sections. If layers 7-8-9 are scanned in one sweep, thick layer 6 in another, and layers 2 through 4 in a third, some five to seven minutes are required for inspecting each section. Obviously, one cannot focus on each individual nucleus, but with even limited experience the non-standard profiles of pyknotic nuclei stand out. These can then be focused upon, and determination made as to whether or not the nucleus is pyknotic. Frequently, tinctorial differences appear, particularly if the nucleus has more than the usual very thin rim of cytoplasm surrounding it. Of the 6,000 cells per side per section, at the time of maximum cell death, only about three nuclei will be identified as pyknotic. Pyknoses, however, are not limited to the advanced larval stages, but are present even at stage IV or earlier (ca. 30 per side). Their numbers increase gradually to a flat peak of about 300 per side at stages XV through XX, and then decline slowly, with cell death continuing at decreasing rates for about the first three postmetamorphic weeks (Fig. 4). The structural alterations which accompany pyknosis in large neurons make them easy to identify, and at 20°C they are identifiable for about three hours (lateral motor column cells in Xenopus -- Hughes, 1961; mesencephalic fifth nucleus cells in R. pipiens -- Kollros, 1984). The much smaller cells and nuclei of the optic tectum, however, make the positive identification of early phases of pyknosis less certain. Hence, estimates of the time required for cell degeneration appear to be much reduced, i.e., to from 50 to 80 minutes (Kollros and Thiesse, 1988). The actual period of time for cell degeneration is not known, but other methods of obtaining this information may yield somewhat longer intervals for these small cells. While no attempt was made to duplicate the work of Currie and Cowan (1975) in establishing the spread of optic nerve fibers over the tectum, it was evident that cell death in control tecta was strongly limited to the areas already reached by optic nerve fibers. Thus at early larval stages, at least the posterior one-third of the tectum failed to display pyknotic cells. With advancing stage ever larger fractions of this region did show cell death, until in late metamorphic climax and postmetamorphically all tectal levels showed some cell death.

When larvae were enucleated unilaterally in stages IV through XXV, there was increased cell death in the contralateral tectum which was always evident as early as 24 hours after the operation. At the earlier larval stages the peak of increased cell death was evident at two or three days, returning to about control levels by the ninth day or soon thereafter. Inasmuch as the deprived tectum already had a significantly smaller cell number than the control tectum, the percentage of cells in pyknosis remained uniformly above control values. At the later larval stages the peak of cell death tended to be one day later, and was of greater magnitude, i.e., up to seven-fold times control values rather than four-fold (Kollros and Thiesse, 1988). Further, differences in absolute numbers of dying cells tended to persist longer than for younger stages.

Recent studies of Hyla show similar results, i.e., 50 or fewer pyknotic cells in control tecta at stage V, rising gradually to between 400 and 500 cells, generally, in stages XV through XXI, with a decline to one-half of those numbers by stage XXV (Kollros, unpubl.). The highest individual values seen, 800 to 900, were at stages XX and XXI, distinctly greater values than in the larger but more slowly developing R. pipiens.

Cell Numbers

Cell numbers in the tecta, are, of course, the result of the differences between cell production and cell death. Even though cell death is evident at all larval stages observed, cell numbers in the R. pipiens tecta probably increase continuously through stages XVIII or XIX. Because of the substantial spacing between cells in layers 7-8-9, individual nuclei can be counted, and the Abercrombie (1946) correction can be applied to obtain "true" cell numbers in those layers. At stages V, X, XV, XX and XXV those numbers are respectively, on average, about 10,000, 60,000, 150,000, 205,000 and 165,000. Since cells in the deeper layers are more densely packed, with extensive overlay of nuclear profiles, accurate counts of their numbers in 10 µm sections would be impossible, or at best very tedious; hence, thin plastic sections (1 µm or less) were made, nuclear counts were performed for all of the individual layers, and numbers in the deeper layers could then be calculated from the counts of nuclei in layers 7-8-9. Cell numbers in layer 6 exceeded those in 7-8-9 by 3.15 times at stage VI, with differences gradually reducing to 2.15 times at stages XX and XXV. Numbers in layers 2 and 4, together, exceeded those in layers 7-8-9 by 2.35 times at stage VI, and gradually reduced to just 0.95 times at stage XX and 0.9 times at stage XXV. It can thus be seen that there is a continuing gradual shift of cells from deeper to more peripheral layers, and as cell production lags after stage X, a substantial depletion of cells from the deepest layers. Over the five sets of stages listed above for cell populations in layers 7-8-9, the deeper populations, i.e., in layers 2 through

6 combined, would be 55,000, 267,000, 548,000, 625,000 and 480,000. Overall, layers 7-8-9 gradually increase their percentage of the total cell population from 15 or 16% at stage V to about 25% at stage XXV. The greatest relative loss is seen in layers 2 and 4, i.e., from about 40% of the entire cell population at stage V to 22 or 23% at stage XXV. These same trends are seen in all of the anuran species studied.

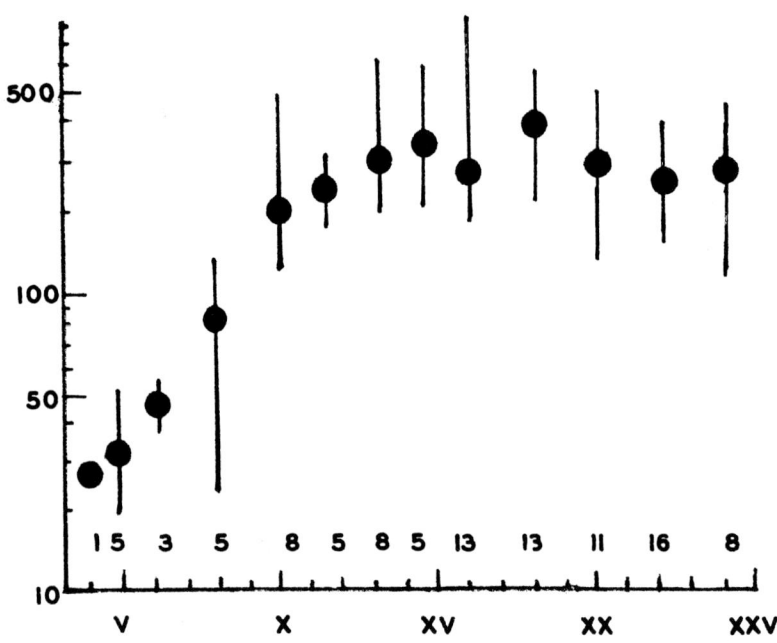

Figure 4. Numbers of pyknotic cells (means and ranges) in Rana pipiens larvae, in all tectal layers combined. Postmetamorphically cell deaths decline, almost to zero, by three weeks after stage XXV.

When one determines cell numbers in animals deprived of one eye in embryonic stages, differences in cell number are seen to increase progressively during development. By stage XXV, when 640,000 to 650,000 cells are present in control tecta, only about 370,000 are present in the deprived tecta. In layers 7-8-9 the differences amount to close to 50%, whereas for the deeper layers the differences come to only 40% or so. The 650,000 figure is about 15% greater than the value given by Eichler (1971), probably because our animals were substantially larger than his. Another estimate of these numbers in R. pipiens is 250,000 (Maturana et al., 1960), whereas for R. esculenta it is about 500,000 (Lázár and Székely, 1967; Kemali and Braitenberg, 1969).

Relatively few studies have dealt extensively with cell production and growth postmetamorphically. There is an assumption, from the very limited mitotic activity at the end of metamorphosis, that new cell production has terminated. Hitchcock and Easter (1988) state so quite bluntly, even though one of their references (Grant and Keating, 1986) demonstrates limited cell addition to the postmetamorphic Xenopus tectum, and provides cell number counts which are consistent with the addition of 3 or 4% of cells in layers 6 and 7 to 8% in layers 7-8-9; they have no information as to whether these newly labeled cells are neurons or glia.

Tectal Growth Patterns

All reports on cell production in the larval anuran tectum agree that cell division rates are consistently highest near the caudal pole and lowest near the rostral pole, with a gradient of activity between these two poles. Further, there is substantial evidence that cell divisions tend to be more common near the midline than more laterally. Straznicky and Gaze (1972), in an autoradiographic study, concluded that cell addition to the tectum was best characterized as the production of "wedges" of full-thickness tectum at the midline, with the broad end of the "wedge" caudad. As new cells were produced each old "wedge" displaced the previously produced tectum laterad and rostrad. They saw some labeled cells which failed to agree with such an interpretation, but they did not modify their schema to account for these. Later investigators appear to have agreed with them, e.g., Currie (1974), Currie and Cowan (1974), Reh and Constantine-Paton (1984), Grant and Keating (1986) and Hitchcock and Easter (1988). Nonetheless, the distribution of mitoses in a stage XIV R. pipiens, figured in Currie and Cowan (1974), clearly displays a very large number of cells lying rostrad and laterad of any possible mediocaudal strip of dividing cells; the Straznicky-Gaze pattern was not displayed. Grant and Keating (1986), in their Fig. 14, show distributions of dividing tectal cells which are virtually random at stages 64-66 in Xenopus, and at three months postmetamorphosis; they conform to neither the Straznicky-Gaze pattern, nor to the pattern of greater numbers caudad than rostrad. Below (Figs. 5-8) are examples from several species, at several different stages, all following removal of one eye. Differences in division rates between the two sides are clear, and what is additionally clear is that a pattern such as that proposed by Straznicky and Gaze is absent from either side. There is some concentration of dividing cells near the midline, but many lateral cells are also dividing, as are cells near the frontal pole. Inasmuch as this kind of pattern is evident throughout the larval period, I propose that the pattern of successive "wedges" of new cells produced near the midline, be at least modified to recognize that day after day, stage after stage, for much or all of the larval period, cells are being added to rostral and lateral regions of the tectum (those areas which would represent the earliest, i.e., oldest "wedges") so that a large fraction of the definitive tectal cells in those regions would have been added by insertion into the tectum, from the underlying ependyma. Inasmuch as the proposal of Gaze et al. (1979) that retinotectal relationships were undergoing constant reorganization during larval development, with elimination and phagocytosis of old synaptic terminals and development of new ones, now has substantial support from the work of others, including shifting of terminals even postmetamorphically (Hitchcock and Easter, 1988), there need be no problem to consider that the cells newly introduced into older tectal areas might well obtain synaptic contacts appropriate for their position, and thus would be fully integrated into the retinotectal map. Tritiated-thymidine labeling of larval tectal cells has shown that such cells are later located in all of the several tectal laminae (Eichler, 1971; Kollros, unpubl.). As yet, we have too little information as to the proportions of cells produced in any given stage which settle into any given cell layer, and whether such settling is greater medially or laterally. But the possibility that such studies can be carried out exists, and such studies could also give us further information as to the rate, extent and loci of migration of cells from deep to superficial layers. Properly conducted, such studies could also give us information as to the proportion of "old" and "new" cells which survive in any particular tectal area.

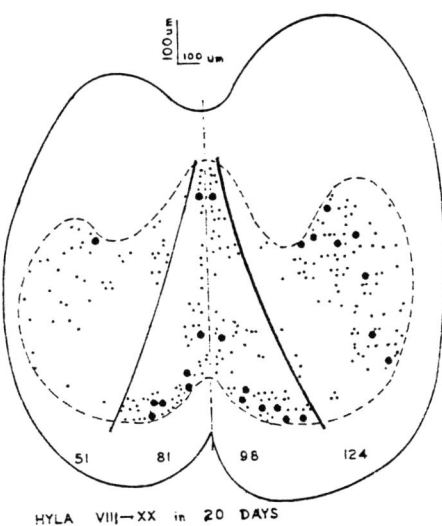

Figure 5. Hyla versicolor tecta represented in outline from above to show positions of dividing cells. Dashed lines represent the ventricular border. Each small dot represents one mitotic figure, and each large dot represents four mitotic figures, closely bunched. On the left are 132 mitoses vs. 222 on the right, i.e., 59.5%. The left ependyma has 80% of the area of the right. The right eye was removed at stage VIII, and fixation was 20 days later at stage XX. Note the greater discrepancy of mitotic numbers laterally than medially. The slanted lines from front to rear suggest delineation of medial from lateral areas. The scale lines show that the lateral dimensions of the tectum are compressed, compared to the antero-posterior dimensions.

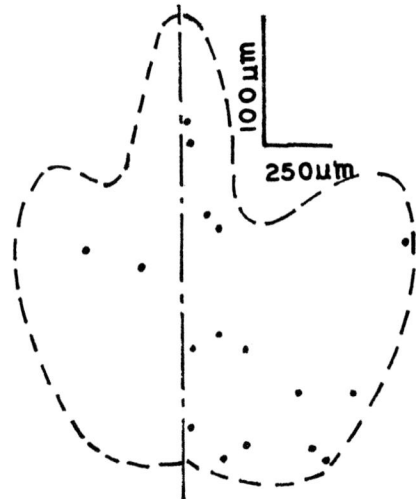

Figure 6. Xenopus laevis tectum represented only in ventricular outline from above. The right eye was removed at stage 47, and fixed 54 days later at stage 63. Each dot represents a mitotic figure (2 on left, 15 on right, or 13%). The ependyma extends from section 16 through section 50, of 90 sections. Its area on the left is 81% of that on the right. Note: There is no apparent pattern to the position of the mitoses, much as in Grant and Keating (1986) at the same stage.

In both Figs. 7 and 8 below, one sees the greatest concentration of mitotic figures near the midline, somewhat more broadly spread caudad than rostrad, but also very many divisions lateral and rostral to such medial concentrations.

Neurons Versus Glia

Substantial evidence exists that glial cells tend to be produced later in development than are neurons in the same brain regions (Jacobson, 1978). However, in some mammals at least, glial production can be quite

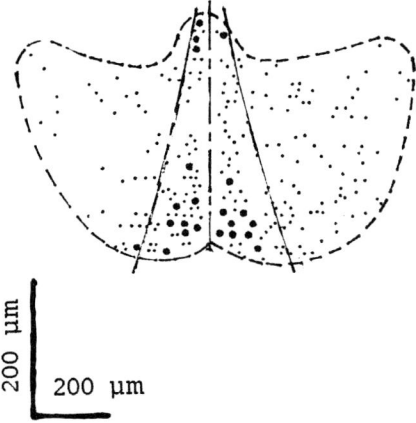

Figure 7. Pseudacris triseriata tectal outlines viewed from above, to show positions of mitotic figures (each small dot equals 1 division figure; each large dot equals 5), in relationship to the ependymal margins (dashed lines). The right eye was removed at stage XX. Ependymal area on the left is 81% that of the right, while the left has 82% as many mitoses as the right (146 vs. 177). Curved slanted lines divide the medial from lateral areas. Note distinctly more lateral mitoses on the right.

early (at 28% of the gestational period in the rhesus monkey -- Levitt and Rakic, 1980), and commitment to glial rather than to neuronal lines can exist even in the ventricular zone (Levitt et al., 1981). The early appearance of glial processes has been noted (Gaze et al., 1979) in the Xenopus tectum at stages equivalent to IV⁻ of R. pipiens, though whether these are mainly from neuroglial or ependymoglial cells is not established. Currie and Cowan (1974) contended that differences in cell production in R. pipiens tecta following removal of one eye reflected exclusively glial production, since the "majority of tectal neurons" are formed "at late embryonic or early larval stages", though they defined

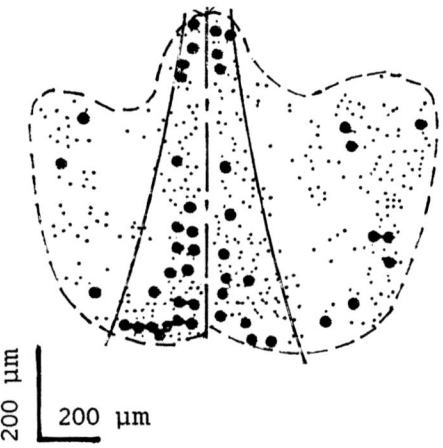

Figure 8. Rana sylvatica tectal outlines, as for Fig. 7. The right eye was removed at stage XII$^+$ and the animal was fixed 10 days later at stage XV$^+$. The ependymal area on the left is 86% of that on the right, whereas the mitotic figures are but 76% (263 vs. 346). There are many more mitoses in the right lateral area than in the left. Curved slanted lines and dot representations as for Fig. 7.

neither "early" nor "late". As was shown in the section on Mitotic Activity above, substantial numbers of tectal cells are still formed after stages X or XII. Further, their identification of glial cells is inadequately described, and they state "Our evidence on this point is not entirely conclusive, mainly because of the difficulty in identifying cell types in heavily labeled autoradiographs of thick sections." They provided no information as to the fraction of the tectal cell population which might be glial. Székely and Lázár (1976), dealing with this issue, estimate the figure to be less than 1% in R. esculenta. In juvenile Xenopus, values of 8% and 2% have been given by Fujisawa and Jacobson (1980). In our laboratory, using electron micrographs in stages of metamorphic climax, we find a range of from less than 2%

to less than 6% in R. pipiens (Thiesse and Kollros, unpubl.). As these values are about an order of magnitude different from the differences in cell counts in tecta after early enucleation, one must conclude that such differences in cell numbers as do occur represent mainly neurons rather than glia.

SUMMATION

The anuran optic tectum has its cell population determined by a balance between cell production and cell death. The influence of the eye accounts for approximately 50% of the tectal cell population at metamorphosis, with the impact on layers 7-8-9 being greater than on the deeper layers. Following eye removal early in development, the main adjustment is via restricting cell production. The amount of alteration between the two sides increases progressively with stage as increasing portions of the control tectum become covered with optic nerve fibers. In contrast, if eye removal occurs late in larval development, though it still results in reduced cell production within three days, relatively few cells remain to be produced. The major impact is evidenced through a large increase in cell death, seen within one day, peaking at three or four days, and remaining at above control levels for essentially all of the remaining time when cell death occurs, i.e., up to three or four weeks after metamorphosis. The small fraction of cells which can be identified as glial ensure that a very large fraction of the cell number adjustment, however occurring, must involve neurons or prospective neurons.

Growth of the tectum from the earliest larval stages onward proceeds more rapidly at the caudal pole than the rostral one. The pattern of cell divisions near the midline, somewhat broader caudad than rostrad, implies that tectal segments which are first formed become displaced laterad and rostrad by the newly forming cells. Since many cell divisions also occur in lateral and rostral positions, away from the midline, tectal growth must also involve interpositioning of the new cells into the previously formed tectal regions. Their integration in these positions can be expected to occur through disestablishment of older synaptic contacts, and establishment of new ones, over the entire period of tectal formation, as proposed by Gaze et al. (1979).

The ways in which retinotectal connections are established with great precision have yet to be fully elucidated. Their consideration has been beyond the scope of this paper. What yet needs exploration is the series of changes in the period near and after metamorphic climax which results in a failure of cell death following eye removal. The possibility that the establishment of indirect ipsilateral eye connections are involved must be considered, as well as the possible role of other connections which are being made at that time (Gaze and Jacobson, 1963; Grobstein et al., 1980; Hoskins and Grobstein, 1985).

While the present paper has dealt with at least three families of anurans, all sharing some common features in the control of tectal cell number, it is by no means certain that the range of adjustments, or the possible mechanisms, have all yet been seen. The utilization of a more diverse group of anurans, and urodeles, might provide added insights.

ACKNOWLEDGMENTS

The studies reported here, and unpublished, have been supported by USPHS grant NS15350 from the National Institute of Neurological and Communicative Disorders and Stroke.

REFERENCES

Ambercrombie M (1946). Estimation of nuclear population from microtome sections. Anat Rec 94:239-247.
Cowan WM (1981). The development of the vertebrate central nervous system: an overview. In Garrod DR, Feldman JD (eds): "Development in the Nervous System." Cambridge: Cambridge University Press, pp 3-33.
Currie JR (1974). Some observations on the development of the visual system in the frog, Rana pipiens. Ph.D. Thesis, Washington University, St. Louis, Missouri, USA.
Currie JR, Cowan WM (1974). Some observations on the

early development of the optic tectum in the frog (Rana pipiens), with special reference to the effects of early eye removal on mitotic activity in the larval tectum. J Comp Neurol 156:123-141.

Currie JR, Cowan WM (1975). The development of the retinotectal projection in Rana pipiens. Develop Biol 46:103-119.

Dürken B (1913). Über einseitig Augenexstirpation bei jungen Froschlarven. Zeit wiss Zool 105:192-243.

Dürken B (1930). Zur Frage nach der Wirkung einseitiger Augenexstirpation bei Froschlarven. Biol Generalis 6:511-552.

Eichler V (1971). Neurogenesis in the optic tectum of larval Rana pipiens following unilateral enucleation. J Comp Neurol 141:375-393.

Filogamo G (1950). Conseguenze della demolizione dell 'abbozzo dell'occhio sullo sviluppo del lobo ottico nell 'embrione de pollo. Riv Biol 42:73-80.

Fujisawa H, Jacobson M (1980). Transsynaptic labeling of neurons in the optic tectum of Xenopus after intraocular [^{3}H] proline injection. Brain Res 194:431-441.

Gaze RM, Jacobson M (1963). The path from the retina to the ipsilateral optic tectum of the frog. J Physiol (Lond) 165:73-74P.

Gaze RM, Keating MJ, Östberg A, Chung S-H (1979). The relationship between retinal and tectal growth in larval Xenopus: implications for the development of the retinotectal projection. J Embryol Exp Morphol 53:103-143.

Glücksman A (1951). Cell deaths in normal vertebrate ontogeny. Biol Rev 26:59-86.

Grant S, Keating MJ (1986). Ocular migration and the metamorphic and postmetamorphic maturation of the retinotectal system in Xenopus laevis: an autoradiographic and morphometric study. J Embryol Exp Morphol 92:43-69.

Grobstein P, Comer C, Kostyk S (1980). The potential binocular field and its tectal representation in Rana pipiens. J Comp Neurol 190:175-185.

Hamburger V, Oppenheim RW (1982). Naturally occurring neuronal death in vertebrates. Neurosci Commentaries 1:39-55.

Hoskins SG, Grobstein P (1985). Development of the ipsilateral retinothalamic projection in the frog Xenopus laevis. III. Role of thyroxine. J Neurosci

5:930-940.
Hughes A (1961). Cell degeneration in the larval ventral horn of Xenopus laevis (Daudin). J Embryol Exp Morphol 9:269-284.
Hitchcock PF, Easter SS Jr (1987). Evidence for centripetally shifting terminals on the tectum of postmetamorphic Rana pipiens. J Comp Neurol 266:556-564.
Jacobson M (1978). "Developmental Neurobiology, 2nd ed." New York: Plenum Press.
Kemali M, Braitenberg V (1969). "Atlas of the Frog's Brain." Berlin: Springer-Verlag.
Kollros JJ (1953). The development of the optic lobes in the frog. I. The effects of unilateral enucleation in embryonic stages. J Exp Zool 123:153-187.
Kollros JJ (1982). Peripheral control of midbrain mitotic activity in the frog. J Comp Neurol 205:171-178.
Kollros JJ (1984). Growth and death of cells of the mesencephalic fifth nucleus in Rana pipiens larvae. J Comp Neurol 224:386-394.
Kollros JJ, Thiesse ML (1988). Control of tectal cell number during larval development in Rana pipiens. J Comp Neurol (in press).
Larsell O (1929). The effect of experimental excision of one eye on the development of the optic lobe and opticus layer in the larvae of the tree frog (Hyla regilla). J Comp Neurol 48:331-353.
Larsell O (1931). The effect of experimental excision of one eye on the development of the optic lobe and opticus layer of the tree frog (Hyla regilla). II. The effect on cell size and differentiation of cell processes. J Exp Zool 58:1-20.
Lázár G (1984). Structure and connections of the frog optic tectum. In Vanegas H (ed): "Comparative Neurology of the Optic Tectum." New York and London: Plenum Press, pp 185-210.
Lázár G, Székely G (1967). Golgi studies on the optic center of the frog. J Hirnforsch 9:329-344.
Leghissa S (1951). A proposito dello svilluppo del tetto ottico nei teleostei (Salmo fario). Bol Zool 18:355-365.
Levitt P, Rakic P (1980). Immunoperoxidase localization of glial fibrillary acidic protein in radial glia cells and astrocytes of the developing rhesus monkey brain. J Comp Neurol 193:815-840.
Levitt P, Cooper ML, Rakic P (1981). Coexistence of neuronal and glial precursor cells in the cerebral

ventricular zone of the fetal monkey: an ultrastructural immunoperoxidase analysis. J Neurosci 1:27-39.
Maturana HR, Lettvin JY, McCulloch WS, Pitts WH (1960). Anatomy and physiology of vision in the frog (Rana pipiens). J Gen Physiol Suppl 43:129-175.
Pflugfelder O (1952). Weitere volumetrische Untersuchungen über die Wirkung der Augenexstirpation und der Dunkelhaltung auf das Mesencephalon und die Pseudobranchien von Fischen. Arch Entwmech 145:549-560.
Purves D, Lichtman JW (1985). "Principles of Neural Development." Sunderland, Mass.: Sinauer Assoc. Inc.
Reh TA, Constantine-Paton M (1984). Retinal ganglion cell terminals change their projection sites during larval development of Rana pipiens. J Neurosci 4:442-457.
Steinitz E (1906). Über den Einfluss der Elimination der embryonalen Augenblasen auf die Entwicklung des Gesamtorganismus beim Frosche. Arch Entwmech 20:537-578.
Straznicky K, Gaze RM (1972). The development of the tectum in Xenopus laevis: an autoradiographic study. J Embryol Exp Morphol 28:87-115.
Székely G, Lázár G (1976). Cellular and synaptic architecture of the optic tectum. In Llinás R, Precht W (eds): "Frog Neurobiology." Heidelberg: Springer-Verlag.
Taylor AC, Kollros JJ (1946). Stages in the normal development of Rana pipiens larvae. Anat Rec 94:7-23.

A NEURAL PATTERN UNFOLDING: PROPERTIES OF RETINOTECTAL DIFFERENTIATION IN FROG TADPOLES

Martha Constantine-Paton

Department of Biology, Yale University,
New Haven, Connecticut 06511

The easy accessibility provided by the external development of the frog tadpole provides an unusual opportunity to describe the dynamic processes of CNS differentiation and to probe them experimentally in mechanistic studies. Moreover, the frog optic tectum represents a cytoarchitectonically laminated, functionally reiterated sensory/motor processing center. It is consequently an excellent experimental system in which to explore issues usually associated with the organization of neocortex such as the interdependence of topographic synaptic fields and columnar organization.

There has been a tremendous amount of work in this area. The "retinotectal pathway" has now been used for nearly four decades in experimental studies of nervous system "specificity" and "plasticity". The majority of these studies deal with rules of topographic organization inferred from changes in afferent termination patterns that are induced by surgical perturbations. These have been covered in numerous reviews (for examples see Gaze, 1978; Constantine-Paton, 1981). Information relating normal patterns of development in the optic tectum and providing evidence of the interaction between retinal neurons and tectal cells has been largely omitted from such surveys. Nevertheless, it is the relatively sophisticated level of understanding of the patterns of development of the tectum and its satellite circuitry, as much as experimental accessibility, that underlies our use of the system in studies of the molecular mechanisms of CNS patterning. Thus the primary goal of this contribution is to provide an integrated description of how this neural pattern unfolds. This hopefully will motivate the hypotheses and ideas concerning the cascade of potentially very general events which are presented in the last section and which may underlie the development of all topographically organized networks in the vertebrate brain.

THE TECTAL PROLIFERATIVE ZONES

Shortly after the cessation of neurulation, the first neurons destined for the optic tectum become post-mitotic in the rostral lateral pole of the presumptive midbrain. The remainder of the roof of the midbrain ventricle maintains a pseudostratified columnar epithelium which is separated from the post-mitotic neurons by a band of rapidly proliferating cells (the caudal-medial proliferative zone). By the time the lens and cornea of the embryonic eye have cleared and the axons of the first retinal ganglion cells have reached the mesencephalic-diencephalic junction, the tectal neuroblasts from this proliferative zone have migrated into the subpial mantle layer to initiate the formation of the mature cellular lamination pattern (Currie, 1974; Currie and Cowan, 1975).

The caudal-medial proliferative zone and the pattern of cell genesis in the optic tectum was initially established in material stained for chromatin and examined for densities of the periventricular mitotic figures (Kollros, 1953; Eichler, 1971). Within the past two decades a variety of workers using ^{3}H-thymidine pulsing of amphibian tadpoles in conjunction with staggered survival times have supported the initial observations by demonstrating that the caudal-medial proliferative zone gradually retracts during larval life laying down differentiated tectal lamination at its most rostrolateral border (Straznicky and Gaze, 1972; Currie, 1974). Thus, many tectal neurons are added in an age-grouped series of bands that stretch mediolaterally across the expanding tectal surface. This pattern can be seen in the two-dimensional computer reconstructions of ^{3}H-thymidine labeled cell positions shown in Fig. 1a and b. In the reconstructions, the band of heavy label marks the region of tectum that was at the rostral

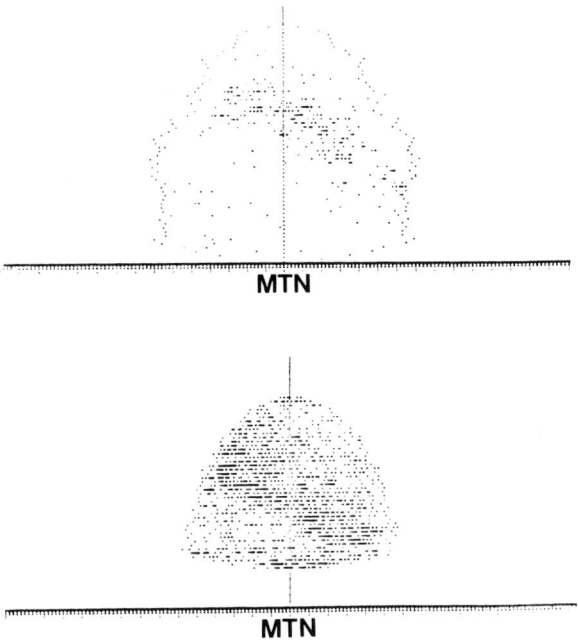

Figure 1. Two-dimensional computer reconstructions of the distribution of ^{3}H-thymidine labeled nuclei in sections through the left tectal lobes of two tadpoles. Each line in the reconstruction represents the length of the dorsal border of tectal layer 6 in consecutive 10 µm coronal sections through the entire midbrain. Each dot in the reconstruction (with the exception of the two representing the ends of each line) represents the position of at least one ^{3}H-thymidine labeled nucleus projected onto the layer 6 border. Distances are equivalently scaled along the x and y axes. One division on the x axis equals 10 µm. a) Tadpole injected with ^{3}H-thymidine at Taylor and Kollros stage V and killed at stage X. b) Tadpole injected at Taylor and Kollros stage IV and killed at stage VII. Increased labeling in this animal is most likely a function of a longer autoradiographic exposure time and/or a larger effective dose of ^{3}H-thymidine. Rostral is down and medial is to the right in both reconstructions. MTN = middle of the tectal neuropil.

boundary of the caudal-medial proliferative zone where most cells were undergoing their last round of DNA synthesis when the radioisotope was administered. With successively longer survival times following a single pulse of ^{3}H-thymidine more unlabeled tectal cells will be laid down behind the age-labeled cohort of heavily labeled cells. Thus, when the labeling patterns of tecta are compared between animals surviving ^{3}H-thymidine injections for long (Fig. 1a) versus shorter (Fig. 1b) intervals, the animals surviving for longer intervals exhibit the labeled band of cells at positions proportionately closer to the tectum's rostral pole.

Superimposed on this rostrolateral to caudomedial spatiotemporal pattern of cells withdrawing from the mitotic cycle is a radial pattern of cell settling. Two generalizations concerning radial patterns of settling can be made about most vertebrate brain regions: first, that larger, long distance projection neurons originate first (Jacobson, 1975); second, that, in cortical regions, deeper lying neurons originate prior to more superficial neurons so that the later generated cells must migrate past their older neighbors (Rakic, 1974). In mammalian neocortex these two patterns merge into one since the deepest lying cortical layer (VI) is also the layer containing the majority of long distance projecting pyramidal cells. Currie (1974) has used a series of tadpoles with staggered survival times to ascertain the sequence with which cells take up their positions in differentiated tectal laminae. She has found that the overall pattern is quite similar to that observed in many cortical regions of mammals with an interesting qualification: in the tectum there are two distinguishably different patterns of neurogenesis. That is, the larger projection neurons of the superficial tectal laminae (tectal layers 6 and 7) originate first, followed by the smaller neurons distributed throughout the depths of the tectum (layers 4, 6, 8 and 9). Within this second phase of small neuron migration, cells within the deeper laminae (tectal layers 4 and 6) originate earlier than cells in the more superficial laminae (tectal layers 8 and 9).

The rostrolateral to caudomedial gradient of tectal differentiation has already been established by the end of embryonic life, and it dominates the differentiation of the tectum and its satellite structures throughout the larval period. The gradient of cytoarchitectonic differentiation is apparent in the photomontage of Fig. 2 which shows a section of tectum cut parallel to the rostrolateral-caudomedial axis. The tissue in the figure has been reacted with an antibody raised against the inhibitory transmitter gamma-amino butyric acid (GABA). GABA immunoreactivity (GABA-IR) is one of the earliest expressed markers of a neuronal phenotype. Consequently, with this label it is possible to see the tectal lamination pattern emerge. The first postmitotic neuroblasts are only slightly displaced from the dense proliferative zone (P.Z.) in the most caudal tectal regions. However, in many cases, a process (presumably a young axon) can be traced into a fiber tract of the developing mantle region. In progressively more rostral regions of tectum this fiber tract merges with lamina 7. Differentiating neuroblasts destined for the superficial layers 8 and 9 migrate across this axon-rich lamina to take up their mature positions in a pattern quite reminiscent of cortical neuron migration across the intermediate zone of developing neocortex. The small size of cell bodies and their dense packing makes it impossible, in fixed tissue, to ascertain the degree of active neuroblast migration and rearrangement along the most dorsal border of the tectal proliferative zone. From the ^{3}H-thymidine data, we know that eventually there will be an inside out assortment of cells as a result of activity in this region. Nevertheless, when regarded as a sequence along the age gradient, cytoarchitectonic differentiation of the tectum appears much more analogous to differentiation in mammalian thalamus than neocortex. Thus layer 6, the most cell dense zone

---

Figure 2. Photomontage of a sagittal cryostat section through a tadpole tectum showing the developmental gradient of cytoarchitectonic differentiation. The section has been incubated with a rabbit antiserum raised against BSA-conjugated GABA. Binding of this antibody to tissue sections can be blocked by preabsorption with excess GABA-BSA. Visualization of primary antibody binding is with a FITC conjugated second antibody. The arrow indicates the caudalmost extent of the retinal projection. P.Z. = proliferative zone. (See overleaf for Fig.2.)

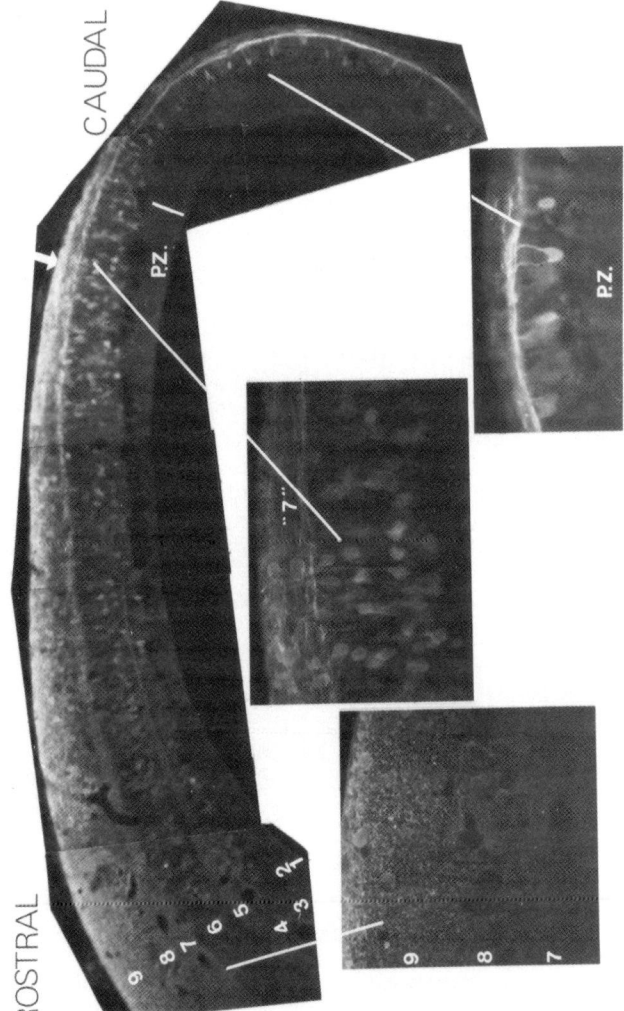

Fig. 2. See page 235 for legend.

of mature tecta as well as the deeper cellular laminae 4 and 2 appear to simply delaminate from the upper region of the proliferative zones: their identity as separate functional cell groups becoming obvious initially only as a result of the appearance of the cell-free plexiform layers 5 and 3.

Longitudinal sections of the tectum provide a "timeline" with which to assess the relative appearance of different cell types. This plane of section in conjunction with immunocytochemistry has revealed that the pattern of GABA-IR is not generalizable to all phenotypic markers. For example, immunoreactivity to an antibody raised against Substance P, a cotransmitter in many vertebrate neurons, only appears relatively late in tectal morphogenesis in a well-differentiated subset of neurons of layer 6 in rostral tectum. A monoclonal antibody raised in my laboratory against frog oligodendrocytes (Steen et al., 1987) reveals that these cells have yet a different pattern of expression. It is fairly well established that myelination in all vertebrate brains is triggered by the presence of axons of sufficient maturity. The histological and GABA studies suggest that one of the first tracts to be laid down in the tectum is the efferent fiber layer 7. It is not surprising, therefore, that staining with the oligodendrocyte antibody reveals myelination well underway in layer 7 even in undifferentiated caudal tectal regions well before the neurons of all other laminae have begun to myelinate. The process of myelination continues throughout tectal differentiation and for any given radial slice of tectum, glia are being generated in different layers at different times. For example, oligodendrocytes appear in the deepest regions of retinorecipient layer 9 well after it becomes cytoarchitectonically distinct. The latency presumably reflects the time necessary for the large caliber retinal ganglion cell axons to reach a level of maturity sufficient to stimulate myelination. Observations such as this defy the simple scheme often proffered by students of CNS differentiation and an earlier source of controversy in the tectal literature (Kollros, 1953; Currie and Cowan, 1974) in which proliferation zones are believed to give off neurons initially and only later produce glia.

The caudomedial proliferative zone was historically

the first midbrain proliferative zone recognized. It also appears to be the primary source of all cells in the midbrain roof, but it is not the only source of new cells in the tectal lobe (see Kollros, this volume). As the caudomedial zone withdraws, it leaves behind it, in relatively differentiated rostral regions, two zones in which cells label with ^{3}H-thymidine even after short survival times (1/2 hour). One of these zones is in the periventricular ependymal layer where cell bodies of the radial glia, the dominant glial cell type of the tectal lobe, are localized. Even after survival times of a week to a month, ^{3}H-thymidine label in the somata of these ependymal glia cells is always displaced quite rostrally relative to the contiguous band of tectal neurons that are given off by the caudomedial proliferative zone shortly after a single ^{3}H-thymidine injection (Currie and Cowan, 1974; Cline and Constantine-Paton, 1986). Thus, it appears that the periventricular ependymal layer maintains a population of stem cells into relatively late stages of tectal differentiation, and that the cells which differentiate in this zone continue to increase the tectum's radial glial population.

It also appears, however, that as the caudomedial proliferative zone recedes it leaves behind a third stem cell population which can be distinguished by ^{3}H-thymidine uptake after very short survival times in differentiated tectal laminae. These cells either migrate to differentiated tectal laminae along with the major wave of tectal neuroblasts from the caudomedial proliferative zone, or they migrate out of the rostral periventricular proliferative zone into the fully differentiated tectal laminae. We cannot, at present, distinguish between these two possibilities. This third proliferative zone is much smaller than the other two. It is distinguished by perhaps three or four labeled cells per tectum after a single ^{3}H-thymidine pulse and a short (1/2 hour) survival time. It is easily missed in normal animals because of its small size. In fact, all of our current information on this zone derives from studies in animals with artificially elevated cell proliferation as a result of thyroxin treatment. When thyroxin is supplied to young larvae this zone stands out as a distinct region of ^{3}H-thymidine uptake in the upper laminae (predominantly layers 6 and 7) of differentiated rostral tectum (Constantine-Paton and Cline, 1987).

Double-label experiments with ^{3}H-thymidine to identify this late dividing population, retrograde transport of HRP from tectal projection zones and immunocytochemical markers for Substance P, GABA and oligodendrocytes are presently underway to determine if this zone is pluripotential, giving rise to both neurons and glia. The answer to this question is an important one because the existence of a late-generated neuronal population would raise two very general questions. Can late addition of new cells contribute new functional properties to already differentiated CNS circuitry? Are late-generated cells under differentiation control mechanisms distinct from those controlling the phenotype of cells arising directly from the primary proliferative zone?

THE COORDINATION OF TECTAL DIFFERENTIATION WITH THE DIFFERENTIATION OF ITS INPUTS

Like all major integrating centers in the vertebrate brain, the optic tectum has numerous reciprocal connections with both visual and non-visual centers. Several studies indicate that neurogenesis in the tectum, and its major inputs and target zones, is a stereotypically orchestrated sequence of both independent and interactive events.

Recent work in my laboratory using small rhodamine-labeled beads as retrograde fluorescent tracers has begun to examine the complex sequences in which the major nonretinal inputs to the tectum differentiate. It is clear from this work that large numbers of neurons in the differentiating thalamus, midbrain tegmentum and isthmi region of the brainstem have well-established axons in the rostral differentiated tectal laminae by larval stage VI (Debski, personal communication). Exactly when the first of these nonretinal projections reach the tectum, and if they proceed or follow the initial invasion of retinal ganglion cell axons, is yet to be determined. However, we do know that, at least for one of them, the ipsilateral isthmiotectal projection, the topography of its tectal connection is relatively independent of the much larger retinal input.

When both eyes of Rana embryos are removed in tail-bud stage embryos, the tecta undergo a marked decrease in volume. This amounts to a roughly 70% reduction in the superficial neuropil (layers 7 to 9). Nevertheless, the isthmiotectal axons, which usually terminate along with the retinal axons in the neuropil, are able to form a normally aligned topographic distribution of their axon terminals that is maintained throughout larval life and in young post-metamorphic frogs (Constantine-Paton and Ferrari-Eastman, 1981).

The overview above has attempted to demonstrate that the tectal cell population is not a simple assembly of undifferentiated cells upon which the massive retinal projection imposes its order. It is important to make this point since many of the theories and experiments in retinotectal map formation have tended to treat the tectum as if this were the case. The tectum has been surgically sliced and reconstituted without consideration for intrinsic circuitry or nonretinal inputs. The inherent complexity of the tectum is also important to highlight, prior to any treatment of the interactions between retinal axons and tectal cells. This is because there is a gradually developing consensus that one of the major ways in which the retina influences visual pathway development in all vertebrates is through the temporal patterning of synaptic activity. The latter process depends on the interaction of retinal activity with the myriad of nonretinal inputs that impinge on the same tectal cells. Thus, the formation of a functional visual pathway is just as likely to be dependent on autonomous processes of tectal differentiation as it is on the more intensively studied properties of retinal axon growth.

THE DEVELOPMENT OF RETINAL INNERVATION IN THE TECTAL LOBE

Dr. Kollros in this volume has reviewed the now considerable evidence that the retinal ganglion cell input modulates mitotic activity in the tectal lobe. However, despite this means of coordination there are several incongruities between the growth of the retinal ganglion cell population and its tectal target zone which have important implications for synaptic specificity and competition in this system. One incongruity is a simple size matching. The retina differentiates and grows proportionately more rapidly than the tectal neuropil within which it terminates. For example, between Taylor and Kollros (1946) stage VI and the young frog (stage XXV), the ratio of tectal neuropil volume per ganglion cell increases nearly threefold from 1.1×10^3 µm³/ganglion cell to 3.0×10^3 µm³/ganglion cell (Reh and Constantine-Paton, 1983). On a cellular level, this implies that, in this developing synaptic zone, throughout tadpole life available afferent inputs generally pre-date differentiated tectal dendrites. A second incongruity is produced by the distinctly different patterns of retinal and tectal growth: during the larval period the retina grows as an expanding circle (Hollyfield, 1968, 1971; Straznicky and Gaze, 1971; Reh and Constantine-Paton, 1983), whereas the caudomedial proliferative zone produces a retinal target zone which adds the largest proportion of new neuropil only at its caudomedial border. Nevertheless, a well-aligned retinal projection is maintained throughout this period because the oldest retinal ganglion cells, in central retina, gradually shift the sites of their terminal arbors toward newer post-synaptic cells in the caudomedial sections of the tectal lobe (Gaze et al., 1979; Reh and Constantine-Paton, 1984). Thus, synapses in the larval tectum must be considered highly dynamic structures with relatively short lifetimes.

The problem of dynamic, developing synapses is, by its very nature, two-sided. The mechanisms of synaptogenesis in the tectum must, in some way, continually maintain a high-fidelity, coherent retinal projection among a population of constantly shifting pre-synaptic boutons. The same processes must allow tectal neurons to differentiate functionally effective circuitry in the face of major afferent inputs that are constantly changing. It is important to recognize, in this context, that tectal neurons first begin to elaborate their processes at the rostral border of the caudomedial zone (Lázár, 1973). This is an extremely complex microenvironment. The new tectal neurons are situated at the low end of a gradient of synaptic innervation densities that is highest in rostral tectum. Rostral to the young neurons lies a relatively differentiated neuropil containing a high-fidelity dense retinal projection. By contrast, immediately behind the zone in which tectal neurons are generated, lies a relatively undifferentiated mantle layer containing a low density of "new" nasal retinal ganglion cell axons that have recently invaded the caudal tectal boundary. We have recently examined the morphology of neurons in layers 6, 7 and 9 of tadpole tecta by flattening living tectal lobes in a tissue slice chamber and filling individual cells, after impalement, with Lucifer Yellow (Katz and Constantine-Paton, 1988). The study revealed a structural bias in tadpole tectal cell dendritic morphology which may reflect the rostral-caudal dichotomy in which the cells differentiate: most tectal neurons have dendritic arbors that are highly biased toward either the zone lying rostral or caudal to the position of the cell body. The majority of cells show a rostral bias: 22 neurons exhibited a rostral bias as opposed to nine cells with a caudal bias. In only 11 cells was the envelope of the dendritic arbor lying rostral to the cell body and the envelope of the dendritic arbor lying caudal to the cell body roughly equal (e.g., differing from each other by less than two to one). It has recently been shown, in experimental studies of mammalian retina (Perry and Linden, 1982) and insect sensory interneurons (Murphey et al., 1974; Hoy et al., 1984), that the growth of dendrites can be influenced by the availability of appropriate inputs. In these systems dendritic trees appear to shift their zone of arborization toward the region of high density innervation or the zone where competition for inputs with other dendrites is at a minimum. Tectal dendrites could be responding in much the same way. This would imply that the post-synaptic dendrites in the retinotectal pathway, like the retinal afferents themselves, are highly dynamic structures. Dendrites could compete with each other for inputs and have the direction of their subsequent growth altered depending upon when they encounter the largest number of effective afferents.

These phenomena raise fundamental mechanistic questions. Namely, what interactions drive the shifting of retinal-tectal connections, maintain the coherence of the afferents and modulate dendritic morphology?

There is now considerable evidence, in frog tectum (Reh and Constantine-Paton, 1985), in the goldfish tectum (Meyer, 1983; Schmidt and Edwards, 1983), in the kitten geniculocortical pathway (Dubin et al., 1986;

Stryker and Harris, 1986; Stretavan et al., 1987) and in the mammalian neuromuscular junction (Brown et al., 1981) that a critical parameter in at least one of these functions is the pattern of action potential activity carried by the inputs. In mammalian skeletal muscle, for example, blocking synaptic activation of muscle, by either tetrodotoxin (TTX) cuffs on muscle nerves or nicotinic receptor block, produces sprouting of all motor nerves in the vicinity of the silenced muscle fibers; direct electrical stimulation of the silenced muscle in a particular pattern will inhibit this sprouting. Thus, it appears that ineffectively innervated muscle fibers can, in some way, induce sprouting of prospective inputs (Brown et al., 1981). In the amphibian tadpole tectum and in the fetal cat lateral geniculate nucleus, TTX treatments that silence retinal ganglion cell activity and effectively decrease synaptic activation of the target cells also cause pronounced "sprouting" of the retinal ganglion cell terminals. It is therefore possible that developing CNS neurons, like muscle, may use activity to achieve an effective innervation level. When innervation is low or ineffective, as in TTX treatment, the cells essentially recruit more inputs by inducing available inputs to sprout. When sufficient levels of innervation are achieved the cells cease or down regulate this recruiting activity. In the tadpole tectum, such a system could be involved in the continual shifting of established retinal ganglion cell synaptic contacts toward newer, relatively poorly innervated tectal neurons in caudal tectum.

The actual chemical signals involved in such an activity-dependent signalling system remain obscure. Evidence has been obtained in several laboratories for a "sprouting" substance that emanates from ineffectively innervated CNS target neurons (Needel et al., 1987) and from silenced skeletal muscle (Gurney, 1984). Alternatively, it has been hypothesized that the relative depolarization of pre-synaptic terminals adjacent to activated post-synaptic membranes may drive Ca^{2+} into the terminal and activate proteases that effectively inhibit renewed sprouting (O'Brien et al., 1982). In addition, denervated frog tecta have been reported to show a marked increase in the extracellular matrix protein, laminin. This could facilitate sprouting by increasing the substrate binding affinity of retinal ganglion cell axons (Liesi, 1985).

Normal patterns of retinal ganglion cell activity also seem likely to be involved in maintaining the coherence and high fidelity of the retinal projection during the early stages of synaptogenesis. In the visual pathway, most investigations of the role of activity in actually patterning the distribution of pre-synaptic axons within a target have used the segregation of inputs onto separate post-synaptic cells. Thus, TTX block of kitten retinas decreases the point-to-point fidelity of the retinal map in the lateral geniculate nucleus and the functional segregation of different ganglion cell types on geniculate neurons (Dubin et al., 1986). In kitten visual cortex, retinal TTX block inhibits the segregation of geniculocortical axons into ocular dominance columns (Stryker and Harris, 1986).

Our work in this area uses a preparation in which, as a result of embryonic microsurgery, a supernumerary retina is forced to compete with a normal retina for terminal space in a tadpole tectal lobe (Constantine-Paton and Law, 1978). In normal free-swimming Rana pipiens tadpoles, once the cell death associated with the initial formation of the eyecup and the retinal laminae is complete (Glücksman, 1940), the retinal ganglion cell layer only adds cells. In this system there is absolutely no evidence that already differentiated retinal ganglion cells die during the formation of their central connections (Reh and Constantine-Paton, 1983). In addition, the competing eyes of three-eyed animals show no signs of cell depletion in their retinal ganglion cell layers. In fact, quantitative morphometric studies in these animals reveal an average 100% increase in the number of innervating ganglion cells and only a modest 33% increase in tectal volume (Constantine-Paton and Ferrari-Eastman, 1987). The synaptic number in these doubly-innervated tectal lobes is characteristic of normal tecta and apparently unrelated to the number of retinal ganglion cells that terminate in the tectal lobe (Constantine-Paton and Norden, 1986).

The most dramatic effects of double-innervation are, however, the pronounced qualitative changes in the normally continuous retinotectal projections from the competing eyes. The terminals from each eye maintain

the normal alignment of each retina's projection within
the tectal lobe, but they sort out from each other to
establish a system of interdigitating eye-specific
stripes. The final pattern is highly reminiscent of the
normally occurring ocular dominance columns of cat and
primate neocortex (Constantine-Paton and Law, 1978). As
has been reviewed elsewhere (Constantine-Paton, 1981;
Constantine-Paton and Reh, 1985), there is growing
agreement that these stripes represent the interaction
of two potentially independent mechanisms. 1) Differentially distributed cell surface cues on retinal axons
and tectal cells: these serve to align the projections
by causing ganglion cells from particular quadrants of
each retina to terminate only in particular quadrants of
the tectal lobe. 2) An activity-dependent synaptic
sorting mechanism: the activity-dependent mechanism
selectively stabilizes only those synapses which arise
from nearest retinal neighbors and converge on the same
post-synaptic target. The cue used in this discrimina-
tion is apparently the degree of temporal correlation in
the action potentials carried by the cells: neighboring
ganglion cells of the same response-type have patterns
of action potential activity that are highly correlated
in time even under conditions of complete dark adaptation. This latter mechanism is likely to be the same
one that increases the point to point fidelity of continuous retinal representations within the brain. In
the case of two separate retinal projections attempting
to terminate in the same target zone, the mechanism
assures that terminals with highly correlated activity
from the same retina aggregate together. In three-eyed
frogs, as in normal kittens, abolishing the activity cue
with TTX effectively abolishes the ability to synapse
selectively along with retinal neighbors and eliminates
eye-specific stripes (Reh and Constantine-Paton, 1985;
Stryker and Harris, 1986).

The striped tectal lobes of three-eyed frogs also
provide a rare opportunity to explore the way in which
the morphologies of individual post-synaptic tectal neurons are modulated by the patterns of activity in their
inputs because each stripe boundary effectively represents an abrupt discontinuity in the activity patterns
carried by retinal ganglion cell axons. We have visualized stripes in living tecta using an anterograde
transport of tetraethylrhodamine isothiocyanate (TRITC).

Individual tectal neuron morphologies were examined in the same tecta using intracellular filling with Lucifer Yellow (Katz and Constantine-Paton, 1988). Stripes are generally 100-150 µm wide and the majority of cells in tadpole tecta have dendritic arborizations that are roughly 50 µm in diameter. Consequently, many of the cells analyzed in this study did not abut stripe boundaries. However, we did observe disruptions of normal dendritic morphology which appeared to represent specific responses to stripe boundaries in instances where cells were positioned at or near these borders. In registration with these boundaries dendrites ended, turned abruptly or branched. The first type of behavior, dendrites that terminated or turned, produced cells with markedly asymmetric dendritic fields as a result of abutting a stripe boundary. The second type of behavior, dendritic branching at stripe boundaries, produced cells in which different sectors of the dendritic tree were completely segregated from each other by the boundary (Fig. 3). These apparent alterations in dendritic arbors were not isolated responses of a specific cell type. We recorded from, filled and analyzed 50 cells in striped tecta. About 60% of the sample were members of classes that either had dendrites entirely restricted to one stripe or appeared to segregate dissimilar inputs on different branches. Twenty-five percent of the cells belonged to classes that altered their dendritic growth patterns at stripe borders with abrupt turns. In general, most dendrites in striped tecta had morphologies suggesting that they either grew or were pruned so as to minimize the amount of mixing of dissimilar inputs on adjacent regions of post-synaptic membrane.

These observations have several implications for the competitive interactions of retinal axons and post-synaptic cells that pattern connections in developing tecta and possibly in all regions of the vertebrate brain. Although the critical cellular signals are still unknown, the activity-dependent sorting mechanism is usually couched solely in terms of a selective stabilization of the pre-synaptic boutons which is believed to be mediated by the post-synaptic cell. On the other hand, growth of tectal dendrites toward regions of higher innervation density could be mediated by a mechanism that is completely independent of activity, by simply the presence of any active afferents or by

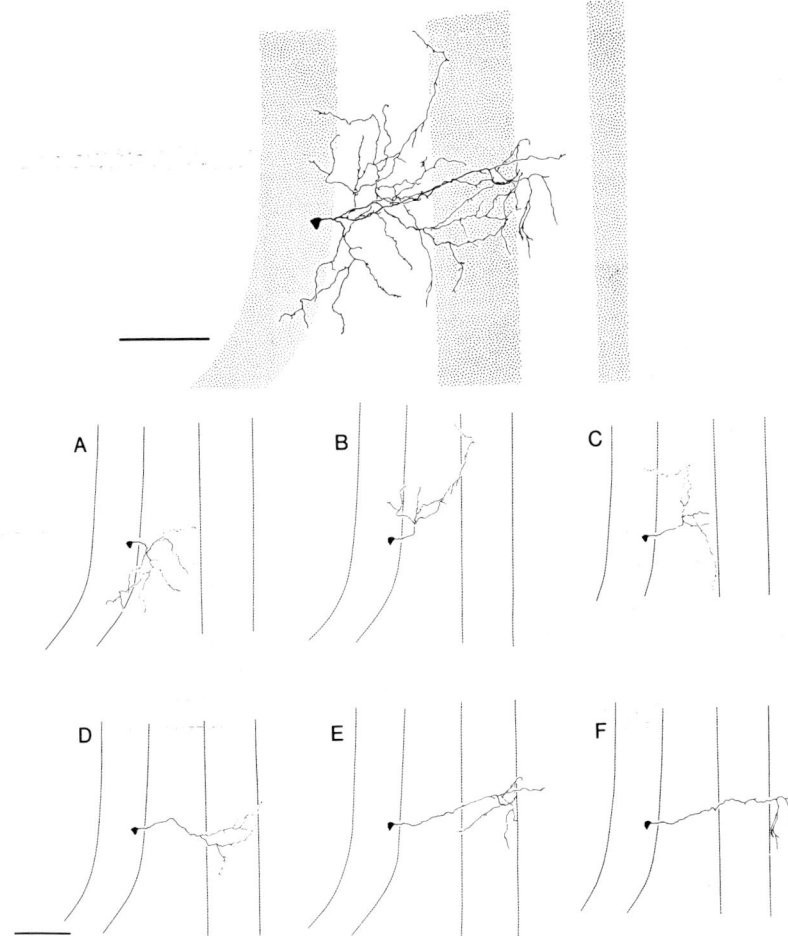

Figure 3. Camera lucida tracing of a tectal cell visualized by intracellular injection of Lucifer Yellow in a flattened in vitro tectal lobe. Eye-specific stripes were visualized in the same tissue following the application and anterograde transport of TRITC to the supernumerary retina. The entire cell and its relation to stripes is shown in the tangential plane at the top of the figure. A-E represent the relationship of individual dendrites to the stripe boundaries. After the primary dendritic branch, each sector of the dendritic tree appears restricted to a single eye's stripe.
Scale bar = 100 µm.

afferents with highly correlated activity. However, the fact that many tectal neurons, when confronted with a stripe boundary, segregate these inputs at the level of the primary or secondary dendrite, highlights three properties relevant to the underlying mechanism. First, that dendrites are not immobile, passive structures in the face of differences in the activity patterns carried by their inputs. Second, that the dendrites appear to respond to, and effectively discriminate, through selective growth or pruning, differences in activity patterns. Third, that the dendritic branch, and not the entire cell, is the unit of post-synaptic integration. These observations suggest that inputs with correlated activity, not just random activity, facilitate the maintenance or continued growth of the contacted dendrite. They raise the possibility that perhaps one of the primary effects of correlated activity is to increase the post-synaptic surface area available to the terminals that are responsible for the correlated signals. If, as has been suggested for the neuromuscular junction, changes in ionic concentrations in active terminal regions are involved in stabilizing synapses, then, increased post-synaptic contact regions and attendant increases in post-synaptic current might serve directly to increase the inherently short lifetimes of developing synapses. Alternatively or in addition, these post-synaptic increases could act indirectly on the pre-synaptic terminals through an increase in some secondary set of interactions which might be proportional to the area of pre- to post-synaptic apposition.

This reasoning is particularly attractive in light of recent evidence supporting a molecular mechanism for activity-dependent sorting of terminals that is based on the properties of the N-methyl-d-aspartate (NMDA) glutamate receptor (Kleinschmidt et al., 1987; Raushenker and Hahn, 1987). The retinotectal projection in goldfish and frogs now appears to be predominantly glutaminergic (Langdon and Freeman, 1986; Debski et al., 1987) and blocking the NMDA receptor results in complete reversible desegregation of frog tectal stripes (Cline et al., 1987). The data on NMDA channel physiology and pharmacology indicate that this channel could mediate competition in local regions of the post-synaptic membrane in the following way. Depolarization of a single dendrite by activity in a subset of converging synapses would allow glutamate to activate the NMDA conductance locally and admit Ca^{2+} (Mayer et al., 1984; Ascher and Nowak, 1987) to only a restricted domain of the post-synaptic cell. This local influx of Ca^{2+} could work directly or indirectly on the cytoskeleton of a differentiating dendrite (Lynch and Baudry, 1984; Aoki and Siekovitz, 1985; Freeman et al., 1985). In short, dendrites of developing tectal neurons may show selective responses to afferent zones of correlated synaptic activity because the resulting increase in internal Ca^{2+} in some way stabilizes or facilitates the polymerization of cytoskeletal elements that are necessary to the maintenance of dendritic sprouts and the elaboration of post-synaptic membrane.

Most of the ideas presented above are speculative, and they may soon be replaced or modified by alternative or more specific molecular hypotheses. Nevertheless, the observations on the dynamic aspects of the differentiating tectal target cannot be readily dismissed. Indeed, for all regions of the vertebrate CNS where sufficiently detailed data are now available, initial synapses appear labile, and the cellular composition as well as the shape and overall dimensions of target regions undergo continuous remodeling as development proceeds. Thus the emergence of post-synaptic dendritic morphologies and the active responses of a heterogeneous population of target cells, as well as the long recognized ingrowth of afferent axons, play a role in the structuring and the stabilization of the final patterns of connectivity.

REFERENCES

Aoki C, Siekovitz P (1985). Ontogenic changes in the cyclic adenosine 3'-5' monophosphate-stimulatable phosphorylation of cat visual cortex proteins particularly of microtubule associated protein 2 (MAP2): effects of normal and dark rearing and of the exposure to light. J Neurosci 5:2465-2483.

Ascher P, Nowak L (1987). Electrophysiological studies of NMDA receptors. Trends Neurosci 10:284-287.

Brown MC, Holland RL, Hopkins WG (1981). Motor nerve sprouting. Ann Rev Neurosci 4:17-42.

Cline HT, Constantine-Paton M (1986). Thyroxin effects

on the development of the retinotectal projection. Soc Neurosci Abstr 12:437.

Cline HT, Debski E, Constantine-Paton M (1987). N-methyl-D-aspartate receptor antagonist desegregates eye-specific shapes. Proc Natl Acad Sci USA 84:4342-4345.

Constantine-Paton M (1981). Induced ocular-dominance zones in tectal cortex. In Schmitt FO, Worden FG, Adelman G, Dennis SG (eds): "The Organization of the Cerebral Cortex." Cambridge, Massachusetts: MIT Press, pp 47-67.

Constantine-Paton M (1982). The retinotectal hook-up: the process of neural mapping. In Subtelny S, Green PG (eds): "Developmental Order: Its Origin and Regulation." New York: Alan R. Liss, pp 317-349.

Constantine-Paton M, Ferrari-Eastman P (1981). Topographic and morphometric effects of bilateral embryonic eye removal in the optic tectum and nucleus isthmus of the leopard frog. J Comp Neurol 196:645-669.

Constantine-Paton M, Ferrari-Eastman P (1987). Pre- and post-synaptic correlates of interocular competition and segregation in the frog. J Comp Neurol 255:178-195.

Constantine-Paton M, Law MI (1978). Eye-specific termination bands in tecta of three-eyed frogs. Science 202:639-641.

Constantine-Paton M, Norden JJ (1986). Synapse regulation in the developing visual system. In Hilfer SR, Sheffield J (eds): "Cell and Developmental Biology of the Eye." New York: Springer-Verlag Bol, pp 1-14.

Constantine-Paton M, Reh TA (1985). Dynamic synaptic interactions during the formation of a retinotopic map. In O'Lague P (ed): "Neurobiology: Molecular Biological Approaches to Understanding Neuronal Function and Development." New York: Alan R. Liss, pp 151-168.

Currie JR (1974). Some observations on the development of the visual system of the frog, Rana pipiens. Ph.D. Thesis, Washington University, St. Louis, Missouri, USA.

Currie JR, Cowan WM (1974). Some observations on the early development of the optic tectum in the frog (Rana pipiens) with special reference to the effects of early eye removal on mitotic activity in the larval tectum. J Comp Neurol 156:123-142.

Currie JR, Cowan WM (1975). The development of the retintotectal projections in Rana pipiens. Develop Biol 46:103-119.

Debski EA, Cline HT, Constantine-Paton M (1987). Kynurenic acid blocks retino-tectal transmission in Rana pipiens. Soc Neurosci Abstr 13:1691.

Dubin MW, Stark LA, Archer SM (1986). A role for action potential activity in the development of neuronal connections in the kitten retinogeniculate pathway. J Neurosci 6:1021-1036.

Eichler V (1971). Neurogenesis in the optic tectum of larval Rana pipiens following unilateral enucleation. J Comp Neurol 141:375-396.

Freeman JA, Manis PB, Snipes GJ, Mayes BN, Samson PC, Wikswo JP, Freeman DB (1985). Steady growth cone currents revealed by a novel circularly-vibrating probe: a possible mechanism underlying neurite growth. J Neurosci Res 13:257-283.

Gaze, RM (1978). The problem of specificity in the formation of nerve connections. In Garrod DR (ed): "Receptors and Recognition." New York: John Wiley and Son, pp 53-93.

Gaze RM, Keating MJ, Östberg A, Chung S-H (1979). The relationship between retinal and tectal growth in larval Xenopus: implications for the development of the retinotectal projection. J Embryol Exp Morphol 53:135-143.

Glücksman A (1940). Development and differentiation of the tadpole eye. Brit J Opthamol 24:153-179.

Gurney ME (1984). Suppression of sprouting at the neuromuscular junction by immune sera. Nature 307:546-548.

Hollyfield JG (1968). Differential addition of cells to the retina in Rana pipiens tadpoles. Develop Biol 18:163-179.

Hollyfield JG (1971). Differential growth of the neural retina in Xenopus laevis larvae. Develop Biol 24:264-286.

Hoy RR, Nolan TG, Casady GC (1984). Dendritic sprouting and compensatory synaptogenesis of an identified interneuron following auditory deprivation in a cricket. Proc Natl Acad Sci USA 22:7772-7776.

Jacobson M (1975). Development and evolution of type II neurons: conjectures a century after Golgi. In Santini M (ed): "Golgi Centennial Symposium Proceedings." New York: Raven Press, pp 147-151.

Katz LC, Constantine-Paton M (1988). Relationships between segregated afferents and post-synaptic neurons in the optic tectum of three-eyed frogs. J Neurosci (in press).

Kleinschmidt A, Bear MF, Singer W (1987). Blockade of NMDA receptors disrupts experience-dependent plasticity of kitten striate cortex. Nature 238:355-358.

Kollros JJ (1953). The development of the optic lobes in the frog. I. The effects of unilateral enucleation in embryonic stages. J Exp Zool 123:153-187.

Kollros JJ (1982). Peripheral control of midbrain mitotic activity in the frog. J Comp Neurol 205:171-178.

Langdon RB, Freeman JA (1987). Pharmacology of retinotectal transmission in the goldfish: effects of nicotinic ligands, strychnine and kynurenic acid. J Neurosci 7:760-773.

Lázár G (1973). The development of the optic tectum in Xenopus laevis: a Golgi study. J Anat 116:347-355.

Liesi P (1985). Laminin-immunoreactive glia distinguish regenerative adult CNS systems from non-regenerative ones. EMBO J 4:2505-2511.

Lynch G, Baudry M (1984). The biochemistry of memory: a new and specific hypothesis. Science 224:1057-1063.

Mayer ML, Westbrook GL (1987). The physiology of excitatory amino acids in the vertebrate central nervous system. Prog Neurobiol 28:197-276.

Meyer RL (1983). Tetrodotoxin inhibits the formation of refined retinotopography. Develop Brain Res 6:293-296.

Murphey RK, Mendenhall B, Palka J, Edwards JS (1975). Deafferentation slows the growth of specific dendrites of identified giant interneurons. J Comp Neurol 159:407-418.

Needel DL, Nieto-Sampedro M, Cotman CW (1987). Affinity chromatography of neurotrophic and neurite-promoting factors from injured brain. Soc Neurosci Abstr 13:1611.

O'Brien RAD, Östberg AJC, Vrbova G (1982). The reorganisation of neuromuscular junctions during development. In Hoffman JH, Giebisch GH, Bolis L (eds): "Membranes in Growth and Development." New York: Alan R. Liss, pp 247-257.

Perry DH, Linden R (1982). Evidence for dendritic competition in the developing retina. Nature 297:683-685.

Rakic P (1974). Neurons in rhesus monkey visual cortex: systemic relation between time of origin and eventual

deposition. Science 183:425-427.
Raushenker JP, Hahn S (1987). Ketamine-xylazine anaesthesia blocks consolidation of ocular dominance changes in kitten visual cortex. Nature 326:183-185.
Reh TA, Constantine-Paton M (1983). Qualitative and quantitative measures of plasticity during the normal development of the Rana pipiens retinotectal projection. Develop Brain Res 10:187-200.
Reh TA, Constantine-Paton M (1984). Retinal ganglion cell terminals change their projection sites during larval development of Rana pipiens. J Neurosci 4:442-457.
Reh TA, Constantine-Paton M (1985). Eye-specific segregation requires neural activity in three-eyed Rana pipiens. J Neurosci 5:1132-1143.
Schmidt JT, Edwards DL (1983). Activity sharpens the map during the regeneration of the retinotectal projection in goldfish. Brain Res 269:29-39.
Steen P, Kalghatgi L, Constantine-Paton M (1987). Antibody markers for axons and oligodendrocytes in the developing frog brain. Soc Neurosci Abstr 13:1691.
Stretavan DW, Shatz CJ, Stryker MP (1987). Prenatal development of retinogeniculate axon arbors in the presence of tetrodotoxin. Soc Neurosci Abstr 13:59.
Stryker MP, Harris WA (1986). Binocular impulse blockade prevents the formation of ocular dominance columns in cat visual cortex. J Neurosci 6:2117-2133.
Straznicky C, Gaze RM (1971). The growth of the retina in Xenopus laevis: an autoradiographic study. J Embryol Exp Morphol 26:67-79.
Straznicky C, Gaze RM (1972). The development of the tectum in Xenopus laevis: an autoradiographic study. J Embryol Exp Morphol 28:87-115.
Taylor AC, Kollros JJ (1946). Stages in the normal development of Rana pipiens larvae. Anat Rec 94:7-23.

NEUROGENESIS OF THE FROG CEREBELLUM

Amos G. Gona, Nándor J. Uray and Kurt F. Hauser

Departments of Anatomy, University of Medicine and Dentistry of New Jersey, Newark, New Jersey 07103 (A.G.G.); Kirksville College of Osteopathic Medicine, Kirksville, Missouri 63501 (N.J.U.); University of Kentucky, Lexington, Kentucky 40536 (K.F.H.)

INTRODUCTION

The cerebellum is known for the simplicity of its stereotyped structure (see Eccles, 1970). Not surprisingly, the developmental neurobiology of the cerebellum has been studied extensively in several species of animals as well as in the human brain (Ramón y Cajal, 1911, 1960; Saetersdal, 1957; Miale and Sidman, 1961; Forstronen, 1963; Mugnaini and Forstronen, 1967; Hanaway, 1967; Kornguth et al., 1967; Phemister and Young, 1968; Rakic and Sidman, 1970; Altman and Bayer, 1978). However, little attention was paid to cerebellar development in the frog, despite the crucial position of the amphibian on the phylogenetic tree in this regard. Ramón y Cajal (1911) had observed immature Purkinje (P.) cells in the frog tadpole. Later, Larsell (1925) noted that the tadpole cerebellum did not acquire a well-defined P. cell zone until late in larval life. More recently, Baffoni (1959) described some of the developmental aspects of the cerebellum in the toad, Bufo bufo. No further studies appeared to have been undertaken on cerebellar development in the frog, although even the ultrastructure of the adult frog cerebellum has been described in great detail (Hillman, 1969; Sotelo, 1969, 1976).

It is said that a clear understanding of a biological system can only be gained by a careful analysis of (1) how it is put together (i.e., its anatomy); (2) how it works (i.e., its physiology); (3) how it develops (i.e., its ontogeny); and (4) how it evolved (i.e., its phylogeny). In the context of the cerebellum, the first three have been extensively studied in the higher vertebrates. For a phylogenetic analysis of the cerebellum, it is essential that we study organisms at different levels of complexity. An ontogenetic study of the frog cerebellum could add significantly in gaining a clear understanding of this particular biological system.

Over the years, we have used the bullfrog, Rana catesbeiana, almost exclusively for our studies on cerebellar development. In this species, the tadpole stage extends for up to three years before the onset of metamorphosis. This protracted larval phase provides a unique system with a temporal separation of larval development and metamorphic transformation. Furthermore, metamorphosis can be induced at will at any time during the prolonged larval development of the bullfrog.

For several years since we initiated our studies in 1970, we focused our attention primarily on the maturational changes of the cerebellum during metamorphosis. Although we made many interesting observations and gained a great deal of understanding of the metamorphic changes in the cerebellum, we became convinced that certain key issues can be resolved only by studying very early development of the tadpole cerebellum. We summarize our findings here, starting with a brief description of the anatomical features of the cerebellum of the premetamorphic tadpole based on our studies.

CEREBELLUM OF THE PREMETAMORPHIC BULLFROG TADPOLE

The cerebellum in the tadpole is a diminutive version of that in the adult frog although there are certain differences. It is a thin plate at the rostral part of the fourth ventricle and just caudal to the optic tectum with which it is continuous at the base. At earlier stages, it is distinctly bi-lobed, united at the midline by a thin membranous portion. The lateral parts are more massive and will continue to enlarge dorsally and medially throughout the premetamorphic period. By the end of this period the two thickened lobes fuse dorsally, but the ventral part of the cerebellar plate

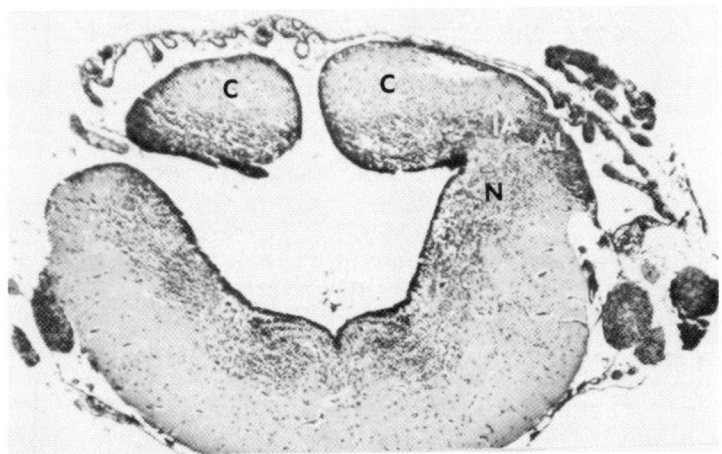

Figure 1. Transverse section through cerebellar region of a premetamorphic tadpole, showing the auricular lobe (AL), corpus cerebelli (C), interauricular granular band (IA) and nucleus cerebelli (N). x60 (From Uray and Gona, 1977.)

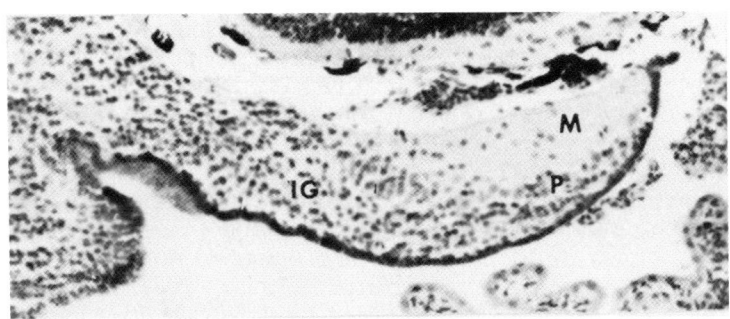

Figure 2. Sagittal section through corpus cerebelli of premetamorphic tadpole. The ventral part is to the left and the dorsal (apical) part is to the right. The pial surface faces the top and the ventricular (ependymal) surface faces the bottom. The dorsal part displays primitive molecular (M), Purkinje cell (P) and incipient internal granular (IG) layers. x120 (From Uray and Gona, 1977.)

which adjoins the isthmus remains membranous. Larsell (1923, 1925, 1967) called the massive lateral parts the auricular lobes and the thinner medial part the corpus cerebelli (Fig. 1). The thickened dorsal part of the corpus cerebelli of the late premetamorphic tadpole together with the auricular lobes form the marginal zone of the cerebellar plate of the adult frog. The cerebellar plate itself is the equivalent of half a folium of the mammalian cerebellum. Its anterior wall, facing the optic tectum, is the pial surface, and the posterior ependymal surface faces the fourth ventricle. A sagittal section through the cerebellar plate shows the dorsal part to be thicker and more organized than the ventral part. Dorsally, a cortical arrangement is evident (Fig. 2), composed of a primitive molecular layer (ML), P. cell layer and primitive internal granular layer (IGL), while the ventral part consists of an amorphous cellular mass.

Larsell (1923, 1967) speculated that the auricular lobes represent a mature cerebellar region associated with the lateral-line and vestibular systems, while the corpus cerebelli is an immature component which later will be associated with the spinocerebellar system. Our studies, however, revealed that the premetamorphic cerebellum consists of an admixture of immature and partially mature components (Gona, 1975, 1978; Gona and Uray, 1980; Hauser et al., 1986a; Uray and Gona, 1977, 1978, 1979, 1982). The bulk of the auricular lobe cells are small and immature. Partially mature P. cells with stunted but clearly identifiable dendritic trees and axons are present in both the auricular lobes and the dorsal thickened part of the corpus cerebelli. In general, these dendritic trees are oriented to intersect incoming, presumably vestibular, fibers (Fig. 3) which run parallel to the pial surface and which comprise a significant part of the primitive ML. These fibers are of small caliber with occasional beads (Uray and Gona, 1977) which form synaptic contacts with dendritic branches of partially developed P. cells (Gona, 1978) and the somata of partially developed stellate cells (Hauser et al., 1986a). Thus, unlike the adult cerebellum where the ML fibers are primarily parallel fibers, fibers of the incipient ML of the premetamorphic cerebellum are mainly of extracerebellar origin. The partially mature P. cells have large somata, conspicuous somatic spines

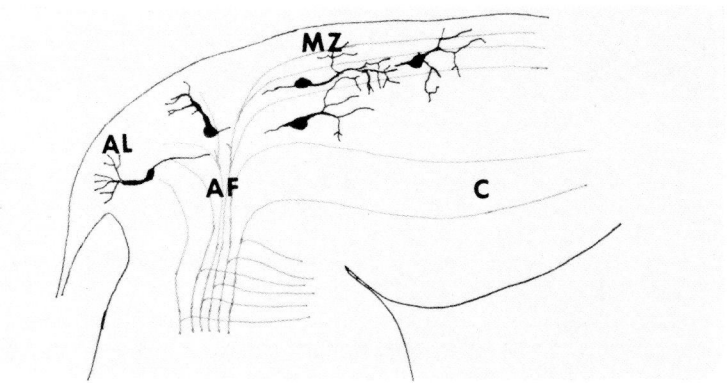

Figure 3. Schematic presentation of partially mature Purkinje cells in the premetamorphic tadpole. Note that the orientation of Purkinje cells corresponds to the course of entering afferent fibers (AF). AL: auricular lobe; C: corpus cerebelli; MZ: marginal zone. (From Uray and Gona, 1977.)

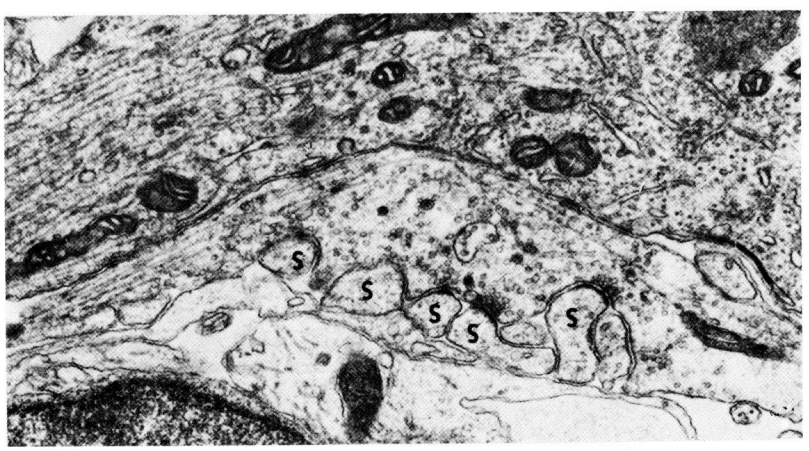

Figure 4. Electron micrograph of a climbing fiber synapse on somatic spines (S) of a well developed Purkinje cell of a premetamorphic tadpole. x24,000 (From Gona and Uray, 1980.)

and massive primary dendrites, and show characteristic synaptic contacts with climbing fibers (Fig. 4), P. cell axon collaterals and stellate cell axons (Gona, 1975; Gona and Uray, 1980; Hauser et al., 1986a). It should be noted that the climbing fibers are in the nid-stage or pre-nid stage at this time.

The stellate cells of the incipient ML are derived from a small external granular layer (EGL) component generated during the premetamorphic period (Uray, 1985). The dendrites of these cells are only partially formed (Uray and Gona, 1977; Hauser et al., 1986a) and are embedded in the primitive ML. These stellate cells are in synaptic contact with the fibers surrounding them and, through their axons, with the somata and primary dendrites of the partially mature P. cells. It should be added that cells which in the adult form the IGL, i.e., granule cells and Golgi cells, are not seen in the pre-metamorphic cerebellum.

EARLY (PREMETAMORPHIC) DEVELOPMENT OF THE BULLFROG CEREBELLUM

During the first four weeks of larval life, the cerebellar primordium consists of bilateral swellings on the metencephalic plates that are united at the midline by membranous tissue (Uray, 1985). The primordium consists of neuroepithelial tissue which continues to proliferate, but has yet to differentiate into histologically demonstrable layers. At six weeks, however, proliferation is accompanied by differentiation in the lateral regions. A cluster of large cells, presumably P. cells, appears in each dorsolateral part of the cerebellar plate. They are apparently generated by the ventricular neuroepithelium and migrate radially. As development continues, successive waves of additional P. cells are similarly generated forming a continuous sheet separating the incipient IGL and the incipient ML. The P. cells do not migrate tangentially, and since each cluster is one to four cells thick, the P. cell layer retains its multilaminar arrangement seen in the adult frog. Concomitant with the expansion of the P. cell layer is an establishment of a fiber system, presumably of extracerebellar origin, running parallel to the pial surface. The ventral boundary of this fiber system

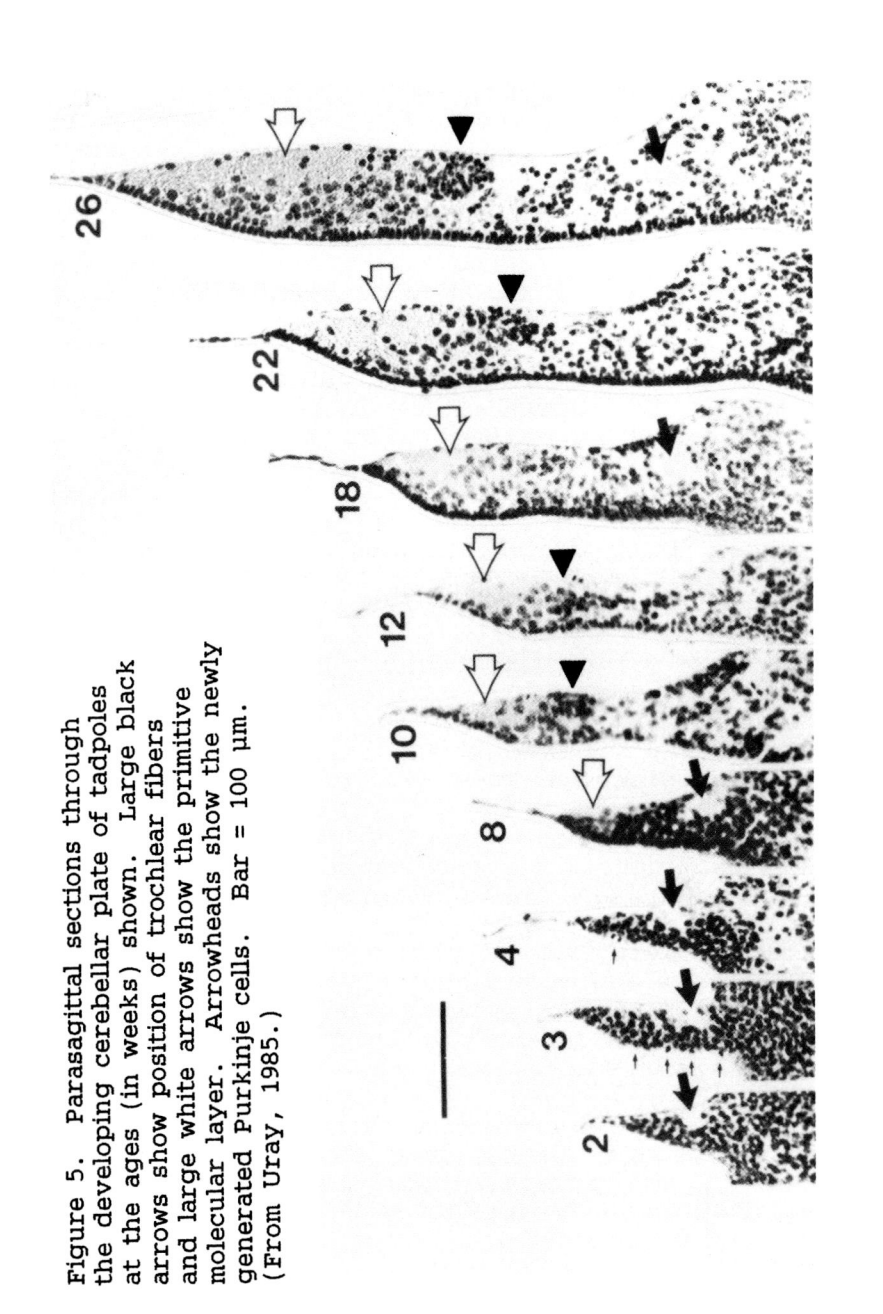

Figure 5. Parasagittal sections through the developing cerebellar plate of tadpoles at the ages (in weeks) shown. Large black arrows show position of trochlear fibers and large white arrows show the primitive molecular layer. Arrowheads show the newly generated Purkinje cells. Bar = 100 μm. (From Uray, 1985.)

within the cerebellar plate corresponds to the position of the most recently generated batch of P. cells (Fig. 5). Continued expansion of the fiber system and the simultaneous addition of new P. cells results in an overgrowth of previously formed P. cell clusters by these fibers, which thus become interposed between the pial surface and the P. cell layer. In a sagittal section, the P. cell layer appears as a diagonal band running from the ventricular surface at the cerebellar apex to the pial surface at its ventralmost part (Figs. 2, 5). The incipient IGL contains a few unidentified fibers and a few small cells, thought to be glia. Ventral to the area of cerebellar differentiation just described, the cerebellar tissue between the neuroepithelium and pial surface appears empty.

Between the eighth and 12th weeks of development the neuroepithelium of the ventrolateral part of the cerebellar plate enlarges to form the neuroepithelial cap (Fig. 6) which produces at least two kinds of small cells, (i) EGL cells and (ii) cells of the interauricular granular band (IAGB). Autoradiographic studies (Uray et al., 1987a, 1988) show that the cells produced by the neuroepithelial cap are generated in several waves with discrete time periods. EGL cell production seems to proceed from about the sixth week until the 24th week. Another wave of EGL cell production starts later and the pace of cell production increases. Throughout this time, the EGL is one cell thick and often discontinuous, its cells migrating underneath the pia. The EGL thus formed is limited to the dorsal, differentiated part of the cerebellum. The ventral, undifferentiated part does not receive EGL cells. These EGL cells migrate into the incipient ML to form stellate cells, and none of them have been seen to migrate past the P. cells. Apparently, the cells derived from these early waves of EGL formation are exclusively ML neurons.

The IAGB cells, which also arise from the neuroepithelial cap, are distinct from the EGL cells in two ways: 1) the generation cycles of IAGB cells are distinct from those of the EGL cells; 2) while the EGL cells migrate to a subpial position first and then tangentially across the cerebellar surface, the IAGB cells migrate radially into the substance of the cerebellum and remain there (Figs. 6, 7). The production of IAGB

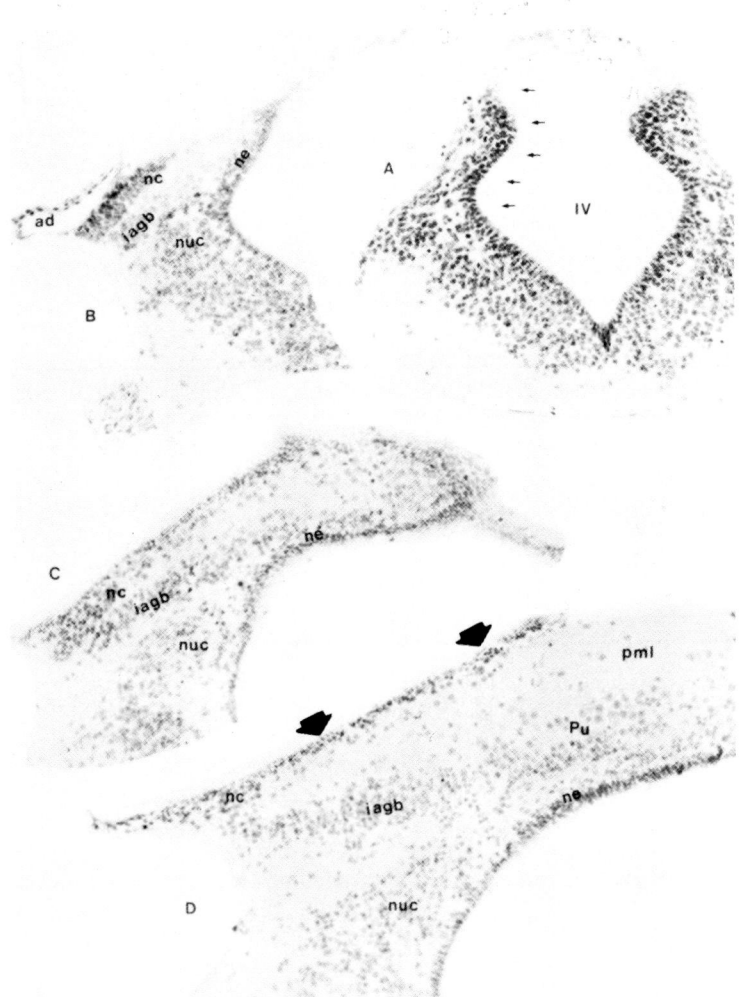

Figure 6. Transverse sections through the cerebellar region of developing tadpoles showing differentiation of various cerebellar components. A: 4 weeks; B: 8 weeks; C: 12 weeks; D: 26 weeks old. Note the two prongs of the neuroepithelial cap (nc) which form the EGL (arrows) and the interauricular granular band (iagb). IV: 4th ventricle; ne: neuroepithelium; nuc: nucleus cerebelli; pml: primitive molecular layer; Pu: Purkinje cell layer. x125 (From Uray et al., 1988.)

cells begins at three weeks of age and reaches peaks at 10 weeks, 16 weeks, 10 months and 11.5 months, with long periods of quiescence between peaks. It should be noted that although the generation of EGL cells and IAGB cells overlaps, the peaks are at different times. We, therefore propose that these two cell groups are distinct populations of neurons derived from different parts of the neuroepithelial cap (Uray et al., 1988).

As a result of the continuous and overlapping process of neurogenesis generating the different cerebellar neurons, the composition and overall appearance of the cerebellum remain essentially the same from 10 weeks to 12 months of age, the time to which it has been studied. However, the numbers of neurons and the area of differentiation in the cerebellum continue to increase as a function of age.

METAMORPHIC CHANGES IN THE BULLFROG CEREBELLUM

The External Granular Layer

The most striking event of metamorphic changes in the frog cerebellum is the appearance of the EGL (Gona, 1972). As described above, the premetamorphic cerebellum lacks a multilayered EGL. A definitive EGL begins to appear as a multilayered bed of cells during the prometamorphic period, a period when metamorphic changes proceed at an accelerated rate (see Etkin, 1968). As some EGL cells migrate down from the pial region, new ones arrive at an ever increasing pace with a net increase in the thickness of the EGL. Maximal thickness of EGL is reached during metamorphic climax when the rate of migration of EGL cells into the IGL begins to outstrip the rate of arrival of new EGL cells and the EGL cells make a dramatic descent as an inverted cone of cell mass (Fig. 8). It should be pointed out that these EGL cells, unlike those of the premetamorphic tadpole, do descend past the P. cells and give rise to the IGL neurons.

We have demonstrated by autoradiographic studies that the source of these EGL cells is a band of ependymal (neuroepithelial) cells along the margins of the

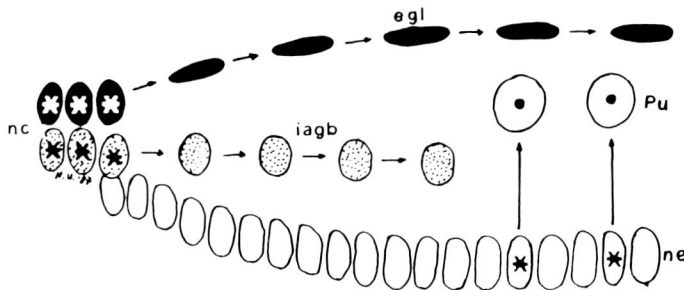

Figure 7. Schematic drawing summarizing the pattern of neurogenesis in the premetamorphic cerebellum. The germinative neuroepithelium has two parts: the ventricular neuroepithelium (ne) which forms Purkinje cells (Pu), and the neuroepithelial cap (nc) which has two subdivisions producing cells of the EGL and iagb, respectively. (From Uray et al., 1988.)

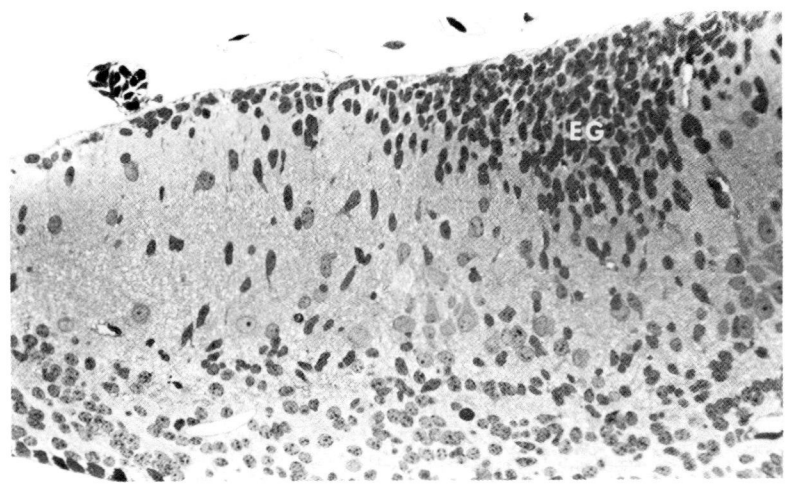

Figure 8. Cerebellum of a climax tadpole showing the dramatic descent of the external granular layer cells (EG) towards the ependymal surface. x250 (From Gona, 1972.)

two lobes of the cerebellar plate (Fig. 9; Gona, 1976). These studies also revealed that, as found later in the premetamorphic cerebellum (Uray et al., 1987a), the EGL of the cerebellum in the metamorphic tadpole is entirely non-proliferative. The fact that these cells take a circuitous route to reach the IGL, in spite of the fact that there is no proliferation while in the EGL, lends support to the possibility suggested by Ramón y Cajal (1960) that there may be an important cell interaction as the EGL cells migrate past the P. cells into the IGL.

Purkinje Cell Maturation

Our initial studies led us to believe that P. cell maturation occurs only during metamorphosis (Gona, 1972). However, it soon became apparent that a small population of P. cells with moderately developed dendritic trees is already present in the dorsal region of the cerebellum of the premetamorphic tadpole (Gona, 1975). Further studies revealed that P. cell maturation in the frog proceeds in two major waves (Fig. 10) as two temporally distinct populations, the first already being present in the premetamorphic tadpole and the second starting during metamorphosis (Uray and Gona, 1977, 1978, 1979, 1982; Gona and Uray, 1980).

The first population of P. cells, distributed partly in the dorsal region of the corpus cerebelli and partly in the auricular lobe of the premetamorphic cerebellum, represents only a small part of the P. cells of the adult. These precociously developed P. cells have stunted dendritic trees and acquire the full extent of arborization later during metamorphosis. The P. cells of the auricular lobe appear more advanced than those of the dorsal part of the corpus cerebelli. Interestingly, the axo-dendritic polarization of the two groups of P. cells are, in general, opposite, with their axonal poles facing each other (Fig. 3), and it is at the boundary between these two P. cell groups that fibers of the vestibulo-lateral line system stream into the cerebellum of the premetamorphic tadpole. It should also be added that electron microscopic studies revealed the presence of parallel fiber-like processes in the incipient ML of the premetamorphic cerebellum showing synaptic connections with dendritic spines of the precociously

Frog Cerebellum / 267

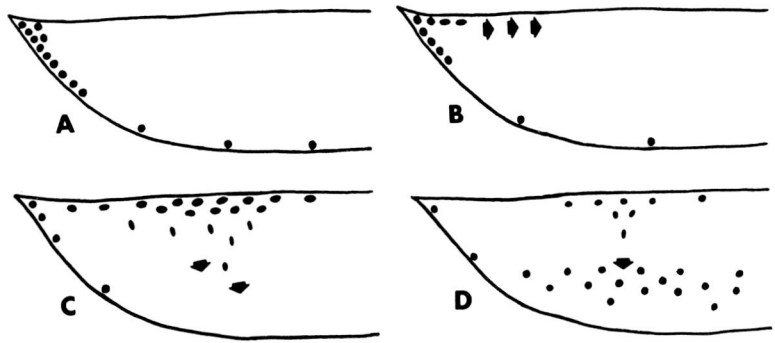

Figure 9. Diagram summarizing the pattern of labeling at various times (A: 3 hrs.; B: 48 hrs.; C: 4 days; D: 14 days) after thymidine-^{3}H injection. Dots indicate sites of labeling. Arrows indicate path of migration. (From Gona, 1976.)

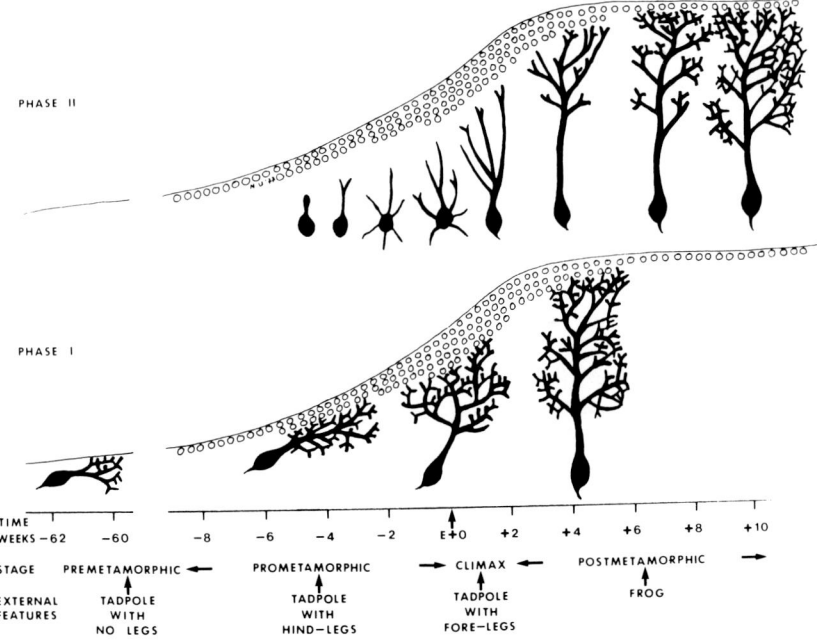

Figure 10. Purkinje cell development in two waves. The first wave begins in premetamorphic tadpoles and reaches maturity around E + 4 weeks; the second begins in prometamorphic tadpoles and reaches maturity around E + 10 weeks. E: foreleg emergence. (From Uray and Gona, 1978.)

developed P. cells (Gona, 1978). These observations suggest the possibility that the afferent fibers of the premetamorphic cerebellum exert an inductive influence which results in the precocious development of the P. cells.

The ventral region of the premetamorphic cerebellum has only immature P. cells with little or no dendritic arborization. Recent immunocytochemical studies showed that only the precociously developed P. cells of the auricular lobe and of the dorsal region of the corpus cerebelli stain positively with the antiserum prepared against vitamin D-dependent calcium binding protein, which is a specific marker for P. cells in the cerebellum (Gona et al., 1986).

Purkinje cells of the second wave appear during metamorphosis and undergo very rapid maturational changes, acquiring elaborate dendritic trees during metamorphic climax and the postmetamorphic period that follows. While the P. cells of the second wave are showing these changes, the precociously developed P. cells of the first wave undergo further maturation (Fig. 10) acquiring dendritic trees of adult proportions (Uray and Gona, 1978, 1979).

THYROXINE-INDUCED CHANGES IN THE BULLFROG CEREBELLUM

Metamorphic Changes

Not unexpectedly, we found early in our studies that thyroxine, administered by injection, induces metamorphic changes in the tadpole cerebellum (Gona, 1973, 1977) as it does in other metamorphic events. It was also found that implants of thyroxine placed in the fourth ventricle of premetamorphic tadpoles induce metamorphic changes in the animal (Gona et al., 1982). Ultrastructural studies showed that the overall changes in the cerebellum are very similar in spontaneous metamorphosis and thyroid hormone-induced metamorphosis (Gona et al., 1982). However, during thyroid hormone-induced metamorphosis, accelerated change is evident in the morphologic differentiation of P. cells (Hauser and

Gona, 1984), stellate cells (Hauser et al., 1986a) and granule cells (Hauser et al., 1986b).

Purkinje cells. When thyroxine is administered to premetamorphic tadpoles, P. cells of both the first wave which are precociously developed and located in the dorsal part of the cerebellum and those of the second wave located in the ventral part undergo rapid maturation. The resultant pattern of thyroid-induced cytodifferentiation in P. cells is similar to that seen in spontaneous metamorphosis, except that the rate of cytodifferentiation is more rapid during induced metamorphosis, rendering the developmental events more synchronized between individual P. cells (Hauser and Gona, 1984).

The greatest maturational response is evident in the immature, ventrally located P. cells of the second wave. These cells lack climbing fiber "nids" in the premetamorphic tadpole. When the premetamorphic tadpole is treated with thyroxine, the rapid invasion of climbing fibers is dramatic, and results in most of these ventrally located P. cells establishing synaptic contacts of the soma with climbing fibers within one week of thyroid hormone treatment. With progressive development, the climbing fiber synapses translocate from their initial contacts with P. cell somatic processes towards their adult positions on the "thorn-like" spines on the proximal parts of the dendritic tree. The dorsally located P. cells also undergo rapid cytological and synaptic maturation in response to thyroid hormone treatment (Hauser and Gona, 1984). However, because these precociously developed P. cells have already attained a moderate level of maturity during the premetamorphic period, thyroid-induced development is less striking and mostly entails changes in the tertiary branching of the dendritic tree and additional synaptic development. It should be emphasized that our studies do not permit a determination of whether the P. cell is a primary target of thyroid hormone action.

Local Circuit Neurons. Generation of the definitive EGL cells which are precursors of granule cells and stellate cells, is dependent on thyroid hormone (Gona, 1973). Unlike mammalian cerebellar development, where thyroid hormone appears to simply modulate the existing rates of ongoing events (Nicholson and Altman, 1972), in frog cerebellar development thyroid hormone has a dramatic effect on EGL cell production. For example, thyroid hormone administration can induce EGL formation one to two years ahead of schedule in premetamorphic bullfrog tadpoles (Gona, 1973; Gona and Gona, 1977), whereas thyroidectomy leads to a permanent cessation of production of EGL cells (Hauser and Gona, 1983). Furthermore, generation of EGL cells will resume in thyroidectomized tadpoles if thyroid hormone is administered (Hauser and Gona, 1983).

Measurements of the rate of increase in the relative volume of EGL and relative number of EGL cells (estimated from increases in cerebellar DNA) indicate a massive increase in the production of these cells which is proportionally greater during thyroid hormone-induced metamorphosis (Hauser et al., 1986b). However, when total EGL cell numbers and absolute measures of cerebellar size are estimated (Hauser et al., 1986b), or when the size of P. cell dendritic arbor is compared (Hauser and Gona, 1984), thyroid hormone treated tadpoles are always deficient as compared with comparably staged, spontaneously metamorphosing tadpoles. It appears that neural development occurring in the absence of thyroid hormone in the premetamorphic phase is essential for maturation to proceed normally during metamorphosis.

The stimulating effect of thyroid hormone is best illustrated in the formation of stellate cells of the ML and granule cells of the IGL. In normal development, there is a temporal separation in the generation of these two cell types; the stellate cells form throughout the extended premetamorphic period while granule cell formation must await the onset of metamorphosis. When development of premetamorphic tadpoles is speeded up by thyroxine treatment, granule cells of the IGL appear within a few days, several months ahead of schedule.

Although it is clear that thyroid hormone has a profound effect on the generation of EGL cells, it is uncertain whether subsequent developmental events, i.e., migration, differentiation and cell death, are thyroid-dependent. Once EGL cells are generated, their further development does not seem to be directly dependent on thyroid hormone. This was demonstrated in tadpoles that were thyroidectomized while undergoing spontaneous metamorphosis (Hauser and Gona, 1983). The EGL cells continued to migrate into the IGL in these thyroidectomized tadpoles. Moreover, differentiation of granule cells and stellate cells from the EGL precursors also appears to occur in the absence of thyroid hormone (Hauser and Gona, unpublished). It is conceivable that migration of EGL cells into the IGL and concomitant differentiation may be dependent on other factors such as the availability of ependymo-glial guides (see Gona, 1978) and/or appropriate input from afferent fiber systems, e.g., mossy fibers (see Hauser et al., 1986b).

Early Development

Very recent studies (Uray et al., 1987b) show that the tadpole cerebellum is responsive to thyroxine treatment at a very early age and undergoes differentiation and maturation prematurely. In the earliest age groups, however, cerebellar development is incomplete, perhaps due to the intrinsic inability to complete maturation at such an early age or as a result of premature death of the animals. In any case, the size of the cerebellum and the extent of cerebellar maturation is dependent on the age of the tadpole when thyroxine treatment is initiated. Thus, the height of the cerebellar plate and the area which shows maturation (as indicated by the presence of EGL, ML, IGL, and P. cell layer) in response to thyroxine treatment for a two week period is greater when treatment begins at the age of 14 weeks than when treatment begins at the age of 12 weeks. Cerebellar height and differentiation in the latter age group, however, is greater than in tadpoles treated at the age of 10 weeks. Apparently, one of the effects of thyroxine treatment is the premature addition of another "strip" of differentiated tissue to the cerebellar plate. One interpretation for these findings is that the increase in the area of cerebellar maturation resulting from thyroid hormone treatment at a given age group is a function of the area of neuroepithelial tissue which is capable of proliferation and differentiation. Progressively older tadpoles have correspondingly larger areas of the neuroepithelial tissue. Thus, in thyroxine-treated tadpoles, as during normal development, cerebellar differentiation proceeds by incremental addition of batches of different cerebellar neurons, except that in thyroxine-treated tadpoles the process is faster and takes place prematurely. It is possible that one of the effects of thyroxine treatment is the elimination of the quiescent periods in neurogenesis which are seen to occur during spontaneous development.

SUMMARY

The cerebellum of the premetamorphic bullfrog tadpole is comprised of a partially formed structure that is diminutive in comparison with the mature form of the adult, and contains only a few partially formed neuronal elements. The dorsal region is partially differentiated and contains two cell types and two fiber systems. Purkinje (P.) cells and stellate cells of this region have partially developed dendrites and axons, and the two cell types are in synaptic contact with each other via their axons. These neurons are also contacted by a fiber system which is extracerebellar in origin and which comprises the bulk of the incipient molecular layer (ML). In addition, the P. cells are contacted by partially developed climbing fibers. Our studies were focused on the origin of the cellular elements present in the cerebellum of the premetamorphic tadpole and the developmental events that transform the premetamorphic cerebellum into the adult cerebellum during metamorphosis.

During differentiation of the cerebellar anlage, the first clearly recognizable differentiated cerebellar tissue consists of a cluster of P. cells in the dorsolateral part of the cerebellar plate seen around the sixth week of larval development, and presumably generated by the ventricular neuroepithelium. As development continues, additional clusters of P. cells are generated through successive waves of proliferation of ventricular neuroepithelium and concomitant differentiation. A continuous sheet of P. cells is thus formed separating the incipient ML and internal granular layer (IGL). The expansion of the P. cell layer from the dorsal toward the ventral region is accompanied by an expansion of the extracerebellar fiber system occupying the primitive ML. Between the eighth and 12th week of larval development, the neuroepithelium of the ventrolateral part of the cerebellar plate enlarges to form the neuroepithelial cap, which gives rise to 1) external granule layer (EGL cells which differentiate into stellate cells of the incipient ML and 2) cells of the interauricular granular band. As these events continue through the protracted premetamorphic phase of larval development, the cerebellar morphology remains essentially unchanged although the size of the cerebellum increases.

With the onset of metamorphosis, cerebellar development is steadily accelerated and entails two major events of neurogenesis: 1) P. cells of a second major wave are generated which undergo maturation at a dramatic pace and give rise to a majority of the adult population of P. cells; 2) ventricular neuroepithelium of the entire margin of the cerebellar plate becomes proliferative and gives rise to a thick bed of EGL cells which, like those of the premetamorphic tadpole, are non-proliferative; however, unlike those of the premetamorphic tadpole, many of them migrate past the P. cells and differentiate into neurons of the definitive IGL.

Thyroid hormone treatment induces rapid developmental changes seen during spontaneous metamorphosis as well as those of early development. While some developmental events are directly dependent on thyroid hormone action, others seem to be independent of this hormone. For example, thyroxine treatment triggers cell proliferation and establishment of EGL. However, the EGL cells migrate even in thyroidectomized tadpoles. Thyroid hormone appears to shorten or eliminate the quiescent periods, especially those seen during the early part of normal development.

REFERENCES

Altman J, Bayer SA (1978). Prenatal development of the cerebellar system in the rat. I. Cytogenesis and histogenesis of the deep nuclei and the cortex of the cerebellum. J Comp Neurol 179:23-48.

Baffoni GM (1959). Osservazioni sulla morfogenesi ed istogenesi cerebellare in un anfibio anuro (Bufo bufo). Rev Neurobiol 5:33-73.

Eccles JC (1970). Neurogenesis and morphogenesis in the cerebellar cortex. Proc Natl Acad Sci USA 66:294-301.

Etkin W (1968). Hormonal control of amphibian metamorphosis. In Etkin W, Gilbert LI (eds): "Metamorphosis: A Problem in Developmental Biology." New York: Appleton-Century-Crofts, pp 313-348.

Forstronen PF (1963). The origin and morphogenetic significance of the external granular layer of the cerebellum, as determined experimentally in chick embryos. Acta Neurol Scand Suppl 139:314-316.

Gona AG (1972). Morphogenesis of the cerebellum of the frog tadpole during spontaneous metamorphosis. J Comp Neurol 146:133-142.

Gona AG (1973). Effects of thyroxine, thyrotropin, prolactin and growth hormone on the maturation of the frog cerebellum. Exp Neurol 38:494-501.

Gona AG (1975). Golgi studies of cerebellar maturation in frog tadpoles. Brain Res 95:132-136.

Gona AG (1976). Autoradiographic studies of cerebellar histogenesis in the bullfrog tadpole during metamorphosis: The external granular layer. J Comp Neurol 165:77-88.

Gona AG (1977). Thyroid-induced maturation of the cerebellar cortex in the frog. In Grave GD (ed): "Thyroid Hormones and Brain Development." New York: Raven Press, pp 107-117.

Gona AG (1978). Ultrastructural studies on cerebellar histogenesis in the frog: The external granular layer and the molecular layer. Brain Res 153:435-447.

Gona AG, Gona O (1977). Local action of thyroxine on cerebellar maturation in frog tadpoles. Exp Neurol 57:581-587.

Gona AG, Uray NJ (1980). Ultrastructural studies on Purkinje cells of the frog tadpole cerebellum. Brain Behav Evol 17:241-254.

Gona AG, Hauser KF, Uray NJ (1982). Ultrastructural studies on Purkinje cell maturation in the cerebellum of the frog tadpole during spontaneous and thyroxine-induced metamorphosis. Brain Behav Evol 20:156-171.

Gona AG, Pendurthi TK, Al-Rabiai S, Gona O, Christakos S (1986). Immunocytochemical localization and immunological characterization of vitamin D-dependent calcium binding protein in the bullfrog cerebellum. Brain Behav Evol 29:176-183.

Hanaway J (1967). Formation and differentiation of the external granular layer of the chick cerebellum. J Comp Neurol 131:1-14.

Hauser KF, Gona AG (1983). Effects of thyroidectomy and

season on the external granular layer of the cerebellum in metamorphosing bullfrog tadpoles (Rana catesbeiana). Exp Neurol 79:265-277.

Hauser KF, Gona AG (1984). Purkinje cell maturation in the frog cerebellum during thyroxine-induced metamorphosis. Neuroscience 11:139-155.

Hauser KF, Uray NJ, Gona AG (1986a). Stellate cell development in the frog cerebellum during spontaneous and thyroxine-induced metamorphosis. J Comp Neurol 244:229-244.

Hauser KF, Uray NJ, Gona AG (1986b). Granule cell development in the frog cerebellum during spontaneous and thyroxine-induced metamorphosis. J Comp Neurol 253:185-196.

Hillman DE (1969). Neuronal organization of the cerebellar cortex in amphibia and reptilia. In Llinás R (ed): "Neurobiology of Cerebellar Evolution and Development." Chicago: AMA/ERF, pp 279-325.

Kornguth SE, Anderson JW, Scott G (1967). Observations on the ultrastructure of the developing cerebellum of Macaca mulatta. J Comp Neurol 130:1-24.

Larsell O (1923). The cerebellum of the frog. J Comp Neurol 36:89-112.

Larsell O (1925). The development of the cerebellum in the frog (Hyla regilla) in relation to the vestibular and lateral line systems. J Comp Neurol 39:249-289.

Larsell O (1967). Anura. In Jansen J (ed): "The Comparative Anatomy and Histology of the Cerebellum from Myxinoids through Birds." Minneapolis: University of Minnesota Press, pp 163-178.

Miale IL, Sidman RL (1961). An autoradiographic analysis of histogenesis in the mouse cerebellum. Exp Neurol 4:277-296.

Mugnaini E, Forstronen PF (1967). Ultrastructural studies on the cerebellar histogenesis. I. Differentiation of granule cells and development of glomeruli in the chick embryo. Z Zellforsch 77:115-143.

Nicholson JL, Altman J (1972). The effects of early hypo- and hyper-thyroidism on the development of the rat cerebellar cortex. I. Cell proliferation and differentiation. Brain Res 44:13-23.

Phemister RD, Young S (1968). The postnatal development of the canine cerebellar cortex. J Comp Neurol 134:243-254.

Rakic P, Sidman RL (1970). Histogenesis of cortical layers in human cerebellum, particularly the lamina

dissecans. J Comp Neurol 139:473-500.
Ramón y Cajal S (1911). "Histologie du Système Nerveux de l'Homme et des Vertébrés." Paris: Maloine.
Ramón y Cajal S (1960). "Studies on Vertebrate Neurogenesis." Guth L (Trans), Springfield: Charles C. Thomas.
Saetersdal TAS (1957). On the ontogenesis of the avian cerebellum, Part IV. Mitotic activity in the external granular layer with a summary of certain aspects of cortical development. Univ Bergen Arbok Naturvitenskap Rekke 4:1-39.
Sotelo C (1969). Ultrastructural aspects of the cerebellar cortex of the frog. In Llinás R (ed): "Neurobiology of Cerebellar Evolution and Development." Chicago: AMA/ERF, pp 327-371.
Sotelo C (1976). Morphology of the cerebellar cortex. In Llinás R, Precht W (eds): "Frog Neurobiology." New York: Springer, pp 864-891.
Uray NJ, Gona AG (1977). The cerebellum of the bullfrog tadpole. J Comp Neurol 176:559-574.
Uray NJ, Gona AG (1978). Golgi studies on Purkinje cell development in the frog during spontaneous metamorphosis. I. General pattern of development. J Comp Neurol 180:265-276.
Uray NJ, Gona AG (1979). Golgi studies on Purkinje cell development in the frog during spontaneous metamorphosis. II. Details of dendritic development. J Comp Neurol 185:237-252.
Uray NJ, Gona AG (1982). Golgi studies on Purkinje cell development in the frog during spontaneous metamorphosis. III. Axonal development. J Comp Neurol 212:202-207.
Uray NJ (1985). Early stages in the formation of the cerebellum in the frog. J Comp Neurol 232:129-142.
Uray NJ, Gona A, Hauser KF (1987a). Autoradiographic studies of cerebellar histogenesis in the premetamorphic tadpole. I. Generation of the external granular layer. J Comp Neurol 266:234-246.
Uray NJ, Pyatt SL, Stuart MD (1987b). Thyroxine-induced cerebellar development in the premetamorphic bullfrog tadpole. Soc Neurosci Abst 13:253.
Uray NJ, Gona AG, Hauser KF (1988). Autoradiographic studies of cerebellar histogenesis in the premetamorphic tadpole. II. Formation of the interauricular granular band. J Comp Neurol (in press).

Index

Acetylcholine receptors, NMJ development, *Xenopus* tissue culture, 105–108
  clustering, 108–112, 117
Acetylcholinesterase, NMJ development, *Xenopus* tissue culture, 106
Action potentials of inputs, retinotectal differentiation, 243
Adult sensory neurons cf. developing sensory neurons, specification, 179–180
  novel targets, 180–181
Ambystoma, spinal ganglia development, 141
  A. mexicanum, 140
Ascending interneurons, transmitter immunocytochemistry, early *Xenopus laevis*, 193–196, 201
Auricular lobes, cerebellum neurogenesis, *Rana catesbeiana*, 257–259
Axogenesis vs. regeneration, hindlimb motor axon innervation patterns, bullfrog, 124, 126
Axon
  extension and limb development, spinal nerve fiber growth and neuronal maturation in vitro, 83–86
    limb innervation patterning, 84–86
    neuronal growth cone, 83–84
  growth, initial, transmitter immunocytochemistry, early *Xenopus laevis* neurons, 200–202
  see also Hindlimb motor axon innervation patterns, bullfrog

Basement membrane, NMJ development, *Xenopus* tissue culture, 104, 108
Body weight and lateral motor column development, 37, 38
Bombinator, 148
Brachial cf. lumbosacral lateral motor column development, 14

Branch points, axon extension and limb development, spinal fiber growth and neuronal maturation in vitro, 85
Bufo americanus
  lateral motor column development, 31
  spinal ganglia development, 139, 148
Bufo bufo, cerebellum, 255
α-Bungarotoxin, 68, 106–108, 111, 114

Calcium
  NMJ development, *Xenopus* tissue culture, 112–113
  retinal innervation in tectal lobe development, 243, 249
Calcium-binding protein, vitamin D-dependent, cerebellum neurogenesis, 268
N-CAM, 86
Carbohydrates, surface, signature, 84
Cat, lateral geniculate nucleus, 242, 244, 245
Cell divisions, optic tectum development, 210
Cell number and death, optic tectum development, 210–211, 215–219, 226
  pyknoses, 215, 216, 218
Cerebellum, *Bufo bufo*, 255
Cerebellum neurogenesis, *Rana catesbeiana*, 189, 255–273
  auricular lobes, 257–259
  external granule cell layer, 260, 262–264, 273
  interauricular granular band (IAGB), 262–264
  internal granule cell layer, 257, 258, 260, 262, 266, 270–273
  larval development, 260–265, 272–273
    pattern, schema, 265
  metamorphic changes, 264–268, 273
    EGL, 264–266
    ependymal cells, 264, 265
    Purkinje cell maturation, 266–268

277

^{3}H-thymidine labeling, 267
molecular layer, 257, 258, 260–262, 266, 270–272
neuroepithelial cap, 263, 264, 273
premetamorphic, 256–260
Purkinje cells, 258–262
  climbing fiber nids, 260, 269, 272
  layer, 257, 258, 260, 271, 272
  orientation, afferent fibers and, 259
  somatic spines, 258, 259, 269
stellate cells, 260, 270, 272
thyroxine-induced changes, 268–273
  early development, 271–272
  EGL cells, 269–271
  at metamorphosis, 268–271
  Purkinje cells, 269
Chemokinetic response, 92–93, 97, 98
Chick cf. frog, 65, 69
  hindlimb motor axon innervation patterns, 123
  lateral motor column development, 5
Choline acetyltransferase, spinal fiber growth and neuronal maturation in vitro, 94–96
Cholinergic blockade prevents motoneuron death, 66, 68, 69
Chondrogenesis, femur, 144
Chromosomal balance, triploid tadpole, lateral motor column development, 13–14
Cinemicrophotography, time-lapse, 90
Cluster formation, NMJ development, 108–112
Colchicine, 150
Collagen type I, 88, 89, 91, 95
  morphologic response to target and substratum, 88–90, 98
  nerve fiber growth rate, 90–92
Commissural interneurons, transmitter immunocytochemistry, early *Xenopus laevis* neurons, 198–201
Competition hypothesis, motoneuron death during development, 53–71
  meritocratic competition, 65–71
    cholinergic blockade prevents motoneuron death, 66, 68, 69
    LMC motoneuron firing, 68, 69
    sensory neuron counts, 70

  musculature and motoneurons, monopodal frogs, 55–65, 70
    myotube number, 63–65
    number of muscle fibers, 57–62
    synapses, 56
  Rana, 57
  Xenopus, 55–57, 66, 69
Con A, NMJ development, 109
Critical choice points, 85
Curare, 68

Decision regions, 85
Dendrites, retinal innervation in tectal lobe development, 246–248
2-Deoxyglucose, 92–94
Developmental pattern, lateral motor column development, 9–10
Differentiative effects, target vs. substratum, spinal nerve fiber growth and neuronal maturation in vitro, 94–96
Dorsal root ganglia, development, 140–142
  growth factors, 152–155
  nerve cell nuclear size, 142
  nerve cell number, 141, 143, 144
  sensory neurons, specification, 162–165, 172–176

Electric organ, *Torpedo*, 109, 111
Ependymal area/cells
  cerebellum neurogenesis, *Rana catesbeiana*, 264, 265
  optic tectum development, 215
EPSPs, spinal sensory neurons, specification during development, 166, 177
External granule cell layer. *See under* Cerebellum neurogenesis, *Rana catesbeiana*
Extracellular matrix, 243
  lateral motor column development, 22
  spinal nerve fiber growth and neuronal maturation in vitro, 88
Eye removal and optic tectum development, 207, 213, 222, 225

Fasciculation, transmitter immunocytochemistry, early *Xenopus laevis* neurons, 201–202
Femur chondrogenesis, spinal ganglia and hindlimb development, 144

Forelimb, forced innervation by thoracic sensory neurons, 172–178
GABA
 retinotectal differentiation, neural patterning, tadpoles, 235–237, 239
 transmitter immunocytochemistry, early *Xenopus laevis* neurons, 191, 193–197, 202
Ganglia, spinal, development, 139–155
 dorsal root ganglion, 140–142
  growth factors, 152–155
  nerve cell nuclear size, 142
  nerve cell number, 141, 143, 144
  sensory neurons, 162–165, 172–176
 hindlimb development, 145–148
  buds, 144, 145
  femur chondrogenesis, 144
  myogenesis, 146, 147
 normal, 140–144
 peripheral change, responses to, 148–152
  hypertrophic ganglia, 149–152
  mitotic activity, 150, 151
  neuronal numbers, 148, 149
 target tissue, 154
Ganglion cell layer, retinal, innervation in tectal lobe development, 244
Gastrocnemius muscle, 58
Glia vs. neurons, optic tectum development, 219, 222–225
Glycine, transmitter immunocytochemistry, early *Xenopus laevis* neurons, 191, 198–200, 202
Goldfish, 242
Granule cell layers, external and internal. *See under* Cerebellum neurogenesis, *Rana catesbeiana*
Growth cone
 spinal fiber growth and neuronal maturation in vitro, 83–84
 transmitter immunocytochemistry, early *Xenopus laevis* neurons, 194–196, 199, 200
Growth factors, 82, 89
 lateral motor column development, 23
 motoneuron (MNGF), 96–98
 nerve (NGF), 152–154
 trophic molecule in *Xenopus* NMJ development, 113–117

Haptochemotaxis, 96, 97
Hindbrain spinal neurons, early *Xenopus laevis* development, transmitter immunocytochemistry
 raphe, 192, 193
 reticulospinal, 193, 195–197, 201
Hindlimb development
 and lateral motor column development, 31, 35–38
 and spinal ganglia development, 145–148
  buds, 144, 145
  femur chondrogenesis, 144
  myogenesis, 146, 147
Hindlimb motor axon innervation patterns, bullfrog, 121–135
 axogenesis vs. regeneration, ^{3}H-thymidine, 124, 126
 cf. chick, 123
 HRP, 122–126, 134
 LMC, 122–126, 134
 perineurial sheath, 135
 Rana catesbeiana, 125
 regenerating motor axons, guidance by distal stump, 127–134
  nerves, listed, 130
  cf. normal, 129, 130, 132
  recordings, 129
  ventral root innervation fields, 128, 133
 vs. sensory pathways, 134
 specificity of neuromuscular connections, 122–123
  development, 122–123
  regeneration after ventral root dissection, 123–127
 Xenopus laevis, 123
Hindlimb muscle fiber number, lateral motor column development, 35–38
Horseradish peroxidase (HRP)
 hindlimb motor axon innervation patterns, bullfrog, 122–126, 134
 sensory neurons, spinal, specification during development, 163, 165, 174–176
Hyla, optic tectum development, 208, 211, 215, 217
 H. regilla, 207
 H. versicolor, 211, 212, 221

Hypertrophic ganglia, spinal ganglia, development, 149–152
Hypophysectomized tadpole, 10–12

Immunocytochemistry. *See* Transmitter immunocytochemistry, early *Xenopus laevis* neurons
Innervation. *See* Hindlimb motor axon innervation patterns, bullfrog
Interactive approach, lateral motor column development, 6–7
Interauricular granular band (IAGB), cerebellum neurogenesis, *Rana catesbeiana*, 262–264
Interindividual variation, lateral motor column development, 31–34, 40, 41, 47–48
Internal granule cell layer. *See under* Cerebellum neurogenesis, *Rana catesbeiana*

Kolmer-Agduhr (spinal) cells, transmitter immunocytochemistry, *Xenopus laevis*, 193–197, 200–202

Laminin, retinal innervation in tectal lobe development, 243
Lateral geniculate nucleus, cat, 242, 244, 245
Lateral motor column development, 3, 5–24, 29–49
  brachial cf. lumbosacral, 14
  Bufo americanus, 31
  cf. chick, 5
  chromosomal balance in triploid tadpole, 13–14
  developmental pattern, 9–10
  hindlimb development and, 31, 35–38
  hindlimb motor axon innervation patterns, bullfrog, 122–126, 134
  interactive approach, 6–7
  lumbar, 29–49
  mechanisms of formation, 8
  motoneuron number
    muscle fiber number and cell death, triploid tadpoles, 43–49
    postsynaptic target size, 40, 43, 44, 48–49
    size of population, 37, 39
    stage 54, 45–48
    stage 66, 44–46, 48
  motoneuron number and metamorphic body size, relation, 33–38
    body weight, 37, 38
    hindlimb muscle fiber number, 35–38
    snout-vent length, 34, 37, 38, 46
  neuron survival in vitro, 18–22
  neuron number, decrease in, 8–10, 12, 14, 16, 18–19, 29–30
    interindividual variation, 31–34, 40, 41, 47–48
    neurite survival related to attachment surfaces, 22–23
    sibling group comparisons, 39–42
    side, right vs. left, 40
    size of prior motoneuron population, 37, 39
    symmetry, bilateral, 31–33, 39, 40, 49
  peripheral target and, 14–19
    limb differentiation and, 16–17
  Rana pipiens, 7, 9–11, 13, 15, 16, 19, 33, 44
  schematic summary, 42
  spinal fiber growth and neuronal maturation in vitro, 84, 85, 87, 93, 95
  thyroxine, 3, 10–12
  Xenopus laevis, 9, 15, 17–19, 29–49
  see also Competition hypothesis, motoneuron death during development
Limb development and axon extensions, spinal fiber growth and neuronal maturation in vitro, 83–86
  limb innervation patterning, 84–86
  neuronal growth cone, 83–84
Limb differentiation and lateral motor column development, 16–17
Limb innervation patterning, spinal fiber growth and neuronal maturation in vitro, 84–86
Lucifer yellow, 242, 246, 247
Lumbosacral cf. brachial lateral motor column development, 14

Mammalian NMJ, 243
Medium
  mesenchyme-conditioned, 88–92

oocyte-conditioned, 116–117
Meritocratic competition, motoneuron death during development, 65–71
Mesenchyme-conditioned medium, 88–92
Metabolic response to target and substratum, spinal nerve fiber growth and neuronal maturation in vitro, 92–93
Metamorphic changes, cerebellum neurogenesis, *Rana catesbeiana*, 264–268, 273
Metamorphic climax, optic tectum development, 209, 224
Microfilaments, NMJ development, AChR diffusion and cytoskeleton in cluster formation, 109
Mitotic activity
   LMC development, 10, 12
   optic tectum development, 211–215, 220–222, 224
   spinal ganglia development, 150, 151
Molecular layer, cerebellum neurogenesis, *Rana catesbeiana*, 257, 258, 260–262, 266, 270–272
Monkey, rhesus, 223
Monosynaptic connections with muscle afferents, spinal sensory neurons, specification during development, 166–167
Morphologic response to target and substratum, collagen type I, 88–90, 98
Motoneuron growth factor (MNGF), 96–98
Motoneuron number changes
   lateral motor column development
      muscle fiber number and cell death, triploid tadpoles, 43–49
      postsynaptic target size, 40, 43, 44, 48–49
      size of population, 37, 39
      stage 54, 45–48
      stage 66, 44–46, 48
   and metamorphic body size, relation, lateral motor column development, 33–38
   see also Competition hypothesis, motoneuron death during development
Motor axon. *See* Hindlimb motor axon innervation patterns, bullfrog
Motor column. *See* Lateral motor column development

Muscle afferents, monosynaptic connections with sensory neurons, 166, 167
Musculature, monopodal frogs, competition hypothesis, motoneuron death during development, 55–65, 70
   myotube number, 63–65
   number of muscle fibers, 57–62
   synapses, 56
Myelination, 237
Myogenesis, spinal ganglia and hindlimb development, 146, 147
Myotomes, NMJ development, *Xenopus* tissue culture, 103, 105–108, 111, 113, 115
Myotube number, competition hypothesis, motoneuron death during development, 63–65

Nerve fiber growth rate, collagen type I, 90–92
Nerve growth factor, dorsal root ganglion development, 152–154
Neural patterning. *See* Retinotectal differentiation, neural patterning, tadpoles
Neural tube formation, 141
Neurite survival related to attachment surfaces, lateral motor column development, 22–23
Neuroepithelial cap, cerebellum neurogenesis, *Rana catesbeiana*, 263, 264, 273
Neuromuscular junction, mammalian, 243
Neuromuscular junction development, *Xenopus* tissue culture, 103–117
   AChR diffusion and cytoskeleton in cluster formation, 108–112
   basement membrane, 104, 108
   calcium role, 112–113
   myotomes, 103, 105–108, 111, 113, 115
   postsynaptic development induction, 105–108, 112
      AChE, 106
      AChRs, 105–108
      polypeptide-coated latex beads, 105–108
   presynaptic development induction, 104–105
      polypeptide-coated latex beads, 104–105
   spinal cords, 103–105, 113

trophic molecule identification, 113–117
  AChR clustering, 113–117
  oocyte-conditioned medium, 116–117
Neuron(s)
  development, specificity, 79
  vs. glia, optic tectum development, 219, 222–225
  maturation. *See* Spinal nerve fiber growth and neuronal maturation in vitro
  numbers
    optic tectum development, 210–211, 215–219, 226
    spinal ganglia development, 148, 149
    see also Motoneuron number changes; *under* Lateral motor column development
  survival in vitro, lateral motor column development, 18–22
Neuronal growth cone. *See* Growth cone
Neurotransmitters. *See* Transmitter immunocytochemistry, early *Xenopus laevis* neurons; *specific neurotransmitters*
NMDA glutamate receptor, retinal innervation in tectal lobe development, 248–249
Nutrient-deficient development, *Xenopus laevis*, 17–19

Oligodendrocytes, 239
Oocyte-conditioned medium, NMJ development, *Xenopus* tissue culture, 116–117
Optic nerve fibers, optic tectum development, 209, 214, 216
Optic tectum development, 189, 207–226
  cell divisions, 210
  cell number and death, 210–211, 215–219, 226
    pyknoses, 215, 216, 218
    wedges, 210, 219–220
  ependymal area, 215
  eye removal, 207, 213, 222, 225
  growth patterns, 219–222, 225
  metamorphic climax, 209, 224
  mitotic activity, 211–215, 220–222, 224
  neurons vs. glia, 219, 222–225
  optic nerve fibers, 209, 214, 216
  Rana pipiens, 209, 211–213, 215–220, 223, 225
  Xenopus laevis, 212, 222

see also Retinotectal differentiation, neural patterning, tadpoles

Patterning. *See* Retinotectal differentiation, neural patterning, tadpoles
Perineurial sheath, hindlimb motor axon innervation patterns, bullfrog, 135
Peripheral change, responses to, spinal ganglia development, 148–152
Peripheral competition hypothesis, 53–54
Peripheral target and lateral motor column development, 14–19
Plasticity, retinotectal differentiation, neural-patterning, tadpoles, 231
Polylysine, spinal nerve fiber growth and neuronal maturation in vitro, 88, 89, 91, 95
Polypeptide-coated latex beads, NMJ development, *Xenopus* tissue culture, 104–108
Postsynaptic contact, spinal fiber growth and neuronal maturation in vitro, 94
Postsynaptic development induction, NMJ development, *Xenopus* tissue culture, 105–108, 112
Premetamorphic cerebellum neurogenesis, *Rana catesbeiana*, 256–260
Presynaptic development induction, NMJ development, *Xenopus* tissue culture, 104–105
Projection organization in adults, spinal sensory neurons, specification cf. during development, 162–164
Pseudacris, optic tectum development, 208, 211, 215
  P. triseriata, 212
Purkinje cells. *See under* Cerebellum neurogenesis, *Rana catesbeiana*
Pyknosis, optic tectum development, 215, 216, 218

Rana
  berlandieri, spinal ganglia development, 143, 144, 151
  catesbeiana
    hindlimb motor axon innervation patterns, bullfrog, 125

sensory neurons, spinal, specification
during development, 162–164,
166
spinal ganglia development, 145, 147,
148
see also Cerebellum neurogenesis,
Rana catesbeiana
competition hypothesis, motoneuron
death during development, 57
esculenta, optic tectum development,
219, 224
optic tectum development, 208, 212, 215
pipiens
dorsal root ganglion, 140–142, 153
lateral motor column development, 7,
9–11, 13, 15, 16, 19, 33, 44
optic tectum development, 209,
211–213, 215–220, 223, 225
retinotectal differentiation, neural patterning, tadpoles, 244
sensory neurons, spinal, specification
during development, 162, 164,
168
spinal ganglia development, 139,
143–149, 151
spinal nerve fiber growth and neuronal maturation in vitro, 86
retinotectal differentiation, neural patterning, tadpoles, 239
spinal ganglia development, 140
sylvatica, optic tectum development, 211,
224
Raphe spinal neurons, hindbrain, transmitter
immunocytochemistry, early *Xenopus
laevis*, 192, 193
Rat, 65
Regeneration
vs. axogenesis, hindlimb motor axon innervation patterns, bullfrog, 124,
126
motor axons, guidance by distal stump,
bullfrog hindlimb, 127–134
nerves, listed, 130
cf. normal, 129, 130, 132
recordings, 129
ventral root innervation fields, 128,
133
specificity, 79

after ventral root dissection, hindlimb
motor axon innervation patterns,
bullfrog, 123–137
Retinal ganglion cell layer, retinal innervation in tectal lobe development, 244
Retinotectal differentiation, neural patterning, tadpoles, 231–249
coordination with input differentiation,
239–240
retinotectal map formation, 240
rhodamine-labeled beads, 239
plasticity, 231
Rana pipiens, 239, 244
retinal innervation in tectal lobe, development, 240–249
action potentials of inputs, 243
sprouting substance, 243
synapses, developing, activity-dependence, 241, 245–249
specificity, 231, 240
tectal proliferative zones, 232–239
GABA, 235–237, 239
rostrolateral–caudomedial spatiotemporal pattern, 232–234
superimposed radial pattern, 234
^{3}H-thymidine labeling, 232–235, 238,
239
thyroxin, 238
timeline longitudinal section, 237
Retinotectal map formation, retinotectal differentiation, neural patterning, tadpoles, 240
Rhesus monkey, 223
Rhodamine-α-bungarotoxin, 111
Rhodamine-labeled beads, retinotectal differentiation, neural patterning, frog tadpoles, 239
Rohon-Beard neurons, 201, 202

Schwann cells, 127
Schwann tubes, 134–135
Semimembranosus muscle, 36, 38, 44, 47
Sensory neuron counts, competition hypothesis, motoneuron death during development, 70
Sensory neurons, spinal, specification during
development, 161–181
adult sensory neurons, 179–180

novel targets, 180–181
dorsal root ganglia, 162–165, 172–176
EPSPs, 166, 177
HRP, 163, 165, 174–176
cf. projection organization in adults, 162–164
Rana
  catesbeiana, 162–164, 166
  pipiens, 162, 164, 168
reflexes elicited from supernumerary limbs, 170–172, 181
  modulation, 170
sensory neuron development, 164–167
  monosynaptic connections with muscle afferents, 166–167
  trunk skin, 166
skin rotation, consequences, 168–170
target signal hypothesis, 161–162
thoracic sensory neurons forced to innervate forelimb muscles, 172–178
  birthdates of TSNs, 178–179
  motoneurons, 177, 178, 180
  schematic of forelimb innervation, 173
ventral neuropil, 175
Xenopus laevis, 164, 172
Sensory pathways vs. hindlimb motor axon innervation patterns, bullfrog, 134
Serotonin, transmitter immunocytochemistry, early *Xenopus laevis* neurons, 191–193, 202
  hindbrain raphe spinal neurons, 192–193
Sibling group comparisons, lateral motor column development, 39–42
Side, right vs. left, lateral motor column development, 40
Signature, surface carbohydrates, 84
Skin rotation consequences, spinal sensory neurons, specification during development, 168–170
Snout-vent length, lateral motor column development, 34, 37, 38, 46
Specificity
  neuromuscular connections, hindlimb motor axon innervation patterns, bullfrog, 122–123
    development, 122–123
    regeneration after ventral root dissection, 123–127

neuronal development, 79
regeneration, 79
retinotectal differentiation, neural patterning, tadpoles, 231, 240
target, spinal nerve fiber growth in vitro, 82, 83
see also Sensory neurons, spinal, specification during development
Spinal cord
  larval frog, diagram, 6
  neuromuscular junction development, *Xenopus* tissue culture, 103–105, 113
  see also Lateral motor column development
Spinal ganglia. *See* Ganglia, spinal, development
Spinal nerve fiber growth and neuronal maturation in vitro, 81–99
  axon extension and limb development, 83–86
    limb innervation patterning, 84–86
    neuronal growth cone, 83–84
  differentiative effects, target vs. substratum, 94–96
    ChAT, 94–96
    postsynaptic contact, 94
  extracellular matrix, 88
  metabolic response to target and substratum, 92–93
  polylysine, 88, 89, 91, 95
  Rana pipiens, 86
  target specificity, 82, 83
Spinal neurons. *See* Sensory neurons, spinal, specification during development
Sprouting substance, retinotectal differentiation, neural patterning tadpoles, 243
Stellate cells, cerebellum neurogenesis, *Rana catesbeiana*, 260, 270, 272
Stochastic walk phenomenon, 97
  biased, 97, 98
Subscapularis muscle, 166, 180
Substance P, 239
Substratum. *See under* Spinal nerve fiber growth and neuronal maturation in vitro

Superimposed radial pattern, retinotectal differentiation, neural patterning, tadpoles, 234
Supernumerary limbs, reflexes, 170–172, 181
  modulation, 170
Surface carbohydrates, signature, 84
Symmetry, bilateral, lateral motor column development, 31–33, 39, 40, 49
Synapses
  competition hypothesis, motoneuron death during development, 56
  developing, activity-dependence, retinotectal differentiation, tadpoles, 241, 245–249
Systems-matching hypothesis, 30

Talin, NMJ development, 110, 111
Target signal hypothesis, sensory neurons, spinal, specification during development, 161–162
Target specificity, spinal nerve fiber growth and neuronal maturation in vitro, 82, 83
Target tissue, spinal ganglia development, 154
Tectum. *See* Optic tectum development; Retinotectal differentiation, neural patterning, tadpoles
Tetrodotoxin (TTX), 243–245
Thoracic sensory neurons forced to innervate forelimb muscles, 172–178
  birthdates of TSNs, 178–179
  motoneurons, 177, 178, 180
  schematic of forelimb innervation, 173
Three-eyed frogs, retinal innervation in tectal lobe development, 245
³H-Thymidine labeling
  cerebellum neurogenesis, *Rana catesbeiana*, 267
  retinotectal differentiation, neural patterning, tadpoles, 232–235, 238, 239
Thyroxine
  lateral motor column development, 3, 10–12
  retinotectal differentiation, neural patterning, tadpoles, 238
Thyroxine-induced changes, cerebellum neurogenesis, *Rana catesbeiana*, 268–273

early development, 271–272
EGL cells, 269–271
at metamorphosis, 268–271
Purkinje cells, 269
Tibialis anterior muscle, 58–64
Tight junctions, 135
Time-lapse cinemicrophotography, 90
Timeline longitudinal section, retinotectal differentiation, neural patterning, tadpoles, 237
Torpedo electric organ, 109, 111
Transmitter immunocytochemistry, early *Xenopus laevis* neurons, 189, 191–203
  axon growth, initial, 200–202
  fasciculation, 201–202
  expression of transmitter, 202
  GABA, 191, 193–197, 202
    ascending interneurons, 193–196, 201
    hindbrain reticulospinal neuron, 193, 195–197, 201
    Kolmer-Agduhr (spinal) cells, 193–197, 200–202
  glycine, 191, 198–200, 202
    commissural interneurons, 198–201
  serotonin, 191–193, 202
    hindbrain raphe spinal neurons, 192–193
Triceps muscle, 164, 166, 177, 178, 180
TRITC, 245, 247
Triturus, spinal ganglia development, 140
Trophic molecule identification, neuromuscular junction development, *Xenopus* tissue culture, 113–117; *see also* Growth factors
Trunk skin, spinal sensory neurons, specification during development, 166

Ventral (anterior) horns, 7
Ventral neuropil, spinal sensory neurons, specification during development, 175
Ventral root innervation fields, guidance of regenerating motor axons by distal stump, 128, 133
Visual system. *See* Optic tectum development; Retinotectal differentiation, neural patterning, tadpoles
Vitamin-D-dependent calcium-binding protein, cerebellum neurogenesis, 268

Wedges, optic tectum development, 210, 219–220

Xenopus laevis
  competition hypothesis, motoneuron death during development, 55–57, 66, 69
  hindlimb motor axon innervation patterns, bullfrog, 123
  lateral motor column development, 9, 15, 17–19, 29–49
  nutrient-deficient development, 17–19
  optic tectum development, 212, 222
  sensory neurons, spinal, specification during development, 164
  spinal ganglia development, 140, 145
  see also Transmitter immunocytochemistry, early *Xenopus laevis* neurons
  optic tectum development, 208, 210, 211, 213, 215, 216, 219, 220, 223, 224
  sensory neurons, spinal, specification during development, 172
  spinal ganglia development, 141, 143, 145–148, 152–153
  see also Neuromuscular junction development, *Xenopus* tissue culture

Y-shaped chambers, 134

Zwischentrang, 140